# TOXICOLOGY STUDIES - CELLS, DRUGS AND ENVIRONMENT

Edited by **Ana Cristina Andreazza and Gustavo Scola**

**Toxicology Studies - Cells, Drugs and Environment**
http://dx.doi.org/10.5772/58714
Edited by Ana Cristina Andreazza and Gustavo Scola

**Contributors**

Cristina Dehelean, Dorina Coricovac, José Custódio, Mariana Ribeiro, Armanda Santos, Donata Favretto, Rossella Snenghi, Daniel Dorta, Omid Mehrpour, Eduardo Rocha, Maria João Rocha, Jalal Pourahmad, Bruno Nunes

**Published by InTech**

Janeza Trdine 9, 51000 Rijeka, Croatia



**Publishing Process Manager** Iva Lipovic

**Technical Editor** InTech DTP team

**Cover** InTech Design team

First published July, 2015

Printed in Croatia

Additional hard copies can be obtained from orders@intechopen.com

Toxicology Studies - Cells, Drugs and Environment, Edited by Ana Cristina Andreazza and Gustavo Scola

p. cm.

ISBN 978-953-51-2140-4

For EU product safety concerns:
IN TECH d.o.o., Prolaz Marije Krucifikse Kozulić 3, 51000 Rijeka, Croatia,
info@intechopen.com or visit our website at intechopen.com.

# Meet the editors

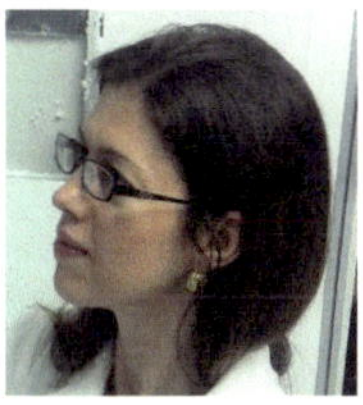

Ana Cristina Andreazza obtained her PhD in Biochemistry from Federal University of Rio Grande do Sul, RS, Brazil in May 2008. Her research interests include the role of biochemical pathways in the pathophysiology of mood disorder, particularly those involving oxidative stress and mitochondrial dysfunction. Specifically, she is interested in exploring the possible connections between molecular mechanisms that lead to synaptic alterations and those which may be potential avenues for therapy. For example, many proteins are targets for oxidative damage in BD, which include dopamine, synaptophysin, cytochrome C, in addition to mitochondrial proteins. Given the clear evidence from multiple sources of increased oxidative stress in BD, Dr. Andreazza's next step is to identify the protein targets for oxidation in BD. Dr. Andreazza has published several research articles in peer reviewed journals and has presented her work at several national and international scientific conferences. Currently, Dr. Andreazza is an Assistant Professor at Department of Pharmacology at the University of Toronto and is cross-appointed as an Independent Scientist at Centre for Addiction and Mental Health in Toronto, Canada, and an Assistant Professor at Department of Psychiatry at the University of Toronto.

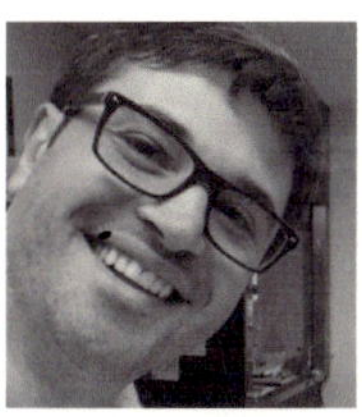

Gustavo Scola is a Postdoctoral Research Fellow at Dr. Andreazza's lab. He is currently working to develop new approaches for the intervention of neuropsychiatric disorders. He obtained his PhD at the Institute of Biotechnology, University of Caxias do Sul, Brazil. His aspirations are to understand the molecular aspects of neuropsychiatric disorders and cancer. Currently, he is developing biomarkers and potential novel therapeutics, mainly natural compounds for the management of these disorders. Dr. Scola is appointed with the Centre for Addiction and Mental Health, the Department of Psychiatry and Pharmacology at the University of Toronto.

# Contents

# Preface

Since the thalidomide tragedy in the 1960s, the theme of toxicology has advanced rapidly over the past decade with emerging innovative toxicity testing protocols, techniques, and regulation being placed. While the discipline of toxicology can be rather complex, having a comprehensive understanding of the principles and mechanisms of foreign substances that can cause toxicity is important for consumers to make decisions about the risks and benefits inherent to issues pertaining to human diseases. Since the bioactivation of many toxins and toxicants and its consequences on human health are not clearly known, special emphasis is devoted by scientists worldwide to understanding how drugs, environmental chemicals and industrial pollutants can cause adverse heath effects. This book provides a unique, integrated approach addressing the theory and mechanisms of toxicity, current cutting-edge methodologies of toxicology, and applications from the latest toxicological studies relevant to human diseases.

Toxicology studies on cell, drug and environment bring the most current state of evidence regarding the role of distinctive toxicants in different living systems. There are three main sections in this book concerning the bases of mitochondrial dysfunction, drug toxicology and environmental toxicology. In the first section, the book puts singular prominence on the effects of toxicants, mainly reactive oxidative species in the cellular level ("Pathological Aspects with Global Impact Induced by Toxicants at Cellular Level") leading to mitochondrial dysfunction induced by anticancer agents ("Mitochondrial Dysfunction on the Toxic Effects of Anticancer Agents— From Lab Bench to Bedside") and drug development targeting the mitochondria ("Mitochondrial Targeting for Drug Development") in the pathophysiology of various diseases.

The second section, entitled "Drug Toxicology", explores the effects of xenobiotics under the forensic perspective ("Forensic Toxicology"), introducing different methods and approaches in biological and non-biological matter. In the same section, the clinical manifestations and life-threatening signs/symptoms of tramadol poisoning are also discussed ("Tramadol Poisoning"), bringing important aspects of drug administration.

Finally, the third section explores environmental toxicology. Three chapters are included in this section about the potential deleterious environmental impacts on human health. The first chapter ("How to Answer the Question — Are Drugs Real Threats to Biological Systems or Overrated Innocuous Chemicals?") explores a wide-spectrum of the effects of substances and its interactions with the biota. The effects of estrogenic endocrine disruptors compounds in water environments are also discussed ("Estrogenic Compounds in Estuarine and Coastal Water Environments of the Iberian Western Atlantic Coast and Selected Locations Worldwide — Relevancy, Trends and Challenges in View of the EU Water Framework

Directive), followed by the impact of pesticides on human health (“Impact of Pesticides on Environmental and Human Health“).

In this book, 20 prominent experts have equally contributed to develop and explore the scientific progress that has been made over the last decades in the toxicology field. We are confident that this book will serve as a guide for researchers and students.

**Ana Cristina Andreazza and Gustavo Scola**
University of Toronto
Canada

Section 1

# Bases of Mitochondrial Dysfunction

Chapter 1

# Pathological Aspects with Global Impact Induced by Toxicants at Cellular Level

Dorina E. Coricovac and Cristina A. Dehelean

Additional information is available at the end of the chapter

http://dx.doi.org/10.5772/59945

## 1. Introduction

In toxicology, the term "toxicant" defines a noxious substance that induces a series of deleterious effects on organs, tissues and biological functions and processes in living organisms. Another term used to describe a toxicant is "poison" [1]. The list of toxicants regardless their origin, of natural sources or ensued from human activities, is quite long.

Some of the main detrimental responses that a toxicant is able to generate at cellular level include: production of reactive oxygen species (ROS) and free radicals. These "basic" processes could be associated with carcinogenesis, immunotoxicity, teratogenesis and genotoxicity. The toxic mechanism of action in such cases is initiated by a terminal toxicant and a target molecule and might involve different types of reactions, including: covalent or non-covalent bonds, hydrogen subtraction, electron transfer, and enzymatic reactions.

The cascade of processes that occur at cellular level and involve ROS is initiated by events like ischemia and lipid peroxidation, which are noticed after the first exposure to reactive metabolites and are considered primary events. As secondary events were described important processes as follows: changes in structure and permeability of membranes, mitochondrial dysfunctions, cytoskeletal and DNA changes, lysosomal destabilization, intervention in apoptosis/necrosis and endoplasmic reticulum destruction. The final step of the cascade is associated with severe pathological destruction on organs level.

In the past decade, the toxicity of heavy metals and their risks on human health has been a subject of high interest, an argument in this regard being the impressive number of publications available (over 2000 articles according to PubMed database). Heavy metals are inorganic elements, natural components of earth's crust, and are labeled as the oldest toxins known by humans [2]. It has been demonstrated that heavy metals induce toxicity at different levels in human body, including: gastrointestinal system, central and peripheral nervous systems, cardiovascular, renal and hematopoietic systems [2]. As regards the toxic mechanism of action of heavy metals, it has been stated that generation of reactive oxygen species represents one of the main mechanisms involved in heavy metals induced-toxicity. It is believed that generation of reactive oxygen species is responsible for the hepatotoxicity, neurotoxicity and nephrotoxicity associated to heavy metals [2, 3].

Free radicals and reactive oxygen species generated by toxicants were described to hold key roles in lipid peroxidation, DNA damage, oxidation of sulfhydryl groups of proteins, depletion of protein, and alteration of calcium homeostasis [2, 4].

Reactive oxygen species (ROS) are oxygen-free radicals that contain one or more unpaired electrons, formed during oxidative metabolism and were characterized as exceedingly active compounds which act by inducing oxidative changes of cellular proteins, lipids and polynucleotides [5-7].

Under normal conditions, ROS play essential functions in cellular homeostasis, as signal molecules in several signaling pathways involved in cell differentiation, organogenesis, stress response and wound healing, and as redox regulators [6]. Oxidative stress represents a status characterized by excessive cellular levels of ROS as a result of an imbalance in the redox homeostasis explained by increased production of ROS or declined antioxidant capacity [2, 6, 7]. A considerable number of studies endorse the fact that oxidative stress is linked to a plethora of pathologies including cardiovascular diseases, atherosclerosis, diabetes, chronic inflammatory processes, neurodegenerative disorders, and mostly to cancer [6-8].

This chapter summarizes an update of available data regarding ROS in physiological and pathophysiological conditions, the roles of ROS in cancer and heavy metals induced toxicity via ROS generation.

## 2. Redox homeostasis and ROS generation

The term "redox" refers to the oxidation-reduction status and is considered a key regulator of several metabolic cellular functions [9] and a fundamental keeper of cellular homeostasis [10].

During redox processes that occur in the cells are generated a variety of reactive oxygen species with functional roles in physiological and pathological conditions dependent on cell's capacity to maintain the ratio between ROS production and ROS disposal in balance. Commonly, the term "redox signaling" is used to express the changes of protein's oxidation status resulted in ROS-mediated events at cellular level [11].

The oxidative stress is characterized by a globally enhancement of intracellular ROS levels appeared from a dysfunction of the mechanisms involved in maintaining redox homeostasis: increased ROS generation or declined capacity of ROS elimination [10]. Mounting evidence suggest that oxidative stress is implicated in various pathologies such as aging, neurodegenerative disorders, development of brain damage, pathogenesis of multiple sclerosis lesions and cancer [10, 12, 13].

ROS are highly reactive molecules, derived from oxygen, ceaselessly generated during oxidative metabolism and exuded into biological systems; outcomes of one or multielectron reductions of oxygen [7, 14]. The balance between ROS production and ROS disposal is ensured by the cell's keepers, antioxidant enzymes (superoxide dismutase – SOD, glutathione peroxidase, catalase and thioredoxin reductase) and non-enzymatic scavengers (ascorbate, tocopherols, tocotrienols, carotenoids, natural flavonoids, melatonin, gluthatione, thioredoxin) [7, 14].

ROS can be generated by multiple endogenous and exogenous sources. The main endogenous source of ROS is mitochondria, which produces reactive species as by-products of normal cell metabolism during the electron leakage that passes in the conversion of molecular oxygen process. Hereupon it might be added the activity of some enzymes, like: membrane-associated NADPH oxidases, cytochrome p450s, P-450-dependent monooxygenases, lipoxygenase, cyclooxygenase and xanthine oxidase [6, 13]. At mitochondrial level responsible for the formation of ROS are complexes I (NADH dehydrogenase (ubiquinone)) and II (succinate dehydrogenase), which produce ROS on the inner side of mitochondrial matrix, and complex III (ubiquinol-cytochrome c reductase) that delivers the generated species (superoxide radical) into the intermembrane space or mitochondrial matrix [14].

Other endogenous sources of ROS are the microsomes and peroxisomes (generate especially $H_2O_2$) and it was, also, demonstrated that immune cells' (neutrophils and macrophages) mechanism of action against invading microorganisms involves ROS [10]. The biosynthesis of prostaglandins, prostacyclins and thromboxane A2 from arachidonic acid, process catalyzed by cyclooxygenases, it is also a source of ROS [13, 15].

As exogenous sources of ROS, there were indicated the following agents: atmospheric pollutants, tobacco smoke, irradiation (UV irradiation, x-ray, gamma-ray), chemicals, iron salts, heavy metals and chemicals [2, 10, 14].

The group of reactive oxygen species comprises two different kinds of species:

**a.** free radicals – possess unpaired electrons in their outer orbitals: superoxide anion radical ($O_2^{\cdot -}$), hydroxyl radical (OH•), hydroperoxyl radical (HOO•), alkoxy (RO•) and peroxy radicals (ROO•), and

**b.** non-radical oxygen species – possess unpaired electrons, too, are very reactive and are able to form ROS radicals: hydrogen peroxide ($H_2O_2$), organic hydroperoxide (ROOH), ozone ($O_3$) and trioxidan (HOOOH) [2, 6, 14].

Free radicals (also known as pro-oxidants) can be recognized by some specific features, like: high instability and reactivity, the presence of unpaired electrons in the outmost orbital of their atoms, the need to acquire equilibrium by bonding with electrons of neighboring atoms, what leads to chain reactions and the ability to react with different cellular molecules [16, 17].

Some of the main ROS species will be presented in Table 1, outlining the generation process and their specific characteristics.

| ROS name | Generation | Characteristics |
|---|---|---|
| **$O2^{\cdot-}$, superoxide anion** | - *at mitochondrial level:* as a side-product of mitochondria formed during aerobic metabolism; there are two sites of mitochondrial ROS production, complex I (NADH – ubiquinone oxidoreductase) and complex III (ubiquinol - cytochrome c oxidoreductase) [10, 18, 19]<br>$O_2 + e^- \rightarrow O_2^{\cdot}$ [20]<br>- *enzymatically:* it is produced is by NADPH oxidase (Nox) expressed in the phagocytes' cell membrane, by cytochrome P450-dependent oxygenases in the endoplasmic reticulum of the liver, lung and small intestine and by the xanthine oxidase (XO) located in the cytosol [14, 16, 18, 19, 21, 22]..<br>- *non-enzymatically*: the generation process consists in the transfer of a single electron to oxygen by coenzymes in reduced form, flavins or iron sulfur clusters or xenobiotics that suffered a reduction reaction [19, 23]. | - is described as the first free radical obtained during mitochondrial electron transfer chain process and it is easily converted to hydrogen peroxide via a dismutation reaction catalyzed by superoxide dismutase (SOD) [6]<br>- it's a short-lived molecule and presents only one reduction equivalent<br>- it cannot be considered a candidate molecule for signal transduction in the cell since the ability of this radical to cross the mitochondrial outer membrane is rather low [14]<br>- at mitochondrial level it is involved in the generation of peroxynitrite ($ONOO_2^{\cdot-}$), a noxious oxidant that induces DNA damage, disruption of mitochondrial integrity, and irreversible modification of proteins [14]<br>- releases $Fe^{2+}$ from iron-sulfur proteins and ferritin [2]<br>is the precursor of most ROS and a mediator in oxidative chain reactions [19] |
| **$H_2O_2$, hydrogen peroxide** | - by direct reduction of $O_2$ [2]<br>-by dismutation from superoxide radical under the action of superoxide dismutases (SOD1 – in mitochondrial intermembrane space and SOD2 – in mitochondrial matrix) [11, 16, 24].<br>$2\,O_2^{\cdot-} \rightarrow H_2O_2 + O_2$<br>-up-to 80% of H2O2 is formed by peroxisomal (eg. D-amino acid oxidase, D-aspartate oxidase or polyamine oxidase) and microsomal (microsomal CYP-mediated ω-oxidation of fatty acids) enzymes [4, 18, 25, 26]. | - presents a two-electron reduction state [2]<br>- is a mitochondrial ROS, a electrophobic molecule able to pass through membranes H2O2 [2, 11].<br>- mitochondrial concentrations of hydrogen peroxide are 100 times greater than that of superoxide anion [11].<br>- it can be regarded as a fundamental ROS in carcinogenesis [18].<br>- its conversion into oxygen and water is mediated by catalases and gluthatione peroxidases [18].<br>- is a strong oxidant, precursor of hydroxy radical (·OH) via Haber Weiss reaction [18].<br>- due to its lipophilic character lightly crosses mitochondrial and plasmatic membranes reaching into the cytosol and extracellular environment where asserts its effects [14].<br>- has the capacity to generate highly reactive hydroxyl radicals via reactions with metals (iron and copper) [20, 27]. |

| ROS name | Generation | Characteristics |
|---|---|---|
| HO•, hydroxyl radical | - via Fenton reaction from hydrogen peroxide [10, 16, 19].<br>$Fe^{2+} + H_2O_2 \rightarrow Fe^{3+} + HO\cdot + OH^-$<br>- by Haber-Weiss reaction - oxidation of superoxide anion radical [19]:<br>$O_2^{\cdot-} + H_2O_2 \rightarrow HO\cdot + OH^- + O_2$<br>-by decomposition of peroxynitrite [2] | - presents a three-electron reduction state [2]<br>- is a extremely reactive specie with a short half-life [2, 18].<br>- induces DNA damage by generating 8-hydroxy 2′-deoxyguanosine (8-OHdG), molecule responsible for DNA mutations, a key factor for the carcinogenic risk [18].<br>- induces changes to other cellular molecules, changes defined by enzymes' denaturation, proteins' structure modifications or peroxidation of polyunsaturated fatty acids [18]. |
| $HO_2^{\cdot-}$, hydroperoxyl radical | - is formed when an oxygen molecule binds to a proton [16]<br>- it can be obtained during the second step of oxygen complete reduction reaction [20]:<br>$O_2^{\cdot-} + H_2O \rightarrow HO_2^{\cdot-} + OH^-$<br>-via Fenton reaction [20]<br>$Fe^{2+} + H_2O_2 \rightarrow Fe^{2+} + OOH^{\cdot-} + H^+$ | - this oxygen-centered reactive specie is capable to abstract H from a lipid molecule (polyunsaturated fatty acid), particularly in the presence of metals like copper or iron, leading to an autocatalytic chain reaction. The result of this process is the formation of a lipid hydroperoxide (or peroxide) [20, 28]. |

**Table 1.** Description of the main ROS species.

## 3. ROS in physiological conditions

Reactive oxygen species are continuously produced in the cells, especially during mitochondrial electron transport chain and eliminated in biological systems, where in physiological conditions (low levels), they play crucial roles in the regulation of different cell's functions, including cell proliferation, apoptosis, transformation, and senescence [7].

The mechanism of action of ROS in activation of cell proliferation or different signal pathways implies the interaction between ROS and cysteine residues leading to the formation of disulfide bonds and activation of signal transducing pathways. The activation of these processes may occur via kinase activation or phosphatase inhibition, and via regulation of proteinases, including matrix metalloproteinases (see Figure 1) [14].

Besides their toxic effects, it was demonstrated that reactive oxygen species interfere in main cellular processes (differentiation, organogenesis, wound healing, cell fate regulation), in the activity of different enzymes (kinases and phosphatase), transcription factors, ionic channels and transporters [6]. Moreover, it appears that ROS acts as an essential cellular messenger alongside with the acknowledged second messengers ($Ca^{2+}$, arachidonic acid, cAMP and IP3) [6].

Pan and coworkers stated that ROS are involved in the microbicidal activity of phagocytes, regulation of signal transduction and gene expression, and act as inducers of oxidative damage to macromolecules (nucleic acids, proteins, and lipids) (see Figure 1) [29].

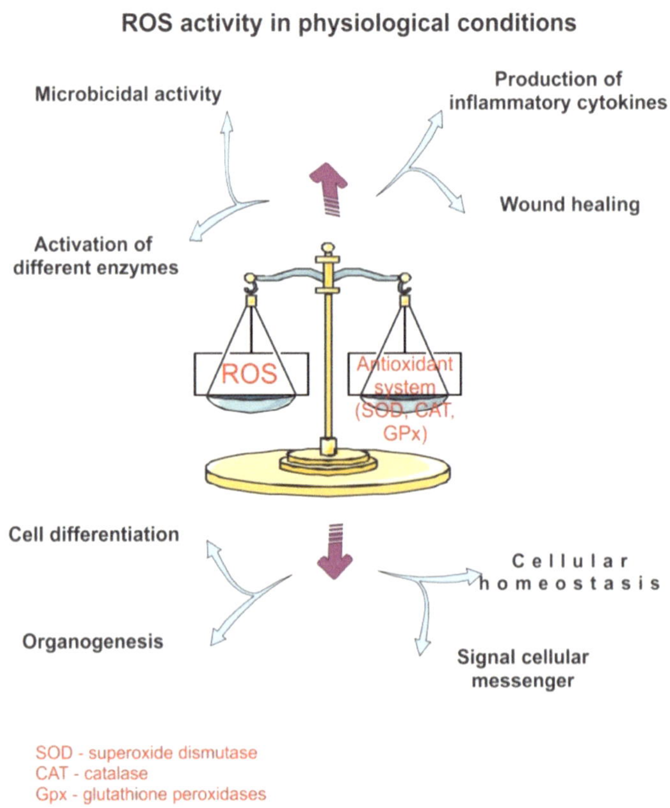


**Figure 1.** ROS cellular functions in physiological conditions (the picture was obtained by using Servier Medical Art templates).

Most of the free radicals generated by various cellular metabolic systems originate from oxygen. The percent of molecular oxygen that is converted into superoxide and hydroxyl radicals at mitochondrial level is 5%. Mounting evidence indicates that the free radicals resulted have major function in the normal metabolism of cells: they are used in the synthesis of prostaglandins, cholesterol and steroidal hormones. Furthermore, the biosynthesis of collagen demands the participation of hydroxyl free radicals [16].

The effects and functions of ROS are distinct and dependent of their concentration, for example: low concentrations of mitochondrial ROS are associated with metabolic adaptation in hypoxic conditions; moderate concentrations are involved in the regulation of inflammatory response and high levels stimulate apoptosis/autophagy pathways responsible of inducing cell death [11].

http://dx.doi.org/10.5772/59945

Other beneficial effects of ROS refer to their involvement in the intracellular killing of bacteria by neutrophil granulocytes, detoxification of the liver and certain cell signaling processes [20, 30].

There is also considerable information regarding the roles of mitochondrial ROS (superoxide anion and hydrogen peroxide) in inflammatory cytokine production and innate immune responses by activation of newly characterized RIG-I-like receptors (RLRs), inflammasomes, and mitogen activated protein kinases (MAPK) [11, 31, 32].

## 4. ROS in pathophysiological conditions

The phenomenon characterized by an impaired balance between ROS generation and ROS elimination is known as oxidative stress. The oxidative damage was frequently associated with different pathologies including: diabetes type II, neurodegenerative disease, atherosclerosis, multiple sclerosis, chronic inflammatory disease, aging and carcinogenesis (see Figure 2). The ability of free radicals to chemically react with most of cell components it was considered a risk, especially for large molecules (nucleic acids, proteins, polymerized carbohydrates - polysaccharides), and lipids, since these components are targets for the oxygenated free radicals [16,20].

The free radical induced-toxicity at cellular level is expressed as lipid and protein peroxidation and damaged nucleic acids (see Figure 2) [20]. The hydroxyl radical is the most reactive free radical molecule capable to cause severe cell damage and to other intracellular structures due to its ability to induce covalent cross-linking of a variety of biological molecules [20].

Superoxide anion is a reactive oxygen molecule that plays important roles in the body because is considered the precursor of the other free radicals that determine cell injury. The toxic mechanism of action of this free radical involves the disassembly of iron-sulphur ([Fe–S]) clusters in proteins via the inactivation of iron regulatory protein-1 (IRP-1), leading to clearing of iron and damage of –SH residues [20,34].

The noxious effects of ROS might be exerted at: DNA level, also known as DNA oxidation what leads to mutations and possibly cancer [20,33]; at protein level causing enzyme inhibition, denaturation and protein degradation, and at lipid level leading to lipid peroxidation [20]. ROS-induced DNA peroxidation inhibits gene transcription and determines gene mutations. The main toxic products resulted from ROS-induced DNA damage are 8-hydroxyadenine (8-OH-Ade), 8-hydroxyguanine (8-OH-Gua), 5,6-dihydroxy-5,6-dihydrothymine (thymine glycol, Tg) [19].

The lipid peroxidation process is a chemical chain reaction that consists of three stages: initiation, propagation and termination [10,20]. During the initiation stage occur the following processes: a ROS (usually a hydroxyl radical due to its high reactivity) reacts with a peroxide-free lipid system in order to remove a hydrogen (H) atom from a methylene group ($-CH_2-$), the result being the generation of free radicals such as conjugated dienes and peroxyl radical [10,20].

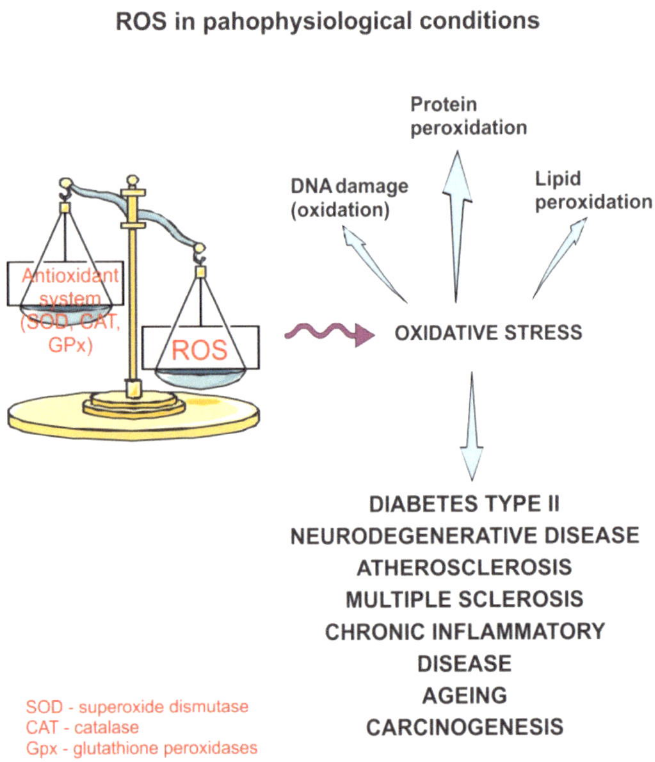


**Figure 2.** ROS cellular functions in pathophysiological conditions (the picture was obtained by using Servier Medical Art templates).

The propagation stage is characterized by the attack of the peroxyl radical resulted during the initiation stage to other lipid molecules (fatty acids) via an autocatalytic chain reaction catalyzed by metals such as iron or copper and it results a lipid hydroperoxide (or peroxide) [10,20]. Polyunsaturated fatty acids are considered easy targets for lipid peroxidation due to the unsaturated chemical structure. The ROS-induced peroxidation end products ($\alpha$, $\beta$ unsaturated reactive aldehydes, such as malondialdehyde - MDA, 4-hydroxy-2-nonenal - HNE, acrolein and isoprostanes) have also deleterious effects on tissues (see Figure 3) [10,20,35].

The injury caused by ROS to membrane phospholipids can affect in a cascade manner the membrane integrity, followed by altered membrane integrity, suppression of enzymes and membrane receptors, an increased tissue permeability, an impaired cellular function and cell death [10,20,29].

The end-products of lipid peroxidation possess a high reactivity and can easily interact with proteins, phospholipids and nucleic acids via different reactions resulting stable products (adduct between proteins and lipid peroxides or glycation products) with potential roles in the pathogenesis of several maladies [20, 36]. The stable products mediate cell death by aggregation of bulky protein complexes which inhibit the activity of 26S and 20S proteosome and determine accumulation of injured proteins (see Figure 3) [10].

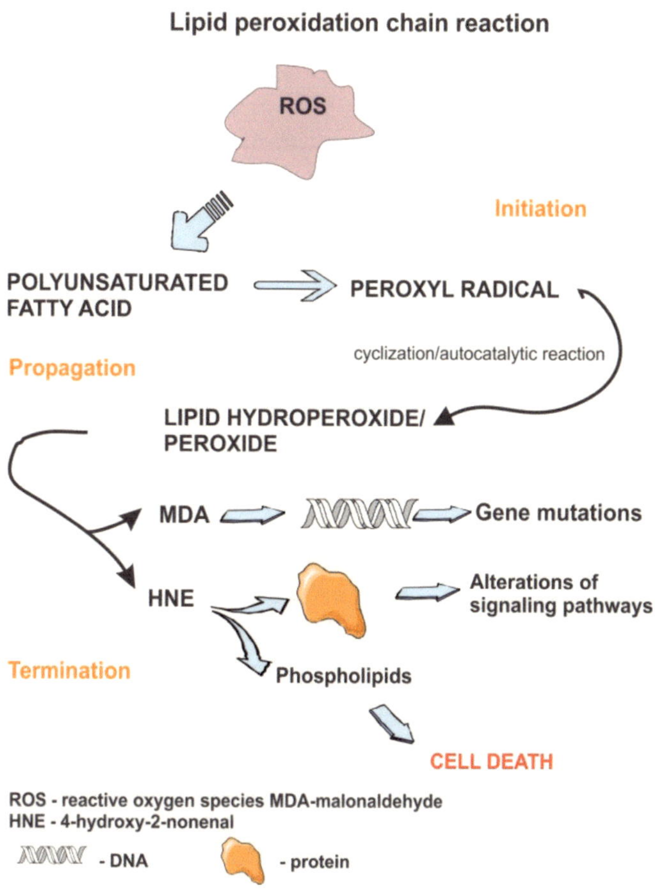


**Figure 3.** ROS-induced lipid peroxidation (the picture was obtained by using Servier Medical Art templates).

Recent studies demonstrated that ROS is involved in the mitochondrial energetically dysfunction associated to ethanol-induced gastric mucosa damage [29,37]. It was stated that impairment of mitochondria and/or up-regulation of NADPH-oxidase complex are linked to various cancers and play major function in establishing the anticancer therapeutic strategies [14].

In the last years, the subject regarding the roles of ROS in cancer gained a lot of interest. The cellular injury initiated by ROS is considered an important step in cancer development. It seems like the signal transduction messenger function of ROS is associated with cancer initiation by activation of different signaling pathways like MAPK, PI3K and NF-κB [7].

The mechanism of action of ROS in ageing is still a matter of debate. There are studies that sustain the fact that elevated ROS levels along with mitochondrial dysfunction and metabolic alterations are features of cellular senescence. Other studies have proposed the hypothesis that ROS is cause and consequence of NF-κB pathway activation during senescence [38].

## 5. ROS and cancer

The imbalance between cellular generation of ROS and its removal leads to oxidative stress which was associated, among other deleterious effects, with the initiation and progression of cancer.

Regarding the carcinogenesis, it is important to note that reactive oxygen species are considered to be regulators of the following major signaling mechanisms: extracellular signal-regulated kinases (ERKs), mitogen-activated protein kinases (MAPKs), phosphoinositide 3-kinases (PI3Ks) and transcription factors such as hypoxia-inducible factors (HIFs). All of these signaling pathways play key roles in cell proliferation, cell growth and cell survival. It was observed that high levels of ROS can induce irreversible oxidative damage in lipids, proteins and nucleic acids. Furthermore, ROS are active in multistage carcinogenesis from initiation to malignant conversion, by inducing oxidative DNA damage and mutations in protooncogenes and tumor suppressor genes, and subsequent activation of signal transduction pathways [14].

In the first stage of carcinogenesis, cancer cells usually express genetic instability and a significant increase in ROS concentration as a consequence of a "vicious circle": ROS induce genetic mutations (especially in mitochondrial DNA), which lead to metabolic dysfunction and additional ROS generation [14].

ROS cause almost all forms of DNA damage, such as changes of the nucleotide bases, strand breakage and DNA protein cross-links, but the end-products depend on the type of ROS. It was mentioned that the mutations induced by specific ROS are implicated in the genesis of cancer. Another mechanism of action of ROS in carcinogenesis was to induce and keep the oncogenic phenotypes of tumor cells. At present, oxidative stress is widely accepted as a key contributor to cancer development [14,29].

Previous studies have demonstrated that oxidative stress is associated with carcinogenesis and is also related to the incidence of cancer [39,40]. During the carcinogenesis process, the imbalance between ROS production and ROS elimination is represented by the increased concentrations of reactive oxygen species in cancer cells and a reduction of antioxidants levels. The increase of ROS in these cells occurs due to the influence of intrinsic or extrinsic factors, resulting in gene mutations and changes in transcriptional processes as well as changes in signaling pathways and, ultimately, the occurrence of cancer [40]. Other contributory factors for the enhanced production of ROS in cancer cells are: cancer-associated fibroblasts (CAFs), cancer-associated macrophages (CAMs), and hypoxia. Cancer-associated macrophages are able to generate ROS via NADPH oxidase in tumor cells [39].

It was also shown that ROS affects the expression of the p53 suppressor gene which is a key factor in apoptosis. In addition, oxidative injury induced by changes in gene expression, cell proliferation, apoptosis, and angiogenesis plays a significant role in tumor initiation and progression [39].

There are recent studies that sustain the idea that ROS induced by oxidative stress might lead to apoptotic or necrotic cell death of skin cells. Especially, the accumulated ROS plays a critical role in the intrinsic aging and photo-aging of human skin in vivo, what leads to the hypothesis that ROS are responsible for different skin cancers and other cutaneous inflammatory maladies. Ultraviolet radiation type B (UVB) is considered a complete carcinogen and generates increased levels of ROS, leading to oxidative damage at skin level. According to several studies, exposure of mammalian skin cells to UVB radiation determines alterations of cellular function via oxidation of macromolecules, DNA damage, generation of ROS, and changes in signaling pathways. As major sources of $H_2O_2$ were described UVB-induced leukocyte infiltration in the skin, and inflammatory leukocytes and it was stated that $H_2O_2$ plays an important role in inflammatory skin diseases and skin cancer [5].

ROS exert key roles in a variety of processes associated with epithelial malignancy such as cell proliferation, epithelial-mesenchymal transition (EMT), angiogenesis, apoptosis evasion and enhancement of metastatic potential [41].

Free radicals in carcinogenesis, ROS and RNS (reactive nitrogen species) contribute in different ways to carcinogenesis and the malignant progression of tumor cells, enhancing their metastatic potential. In fact, they are now considered a distinctive characteristic of cancer. These species lead to genomic damage and genetic instability, and they participate as intermediaries in mitogenic and survival signals via growth factor receptors and adhesion molecules, promoting cell mobility, inducing inflammation/repair and angiogenesis in the tumor microenvironment [16].

## 6. Redox modulation of toxicants — Heavy metals-induced toxicity

The essential metals are very important for the maintenance of cell homeostasis. Among the 23 chemical elements with physiological functions in humans, half of them are metals, including heavy metals [42]. The heavy metals, generally defined as metallic elements with a relative density above 5 mg/ml, have the potential to cause human toxicity; the main examples are: Pb, Hg, Fe, Cd, Tl, Bi, Mn, and As. The intoxications produced by metals, characterized mainly by neurotoxicity, genotoxicity, or carcinogenicity, are widely known [43]. After their absorption into organism, the metals bind to proteins and lead to impaired enzymatic activity; the result being the damage of many organs.

Cellular redox processes are controlled by two systems (thioredoxin, Trx, and glutathione, GSH) [44]. Exposure to ions of heavy metals can amplify the production of reactive oxygen species (ROS), which can react with cellular components followed by the debut of many physiological processes [45]. ROS have a double character as both deleterious and useful compounds: on one hand they act within cells as 2$^{nd}$ messengers in intracellular signaling cascades, inducing and keeping the oncogenic phenotype of cancer cells, and on the other hand, ROS induce the cellular senescence and apoptosis and can be considered anticancer species. The cumulative production of ROS (called oxidative stress) is common for many types of cancer cell which are linked with altered redox regulation of the cellular signaling pathways [46].

Metal-induced formation of ROS causes changes to DNA, increased lipid peroxidation, and altered Ca and -SH homeostasis. Lipid peroxides, formed by ROS attack on phospholipids, can react with redox metals finally producing carcinogenic products [27].

Redox active metals (Fe, Cu, Cr, Co) are part of redox cycling reactions and have the ability to produce ROS. Perturbation of metal ion homeostasis can lead to oxidative stress, a state where increased production of ROS overcome the body antioxidant protection and induces DNA damage, lipid peroxidation, and proteins changes. The action mechanism of these metals involves formation of ROS, finally producing mutagenic and carcinogenic products. Redox inactive metals (Cd, As and Pb) show their toxic effects via bonding to proteins -SH groups and depletion of GSH [47].

Lead (Pb) is a chemical element from group 14, and period 6 (p-block). Pb was removed from alimentary cans, paints, and petrol because it was the most common cause of heavy metal poisoning; an important problem remains the water pipes from older houses, some occupations, and traditional remedies. Pb causes toxicity to mitochondria by depletion of GSH, which results in excessive ROS production and mitochondrial damage. It was discovered that Pb toxicity leads to cellular damage via two pathways: (1) the production of ROS, and (2) the direct reduction of antioxidant reserves. Mitochondrial antioxidant enzymes play an important role in cellular defense mechanism against oxidative damage [48]. A possible molecular mechanism of Pb toxicity is represented by the oxidative stress, which appears when ROS production exceed the capacity of antioxidant defense mechanisms. Pb is capable of causing oxidative damage to heart, liver, brain, and erythrocytes [49].

Mercury (Hg) is a chemical element from group 12, and period 6 (d-block); it is poorly absorbed from bowels and the ingestion is usually harmless. Hg compounds have the ability to provoke cellular damage through an increase of ROS levels (the molecular mechanism involved in its genotoxicity). In response to Hg exposure, the amount of intracellular GSH increase to chelate Hg in order to protect the cells by its antioxidant role. Tchounwou and *colab.* already demonstrated that GSH levels are higher in human populations exposed to methylmercury intoxication by a fish-rich diet [50].

Iron (Fe) is a chemical element from group 8, and period 4 (d-block) and it is one of the most abundant elements in the crust of earth. ROS can play a role in Fe-induced cell toxicity because of its salts' powerful prooxidant activity. In the presence of cellular reductants, Fe from low molecular weight salts can be an initiator of free radical reactions. In Fe overload, hepatocellular Ca homeostasis may be spoiled through mitochondrial damage and microsomal Ca sequestration. DNA has also been reported to be a target of Fe-induced damage in the liver; this may lead to malignant transformation [51].

Due to its oxidation states (3+ and 2+), Fe is considered an intrinsic producer of ROS, leading to neuronal oxidative stress. Paradoxically, Fe redox properties determine its participation in potentially cytotoxic reactions: bivalent form catalyze the formation of hydroxyl radical, considered the most reactive and damaging intermediate of cellular metabolism, while trivalent form can be reduced to $Fe^{2+}$ after reacting with superoxide anion. Both forms are also involved in the propagation of lipid peroxidation, by a complex mechanism; however, it likely involves the direct interaction of Fe with ROS [52].

Cadmium (Cd) is a chemical element from group 12, and period 5 (d-block); it was discovered in the 19th century and the first studies upon its toxicological properties were initiated shortly after. The smoke and food are considered the main sources of Cd. Cd inhibits the activity of antioxidant enzymes; it displaces Zn and Cu leading to a decreased level of these two metals in the enzymes and an increased level in the cytoplasm. Thus appear conformational changes and inhibition of enzyme activity, and deregulation of Cu homeostasis which can lead to ROS production via the Fenton reaction [53].

Thallium (Tl) is a chemical element from group 13, and period 6 (p-block); Tl and its compounds must be manipulated with an increased attention due to their important toxicity. Different authors indicate that Tl induce ROS formation, GSH oxidation, and membrane lipid peroxidation; the liver mitochondria seems to be the main targets of its toxicity because liver is its storage site [54].

Bismuth (Bi) is a chemical element from group 15, and period 6 (p-block); it has a few industrial uses in pigments, ceramics and alloys with low melting points. Bi causes kidney damage and the promotion of a reversible encephalopathy; chelating agents may be used as treatment.

In a few studies of Woods and Fowler there were evaluated Bi effects on organelle structure and heme biosynthetic parameters in liver and cells; their study revealed that action of the metal on membrane enzymes only partially accounts for deterioration of the membrane enzymes' activity. They showed that Bi initial acute effects in liver and kidney cells include deformation of mitochondrial membranes and inhibition of specific heme pathway enzymes. Both effects contribute to deterioration of membrane-associated enzymatic functions [55].

D. Bagchi and *colab.* investigated the effects of acute and chronic stress on the enhanced production of ROS; the precautionary ability of bismuth subsalicylate (BSS) was evaluated against the gastrointestinal mucosal injury induced by oxidative stress. Their findings revealed that BSS decreased chronic stress-induced lipid peroxidation, DNA fragmentation, and membrane microviscosity by approx. 40-50% in gastric and in the intestinal mucosa. It was found that oxidative stress produce gastrointestinal mucosal injury through improved production of ROS, and that BSS protect against gastrointestinal mucosal injury [56].

Manganese (Mn) is a chemical element from group 7, and period 4 (d-block); it is an essential dietary nutrient, but its excess lead to an accumulation with toxic effects (the manganism is a disease associated with Mn accumulation and it is due to ROS production. The bivalent ion is a central component of some enzymes and an activator of many metal-enzyme complexes. On the other hand, the trivalent ion is found in the essential enzymes manganese catalase and Mn-superoxide dismutase (SOD), both of which break down oxidants using the Mn3+ in their reactive catalytic center. The bivalent ion (Mn2+) intends to bind to almost all Ca2+ and Mg2+

binding sites leading to substitutions of these ions in many biological processes; this is due to the similarities of their electron structure [57].

Arsenic (As) is a chemical element from group 15, and period 4 (p-block); it is contained in many minerals, but it also appear as a pure elemental crystal. As inhibits lipoic acid, which is a cofactor for pyruvate dehydrogenase into the citric acid cycle. Another important aspect is the fact that $AsO_4^{3-}$ decouples the oxidative phosphorylation leading to the inhibition of energy-linked reduction of $NAD^+$, mitochondrial respiration, and ATP synthesis. The production of $H_2O_2$ is also increased, which lead to ROS production and oxidative stress. The frequency of human cancers is increased in the case of long term exposure at As probably due to the ROS production [58].

Zhang Z and *colab.* showed that As can activate p47(phox) and p67(phox), proteins which activate NADPH oxidase and it generate ROS in DLD1 cells. It was found that tumor volumes of group treated with As were much larger than those without As treatment. Many researchers found that ROS have a role in the initiation of cellular injury induced by As, which can lead to cancer development. ROS induce direct cellular injury, which may start a set of radical reactions leading to an increase of secondary ROS generation. More than that, the increased ROS production may stimulate the inflammatory processes involving secretion of chemotactic factors, growth factors, proteolytic enzymes, lipoxygenases, and cyclooxygenase, inactivation of anti-proteolytic enzymes, and the release of signaling proteins. NADPH oxidase complex is an important physiological system for ROS production; As is highly capable of activating NADPH oxidase and disrupting of mitochondrias' membrane, leading to the generation of different ROS. It has been generally accepted that ROS are critical regulators for a wide range of cellular responses, from kinase activation, gene expression, DNA damage, cell proliferation, to cell migration in the arsenic treated cells [59].

## 7. Conclusions

Reactive oxygen species (ROS) represented a matter of debate/concern in the last years due to the dual role played by these compounds: beneficial effects at low concentrations (signal molecules, mediators of cellular homeostasis, activators of different enzymes) and deleterious effects at high concentrations (DNA and protein damage, lipid peroxidation and oxidative stress).

The oxidative stress was described as an underlying mechanism in different pathologies, including: neurodegenerative diseases, multiple sclerosis, diabetes, atherosclerosis, ageing, chronic inflammatory diseases and cancer. In cancer development, a possible theory regards the activity of ROS as regulators of major signaling pathways: extracellular signal-regulated kinases (ERKs), mitogen-activated protein kinases (MAPKs), phosphoinositide 3-kinases (PI3Ks) and transcription factors such as hypoxia-inducible factors (HIFs). In addition, it was demonstrated that the toxicity associated to heavy metals (lead, mercury, arsen, cadmium, thallium, bismuth, manganese, iron) is mediated via ROS: ROS generation, mitochondrial injury or inhibition of the antioxidant cellular systems.

## Acknowledgements

Financial support offered by the intern grant PII-C2-TC-2014-16498-10 "Victor Babes" University of Medicine and Pharmacy, Timisoara, Romania.

## Author details

Dorina E. Coricovac and Cristina A. Dehelean*

*Address all correspondence to: cadehelean@umft.ro

Department of Toxicology, „Victor Babes" University of Medicine and Pharmacy, Timisoara, Romania

## References

[1] Manahan SE. Toxicology. In: Manahan SE (ed.) Toxicological Chemistry and Biochemistry 3rd Edition. Boca Raton, Florida: Lewis Publishers; 2003, p134-157.

[2] Sharma B, Singh S, Siddiqi NJ. Biomedical implications of heavy metals induced imbalances in redox systems. BioMed Research International 2014; 2014:640754.

[3] Leonard SS, Harris GK, and Shi X. Metal-induced oxidative stress and signal transduction. Free Radical Biology and Medicine 2004; 37(12):1921–1942.

[4] Valko M, Morris H, and Cronin MTD. Metals, toxicity and oxidative stress. Current Medicinal Chemistry 2005; 12(10):1161–1208.

[5] Narendhirakannan RT, Hannah MA. Oxidative stress and skin cancer: an overview. Indian Journal of Clinical Biochemistry 2013; 28(2):110-5.

[6] Wang X, Fang H, Huang Z, Shang W, Hou T, Cheng A, Cheng H. Imaging ROS signaling in cells and animals. Journal of Molecular Medicine 2013; 91(8):917-27.

[7] Davidson T, Ke Q, and Costa M. Selected Molecular Mechanisms of Metal Toxicity and Carcinogenicity. In: Nordberg GF, Fowler BA, Nordberg M, Friberg LT, (ed) Handbook on the Toxicology of Metals, 3rd Edition, San Diego, California: Academic Press Elsevier; 2007. p79-95.

[8] Bashan N, Kovsan J, Kachko I, Ovadia H, Rudich A. Positive and negative regulation of insulin signaling by reactive oxygen and nitrogen species. Physiological Reviews 2009; 89:27–71.

[9] Das KC, White CW. Redox systems of the cell: possible links and implications. Proceedings of the National Academy of Sciences of the United States of America 2002; 99(15):9617-8.

[10] Trachootham D, Lu W, Ogasawara MA, Nilsa RD, Huang P. Redox regulation of cell survival. Antioxidants & Redox Signaling 2008 ; 10(8):1343-74.

[11] Li X, Fang P, Mai J, Choi ET, Wang H, Yang XF. Targeting mitochondrial reactive oxygen species as novel therapy for inflammatory diseases and cancers. Journal of Hematology & Oncology 2013; 6:19.

[12] Valko M, Leibfritz D, Moncol J, Cronin MTD, Mazur M, and Telser J. Free radicals and antioxidants in normal physiological functions and human disease. The International Journal of Biochemistry & Cell Biology 2007; 39: 44–84.

[13] Ortiz GG, Pacheco-Moisés FP, Bitzer-Quintero OK, Ramírez-Anguiano AC, Flores-Alvarado LJ, Ramírez-Ramírez V, Macias-Islas MA, Torres-Sánchez ED. Immunology and oxidative stress in multiple sclerosis: clinical and basic approach. Clinical and Developmental Immunology 2013; 2013:708659

[14] Ivanova D, Bakalova R, Lazarova D, Gadjeva V, Zhelev Z. The impact of reactive oxygen species on anticancer therapeutic strategies. Advances in Clinical and Experimental Medicine 2013; 22(6):899-908.

[15] Smith WL, DeWitt DL, and Garavito RM. N-glycosylation of prostaglandin endoperoxide synthase-1 and-2 and their orientations in the endoplasmic," Annual Review of Biochemistry 2000; 69:145–182.

[16] Ríos-Arrabal S, Artacho-Cordón F, León J, Román-Marinetto E, Del Mar Salinas-Asensio M, Calvente I, Núñez MI. Involvement of free radicals in breast cancer. Springerplus 2013; 2:404.

[17] Halliwell B. Oxygen and nitrogen are pro-carcinogens. Damage to DNA by reactive oxygen, chlorine and nitrogen species: measurement, mechanism and the effects of nutrition. Mutation Research - Genetic Toxicology and Environmental Mutagenesis 1999; 443(1):37–52.

[18] Henkler F, Brinkmann J, Luch A. The role of oxidative stress in carcinogenesis induced by metals and xenobiotics. Cancers (Basel) 2010; 2(2):376-96.

[19] Li J, O W, Li W, Jiang ZG, Ghanbari HA. Oxidative stress and neurodegenerative disorders. International Journal of Molecular Sciences 2013; 14(12):24438-75.

[20] Aprioku JS. Pharmacology of free radicals and the impact of reactive oxygen species on the testis. Journal of Reproduction and Infertility 2013; 14(4):158-72.

[21] Reed JR, Backes WL. Formation of P450·P450 complexes and their effect on P450 function. Pharmacology & Therapeutics 2012; 133:299–310.

[22] DeLeo FR, Quinn MT. Assembly of the phagocyte NADPH oxidase: Molecular interaction of oxidase proteins. Journal of Leukocyte Biology 1996; 60:677–691.

[23] Turrens JF. Mitochondrial formation of reactive oxygen species. The Journal of Physiology 2003; 552:335–344.

[24] Griendling KK, Sorescu D, Lassègue B, Ushio-Fukai M. Modulation of protein kinase activity and gene expression by reactive oxygen species and their role in vascular physiology and pathophysiology. Arteriosclerosis, Thrombosis, and Vascular Biology 2000; 20(10):2175-83.

[25] Schrader M., Fahimi H.D. Peroxisomes and oxidative stress. Biochimica et Biophysica Acta 2006; 1763:1755–1766.

[26] Yu S, Rao S, Reddy JK. Peroxisome proliferator-activated receptors, fatty acid oxidation, steatohepatitis and hepatocarcinogenesis. Current Molecular Medicine 2003, 3:561–572.

[27] Valko M, Morris H, Cronin MT. Metals, toxicity and oxidative stress. Current Medicinal Chemistry 2005; 12(10): 1161-208.

[28] Catala A. An overview of lipid peroxidation with emphasis in outer segments of photoreceptors and the chemiluminescence assay. The International Journal of Biochemistry & Cell Biology 2006; 38(9):1482-95.

[29] Pan JS, Hong MZ, Ren JL. Reactive oxygen species: A double-edged sword in oncogenesis. World Journal of Gastroenterology 2009; 15(14): 1702-1707.

[30] Victor VM, Rocha M, De la Fuente M. Immune cells: free radicals and antioxidants in sepsis. International Immunopharmacology 2004; 4:327-47.

[31] West AP, Shadel GS, Ghosh S: Mitochondria in innate immune responses. Nature Reviews Immunology 2011; 11:389–402.

[32] Zhou R, Yazdi AS, Menu P, Tschopp J: A role for mitochondria in NLRP3 inflammasome activation. Nature 2010; 469:221–225.

[33] Valko M, Izakovic M, Mazur M, Rhodes CJ, Telser J. Role of oxygen radicals in DNA damage and cancer incidence. Molecular and Cellular Biochemistry 2004; 266(1-2): 37-56.

[34] Schrader M, Fahimi HD. Mammalian peroxisomes and reactive oxygen species. Histochemistry and Cell Biology 2004; 122(4):383-93.

[35] Esterbauer H, Schaur RJ, Zollner H. Chemistry and biochemistry of 4-hydroxynonenal, malonaldehyde and related aldehydes. Free Radical Biology & Medicine 1991; 11(1):81-128.

[36] Dalle-Donne I, Rossi R, Colombo R, Giustarini D, Milzani A. Biomarkers of oxidative damage in human disease. Clinical Chemistry 2006; 52(4):601-23.

[37] Pan JS, He SZ, Xu HZ, Zhan XJ, Yang XN, Xiao HM, Shi HX, Ren JL. Oxidative stress disturbs energy metabolis of mitochondria in ethanol-induced gastric mucosa injury. World Journal of Gastroenterology 2008; 14:5857-5867.

[38] Correia-Melo C, Hewitt G, Passos JF. Telomeres, oxidative stress and inflammatory factors: partners in cellular senescence? Longevity & Healthspan 2014; 3(1):1.

[39] Nourazarian AR, Kangari P, Salmaninejad A. Roles of oxidative stress in the development and progression of breast cancer. Asian Pacific Journal of Cancer Prevention 2014; 15(12):4745-51.

[40] Gao CM, Takezaki T, Wu J-Z, et al. Polymorphisms in thymidylate synthase and methylenetetrahydrofolate reductase genes and the susceptibility to esophageal and stomach cancer with smoking. Asian Pacific Journal of Cancer Prevention 2003; 5: 133-8.

[41] Tobar N, Toyos M, Urra C, Méndez N, Arancibia R, Smith PC, Martínez J. c-Jun N terminal kinase modulates NOX-4 derived ROS production and myofibroblasts differentiation in human breast stromal cells. BMC Cancer 2014; 14(1):640.

[42] Farina M, Avila DS, da Rocha JB, Aschner M. Metals, oxidative stress and neurodegeneration: A focus on iron, manganese and mercury. Neurochemistry International 2013; 62(5):575-94.

[43] Flora SJ, Mittal M, Mehta A. Heavy metal induced oxidative stress & its possible reversal by chelation therapy. Indian Council of Medical Research 2008; 128(4):501-23.

[44] Ueda S, Masutani H, Nakamura H, Tanaka T, Ueno M, Yodoi J. Redox control of cell death. Antioxidants & Redox Signaling 2002; 4(3):405-14.

[45] Ruciñiska-Sobkowiak R. Oxidative stress in plants exposed to heavy metals. Postepy Biochem 2010; 56(2):191-200.

[46] Valko M, Rhodes CJ, Moncol J, Izakovic M, Mazur M. Free radicals, metals and antioxidants in oxidative stress-induced cancer. Chemico-Biological Interactions 2006; 160(1):1-40.

[47] Jomova K, Valko M. Advances in metal-induced oxidative stress and human disease. Toxicology 2011; 283(2-3):65-87.

[48] Patrick L. Lead toxicity part II: the role of free radical damage and the use of antioxidants in the pathology and treatment of lead toxicity. Alternative Medicine Review 2006; 11(2):114-27.

[49] Ahamed M, Siddiqui MK. Low level lead exposure and oxidative stress: current opinions. Clinica Chimica Acta 2007; 383(1-2):57-64.

[50] Crespo-López ME, Macêdo GL, Pereira SI, Arrifano GP, Picanço-Diniz DL, do Nascimento JL, Herculano AM. Mercury and human genotoxicity: Critical considerations and possible molecular mechanisms. Pharmacological Research 2009; 60(4):212-20.

[51] Britton RS. Metal-induced hepatotoxicity. Seminars in Liver Disease 1996; 16(1):3-12.

[52] Jomova K, Vondrakova D, Lawson M, Valko M. Metals, oxidative stress and neurodegenerative disorders. Molecular and Cellular Biochemistry 2010; 345(1-2):91-104.

[53] Nzengue Y, Candéias SM, Sauvaigo S, Douki T, Favier A, Rachidi W, Guiraud P. The toxicity redox mechanisms of cadmium alone or together with copper and zinc homeostasis alteration: its redox biomarkers. Journal of Trace Elements in Medicine and Biology 2011; 25(3):171-80.

[54] Eskandari MR, Mashayekhi V, Aslani M, Hosseini MJ. Toxicity of thallium on isolated rat liver mitochondria: The role of oxidative stress and MPT pore opening. Environmental Toxicology 2013; Aug 30. doi: 10.1002/tox.21900. [Epub ahead of print]

[55] Woods JS, Fowler BA. Alteration of mitochondrial structure and heme biosynthetic parameters in liver and kidney cells by bismuth. Toxicology and Applied Pharmacology 1987; 90(2):274-83.

[56] Bagchi D, Carryl OR, Tran MX, Bagchi M, Garg A, Milnes MM, Williams CB, Balmoori J, Bagchi DJ, Mitra S, Stohs SJ. Acute and chronic stress-induced oxidative gastrointestinal mucosal injury in rats and protection by bismuth subsalicylate. Molecular and Cellular Biochemistry 1999; 196(1-2):109-16.

[57] Martinez-Finley EJ, Gavin CE, Aschner M, Gunter TE. Manganese neurotoxicity and the role of reactive oxygen species. Free Radical Biology & Medicine 2013; 62:65-75.

[58] Klaassen C, Casarett WJ and Doull's. Essentials of Toxicology. McGraw-Hill, 2003, ISBN 978-0-07-138914-3.

[59] Zhang Z, Wang X, Cheng S, Sun L, Son YO, Yao H, Li W, Budhraja A, Li L, Shelton BJ, Tucker T, Arnold SM, Shi X. Reactive oxygen species mediate arsenic induced cell transformation and tumorigenesis through Wnt/β-catenin pathway in human colorectal adenocarcinoma DLD1 cells. Toxicology and Applied Pharmacology 2011; 256(2):114-21.

Chapter 2

# Mitochondrial Dysfunction on the Toxic Effects of Anticancer Agents— From Lab Bench to Bedside

Mariana Ponte Cardoso Ribeiro,
Armanda Emanuela Castro e Santos and
José Barata Antunes Custódio

Additional information is available at the end of the chapter

http://dx.doi.org/10.5772/59488

## 1. Introduction

Cancer will become a major cause of morbidity and mortality in the next decades. It is estimated that the global cancer rate may increase by 75 %, with predicted 22.2 million new cases by 2030 compared with 12.7 million cases in 2008 [1]. The scientific community has made tremendous efforts to develop new therapies to deal effectively with this growing problem. As the recent advances in cancer therapy are improving the cancer patient survival, the toxic effects promoted by anticancer agents have a higher potential impact on long-term outcomes.

Anticancer agents are known to cause severe toxic effects that should be anticipated and carefully monitored. Therapeutic regimens targeting the cell cycle also affect the proliferation of normal cells, such as blood cells in the bone marrow, cells in the digestive tract and hair follicles, resulting in neutropenia, hair loss, and gut toxicity. The side effects observed are dependent on the type of therapy, but they are generally reversible and disappear after the end of the treatment. However, some anticancer agents may also affect, sometimes in a permanent manner, the function of vital organs, such as the heart, kidney, liver and the nervous system. Some of these effects may develop during or shortly after treatment, or may only become apparent a long period after completion of the treatment; if this delay is long enough, it may correspond to the time of progression free survival and affect the benefit-risk balance [2, 3].

Both the liver and kidneys are vulnerable to the toxic effects of cancer therapy and also to the direct impact of cancer itself. The liver has a great capacity to resist injury and to regenerate, but this capacity also makes it susceptible to anticancer drugs toxicity [2]. Indeed, the liver injury induced by anticancer drugs is a significant cause of morbidity and mortality. However, most of these reactions are idiosyncratic and are not typically dose-dependent [2, 4]. Diagnosing liver damage due to anticancer agents is particularly challenging because competing etiologies, such as hepatotoxicity due to the intake of other medications, opportunistic infections, radiation therapy, and pre-existing liver disease, are frequent and greatly affect the host's susceptibility to liver injury [2, 4]. The major mechanisms underlying chemotherapy-related hepatotoxicity are based on the production of reactive metabolites, immunological injury, or mitochondrial dysfunction [4]. On the other hand, the spectrum of cancer-associated renal disease has changed in the last decades, mainly due to the introduction of new chemo-radiotherapy regimens. Nevertheless, renal failure remains an important complication of cancer treatment [5, 6]. Considering that drugs are primarily metabolized in the liver and excreted by the kidneys, hepatic and renal impairment can have an unpredictable impact on the metabolism and clearance of drugs that may ultimately affect the treatment outcome and toxicity.

In addition, cardiotoxicity is a common complication not only related to conventional cancer therapy, such as anthracyclines, but also to new antitumoral targeted therapy, such as trastuzumab. Due to the increasing number of patients treated with these agents, the incidence of cardiotoxicity is continuously growing and strongly affecting the patients' quality of life and overall survival, regardless of the oncologic prognosis [3]. Also, peripheral neuropathy is reported by 30-40 % of the patients and is one of the major reasons responsible for cessation of treatment [7]. Certain structural and functional features of peripheral nervous system make it more vulnerable to the action of anticancer drugs, namely the absence of a vascular barrier and of lymph drainage [7]. Furthermore, mammalian nerves are more susceptible to oxidative stress because of their high content of phospholipids, mitochondria rich axoplasm and weak cellular antioxidant defenses. Moreover, the enhanced free radical production promoted by anticancer drugs causes physical damage to neurons [7].

A thorough understanding of the mechanisms of injury is therefore a matter of great importance since it may contribute to detect toxic mechanisms at an early stage of drug development and, importantly, it can contribute to develop strategies aiming to minimize the toxicity. Mitochondrial dysfunction often underlies drug-induced toxicity and the works published over the last years point out that some of the severe adverse effects promoted by anticancer agents involve the targeting of mitochondria [8-11]. The heart, the kidneys, and the central nervous system, which have high energetic demands and are heavily dependent on oxidative phosphorylation, are more prone to the impact of mitochondrial damage. On the other hand, considering the exposure to high concentrations of drugs, the liver is another common organ showing mitochondrial dysfunction [12].

This chapter aims to provide an overview of the mechanisms of mitochondrial dysfunction induced by anticancer drugs and their involvement in several adverse effects, and particularly liver damage. Finally, possible combinations of therapeutic drugs to minimize the mitochondrial dysfunction promoted by these agents are discussed.

http://dx.doi.org/10.5772/59488

## 2. Methods

We searched literature published in English language included in PubMed for the period of 1970 to 2014. The main keywords searched were "mitochondrial dysfunction", "anticancer drugs and toxicity" and "tissue failure". The remaining papers were found in the reference list of the searched publications.

## 3. Anticancer drugs-induced tissue injury: The role of mitochondrial dysfunction

Mitochondria are dynamic and multifunctional cytoplasmic organelles, which possess a double membrane: an outer membrane (OMM) that is essentially permeable to ions and solutes up to 14 kDa, and an inner membrane (IMM), which is folded, forming the cristae, which is impermeable to ions and polar molecules. In the IMM are located several transporters, including the ATP/ADP and the aspartate/malate transporters, among others that regulate the movements of molecules across the IMM, and also the multisubunit complexes involved in the oxidative phosphorylation. Between the OMM and the IMM is located the intermembrane space (IMS), whereas the space enclosed by the IMM is the matrix (Fig.1). The IMS contains proteins such as the adenylate kinase and the creatine kinase (CK), as well as the cytochrome *c* and the apoptosis-inducing factor (AIF), which translocate to the cytoplasm during the apoptotic process, and other proteins involved in cellular metabolism. The proteins involved in the Krebs cycle, in the fatty acid oxidation, as well as in the synthesis of the heme and steroids, are located in the matrix [8, 9, 12, 13]. The mitochondrial matrix also contains the mitochondrial DNA (mtDNA). Thus, mitochondria are not only responsible for the synthesis of most of the ATP produced in the cell, but they also play a role in the fatty acid oxidation, the synthesis of the heme, steroids, and polypeptides involved in energy generation, as well as in calcium regulation and cell death. Therefore, taken in account the multitude of essential functions of mitochondria in cells, it is expected that their dysfunction might promote tissue failure, as described below.

### 3.1. Disturbance of mitochondrial energy production

The NADH and $FADH_2$ generated in metabolic pathways, including glycolysis, fatty acid oxidation and Krebs cycle are oxidized by complexes I and II of the mitochondrial electron transport chain, respectively. The electrons liberated are then passed to ubiquinone (coenzyme Q) that shuttles electrons to complex III, where it is oxidized; the electrons are then passed to complex IV through cytochrome *c*. The electrons carried by cytochrome *c* are used by complex IV to reduce molecular oxygen to water (Fig.1) [8, 14]. According to Peter Mitchell's Chemiosmotic Theory, complexes I, III and IV are redox-driven proton pumps that harness the energy derived from oxidation-reduction reactions to pump protons into the IMS, in parallel to the electron transfer, creating the electrochemical proton gradient (proton motive force) ($\Delta\mu H^+$), which is comprised of two components: a pH gradient ($\Delta pH$)

and a membrane potential (ΔΨ) (Fig. 1). The complex V (ATP synthase), which consists of the F1 subunit, a soluble portion located in the mitochondrial matrix, and the Fo subunit, bound to the IMM, uses the electrical component ΔΨ to phosphorylate ADP to ATP. Thus, the oxidative phosphorylation is coupled to the ATP requirements and the electron flow along the electron transport chain only occurs when the synthesis of ATP is required. The IMM impermeability ensures that the proton pumping along the respiratory chain is coupled to ATP synthesis [8, 12, 14].

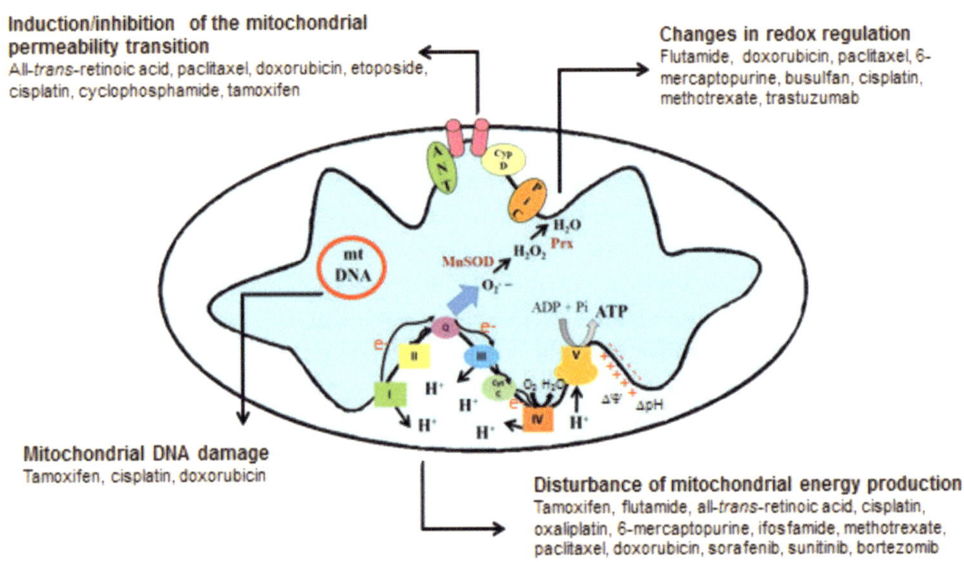


**Figure 1.** Structure of mitochondria and main mechanisms by which anticancer agents affect mitochondrial functions. Drugs can compromise mitochondrial bioenergetic functions by interfering with the generation system of $\Delta\mu H^+$, by dissipating the transmembrane proton gradient and by directly affecting the complex V or the substrate transporters. Drugs can also trigger or inhibit the mitochondrial permeability transition (MPT) by interfering with the proteins that compose or regulate the MPT or by modulating the critical factors to its onset, which may ultimately lead to cell death. Other drugs induce changes in the redox regulation of mitochondrial functions, promoting several deleterious events, including the interference with oxidative phosphorylation, nutrient oxidation and MPT. Drugs can also damage the mtDNA and, indirectly, compromise the ATP synthesis and favor the production of ROS (ANT, adenine nucleotide translocase; CyPD, cyclophilin-D; Cytc, cytochrome *c*; mnSOD, manganese superoxide dismutase; mtDNA, mitochondrial DNA; PiC, phosphate carrier; Prx, glutathione peroxidase; Q, coenzyme Q).

Xenobiotics can affect mitochondrial bioenergetic functions either by interfering with the generation system of $\Delta\mu H^+$or by causing the dissipation of the transmembrane proton gradient, as well as by affecting directly the F1Fo ATPase and the substrate transporters, including the adenine nucleotide translocase (ANT) and the phosphate–hydrogen co-transporter (phosphate carrier) (Fig.1) [14].

In fact, the inhibition of the electron transport chain by drugs may not only lead to ATP depletion, but also hinders the reoxidation of NADH and $FADH_2$ into $NAD^+$and FAD, respectively, which are required for the activity of several dehydrogenases of the Krebs cycle and the mitochondrial β-oxidation [15, 16]. In addition, the inhibition of the electron transport chain favors the accumulation of electrons in the electron transport system complexes that can escape and directly react with oxygen to form the superoxide anion radical [17]. The excessive reactive oxygen species (ROS) production can promote several deleterious events (described in more detail in section 3.3), but it is noteworthy that, in this context, both lipid accumulation and lipid peroxidation are favored [15, 16].

On the other hand, drugs can compromise the impermeability of the IMM to protons and dissipate the proton gradient impairing the production of ATP. The IMM impermeability can be surpassed by drugs that either disrupt the mitochondrial membranes or act as ionophores, uncouplers of the oxidative phosphorylation and inducers of the mitochondrial permeability transition (MPT) [12-14]. Moreover, drugs that interfere with the basic components of the phosphorylative system can also impair the production of ATP. These different effects on mitochondria induce changes in cellular bioenergetics, one of the key hallmarks in tissues.

### 3.2. Mitochondria in $Ca^{2+}$homeostasis: MPT-dependent cell death

Besides serving as the cells' primary energy source, mitochondria are implicated in the maintenance of calcium homeostasis through calcium uptake and release pathways. The rise of mitochondrial matrix free calcium concentration in the presence of a variety of sensitizing factors can lead to the opening of the MPT pore that may serve either the purpose of providing a fast calcium release or can convey both apoptotic and necrotic death signals.

MPT can be defined as an increase in the IMM permeability to solutes with molecular masses up to 1 500 Da, due to the opening of a voltage and calcium-dependent, cyclosporine A (CyA)-sensitive channel [18].

The molecular identity of the MPT pore is still under debate [19] (Fig. 1). Cyclophilin-D is the binding site for CyA, the golden standard of MPT inhibitors, and among the several components that have been proposed to play a role on MPT, cyclophilin-D is probably the most consensual. The ANT and the voltage-dependent anion channel (VDAC) were also considered key components of the MPT pore complex for many years. Knockout mice devoid of cyclophilin-D are resistant to necrosis promoted by ROS and calcium overload and the mitochondria isolated from the liver, heart and brain of these animals are resistant to MPT *in vitro* [20, 21]. Although these results support a central role for cyclophilin-D, MPT can occur even in the absence of cyclophilin-D if the calcium concentration is high enough [22]. Likewise, MPT can occur in mitochondria lacking ANT, although a higher concentration of calcium is required [23] and, therefore, the ANT is now considered a regulatory component of the MPT pore, rather than a structural one. Similar studies have excluded the VDAC as an essential component of MPT pore megacomplex [24].

The phosphate carrier was also proposed to play a key role in MPT [25], but a later study demonstrated that the reduction of phosphate carrier protein expression does not affect the MPT [26]. A more recent work suggested that the MPT pore complex is composed of ATP synthase dimers and pointed out that cyclophilin-D binds the lateral stalk of the ATP synthase at the same site as benzodiazepine 423, increasing the sensitivity to calcium [27]. However, the composition of MPT still remains a contentious issue.

Besides the calcium concentration in the matrix, the level of oxidative stress is possibly the most critical factor regulating MPT pore opening. Indeed, both the ANT and cyclophilin D were shown to be modulated by S-oxidation reactions [28-29]. However, other factors may contribute as well: the depletion of adenine nucleotides and high concentrations of phosphate increase the sensitivity of MPT to calcium, while a low pH and a high (negative) $\Delta\Psi$ inhibit MPT pore opening [30].

Drugs can trigger MPT either by interfering with the proteins that compose or regulate the MPT or by modulating the critical factors to its onset (Fig.1) [8]. As a consequence of MPT pore opening, the IMM loses its impermeability to protons, which allows the movement of solutes between the matrix and the cytosol, the dysregulation of cellular ionic homeostasis and the dissipation of $\Delta\mu H^+$. Moreover, since the protein concentration is higher in the matrix, a high osmotic pressure is generated and may lead to mitochondrial swelling, rupture of OMM, and loss of proapoptotic proteins that may trigger the apoptotic pathway in the cytoplasm [30, 31]. These events, together with the bioenergetic failure and the redox catastrophe, can culminate in cell death; if there are no sufficient levels of ATP, necrotic death may predominate over apoptosis [32]. Thus, depending on the cell type involved, different pathological conditions can occur as consequence of MPT induction.

### 3.3. Changes in redox regulation of mitochondrial functions

During the transfer of electrons along the electron transport chain to oxygen, and particularly at complexes I and III, some of these electrons escape and directly react with oxygen. The univalent reduction of oxygen generates the superoxide anion radical, which is then dismutated by the mitochondrial manganese superoxide dismutase into hydrogen peroxide, a key ROS signaling molecule due to its longer half-life and capacity to diffuse through membranes. The hydrogen peroxide is detoxified into water by the mitochondrial glutathione peroxidase and hence, in normal circumstances, most of the ROS generated by the electron transport chain are neutralized by the mitochondrial antioxidant defenses (Fig.1) [17]. The accumulation of hydrogen peroxide can promote the oxidation of thiolic groups, irreversibly deactivating the protein; likewise, the superoxide anion disassembles Fe–S clusters in several Krebs cycle enzymes and in respiratory complexes, and can combine with nitric oxide to form the highly toxic peroxynitrite. In addition, high levels of ROS can lead to the production of hydroxyl radical, which indiscriminately oxidizes biological macromolecules [33]. Other sources that can contribute to the total mitochondrial ROS include 2-oxoglutarate dehydrogenase, pyruvate dehydrogenase, dihydroorotate dehydrogenase, sn-glycerol-3-phosphate dehydrogenase, electron transfer flavoprotein:ubiquinol oxidoreductase, p66shc/Cytochrome C, Mia40p/ Erv1p, and complex II [33]. When maintained within a certain concentration range, ROS act as important signaling molecules, contributing to the redox balance, which regulates the functions that assist the normal cellular physiology [33]. However, the excessive formation of ROS can promote a series of deleterious events that deregulate key mitochondrial functions, including oxidative phosphorylation, nutrient oxidation and MPT, which may ultimately lead to cell death, tissue failure and have also a key role in disease pathogenesis [33].

### 3.4. Mitochondrial DNA damage

The mtDNA, maternally inherited, encodes 13 polypeptides that are subunits of the complexes I, III, IV and V, which are synthesized in mitochondrial ribosomes. The majority of the other mitochondrial proteins, including the subunits of complex II, are encoded by nuclear DNA, and imported into mitochondria after synthesis on cytosolic ribosomes [8-10].

The mtDNA is particularly vulnerable to the action of drugs, as it lacks histones, similarly to the bacterial DNA. Furthermore, the DNA repair mechanisms are less efficient that those of nuclear DNA. Therefore, and considering the proximity to the sites where ROS are routinely generated, the frequency of mtDNA mutation is much higher than that of nuclear DNA [13]. Mutations of mtDNA can seriously damage the respiratory chain as most of the polypeptides that form the respiratory chain complexes are encoded by mtDNA. As discussed in section 3.1., the impairment of the respiratory chain decreases the ATP synthesis capacity and enhances the production of ROS, which in turn will promote oxidative damage on several biomolecules, including the mtDNA itself, creating a vicious cycle that further enhances the insult [34].

## 4. Anticancer drugs impair mitochondria functions: relevance to tissue failure

In the last decades a large number of anticancer drugs have been reported to induce tissue failure by promoting changes in essential functions of mitochondria. The extent and type of mechanisms underlying the anticancer drug-induced mitochondrial dysfunctions are tissue-dependent and responsible for most of the idiosyncratic adverse drug responses.

In this section, we discuss some examples of the prominent members of different groups of anticancer drugs with evidences for the involvement of mitochondrial dysfunction in tissue impairment induced by these compounds.

### 4.1. Selective estrogen receptor modulators

Tamoxifen has been the endocrine therapy of choice for women with estrogen-receptor positive breast carcinoma over the last decades. Fatty liver is observed in more than 30 % of patients taking tamoxifen, which may persist after the discontinuation of the treatment [35, 36]. Nonalcoholic steatohepatitis, hepatic fibrosis, cirrhosis and hepatic necrosis were also reported [37-39].

Tamoxifen depresses the phosphorylation efficiency and the levels of ATP in a concentration-dependent manner in isolated rat liver mitochondria; these effects were attributed to a decrease in the active ANT content and a partial inhibition of the phosphate carrier [40, 41]. On the other hand, tamoxifen uncouples liver mitochondria respiration [40, 42] and, at higher concentrations, tamoxifen disrupts membrane integrity [43-44], enhancing the proton leak [40]. Tamoxifen also inhibits the electron transfer along the electron transport chain [40, 42] and the flavin mononucleotide site of complex I was identified as the target of tamoxifen [45]. The interaction of tamoxifen with complex III and IV was also shown [42]. The fact that tamoxifen interferes with membrane dynamics [46] may also decrease the diffusional mobility of membrane proteins and the electron transfer along the electron transport chain [40]. Furthermore, an *in vivo* study pointed out that tamoxifen depletes hepatic mtDNA, which further contributes to inhibit mitochondrial electron transport chain activity, and triggers steatose in mouse liver [47]. Therefore, the effects promoted by tamoxifen on mitochondrial bioenergetics may contribute to the liver damage observed in patients taking tamoxifen (Fig.1).

Interestingly, tamoxifen active metabolites, 4-hydroxytamoxifen and endoxifen, which are responsible for the antitumor actions of tamoxifen [48], do not significantly compromise mitochondrial bioenergetics at the concentrations reached in tissues [49, 50]. These results may indicate that the clinical use of tamoxifen metabolites instead of the prodrug may minimize liver damage. As the outcome of tamoxifen treatment seems to rely on its metabolic activation and endoxifen is a promising drug for cancer treatment, the future utilization of tamoxifen metabolites, and especially endoxifen, deserves further investigation. On the other hand, tamoxifen prevents and reverses the MPT induced by several agents [51-55]. Likewise, tamoxifen metabolites 4-hydroxytamoxifen and endoxifen also prevent and reverse the MPT induced by calcium and phosphate [50, 56]. Although the mechanisms underlying the inhibition of MPT by the antiestrogens are still under debate [57], this protective effect of TAM and its active metabolites regarding MPT might be of interest when considering combined anticancer drug therapies since it can decrease the toxicity of the associated drugs, as discussed in section 5.

### 4.2. Antiandrogens

Flutamide is a nonsteroidal anti-androgen used in the treatment of advanced prostate cancer, which has been associated with idiosyncratic drug-induced liver injury [58] and, although the mechanisms underlying liver damage are still unknown, mitochondria are a potential target of flutamide.

Indeed, high-doses of flutamide promote hepatocytes death in heterozygous Sod2(+/-) mice, but not in wild-type animals, suggesting that flutamide may exacerbate underlying mitochondrial abnormality [59]. Flutamide leads to the covalent binding of reactive electrophilic metabolites to proteins and diminishes the reduced glutathione (GSH)/glutathione disulfide (GSSG) ratio, as well as the total protein thiols in isolated rat hepatocytes; these effects are associated with the release of lactate dehydrogenase (LDH) [60]. Similar findings were reported by others, which also demonstrated that flutamide increases the hepatic GSSG/GSH ratio, the protein carbonyl levels, and serum lactate levels, supporting the view that the liver damage promoted by flutamide involves oxidative stress and mitochondrondrial dysfunction [59]. Accordingly, the addition of cysteine increased hepatocellular GSH and decreased LDH release in male hepatocytes [60].

Additionally, flutamide markedly impairs rat liver mitochondrial respiration (mainly at the level of complex I) and decreases the levels of ATP in rat hepatocytes [60]. Moreover, flutamide-treated Sod2(+/-) mice present a decrease in the expression of complexes I and III subunits [59]. Therefore, it seems possible that the increased oxidative stress promoted by flutamide may damage mitochondrial proteins and mtDNA, particularly when the antioxidant system is compromised [59], contributing to liver damage (Fig.1).

### 4.3. Alkylating agents

#### *4.3.1. Platinum analogs*

Cisplatin, which crosslinks DNA, is widely used in the treatment of head, neck, bladder ovarian and testicular cancers, but it has also been used in the management of other malignancies. Unfortunately, cisplatin promotes severe side effects, and particularly nephrotoxicity [61] and neurotoxicity [62].

Peripheral neuropathy is the dose limiting side effect of cisplatin and occurs in 30 % of patients. Dorsal root ganglion neurons treated with cisplatin exhibit mitochondrial vacuolization and degradation both *in vitro* and *in vivo*, suggesting that mitochondrial damage is involved in cisplatin-induced neurotoxicity (Fig.1) [63]. Besides covalently binding to nuclear DNA [64], cisplatin also directly binds to mtDNA, hindering the transcription of mitochondrial genes [63]. Another platinum analog, oxaliplatin, affects both complex I- and complex II-mediated respiration and decreases ATP production in rat peripheral nerve axons [65]. Acetyl-l-carnitine, which inhibits the development of oxaliplatin-evoked neuropathy, prevents oxaliplatin-induced mitochondrial dysfunction, further implicating mitochondria in the etiology of peripheral neuropathy [65].

About a quarter to one third of patients undergoing cisplatin treatment experience nephrotoxicity, which is manifested clinically as lower glomerular filtration rate and reduced serum magnesium and potassium levels [61]. Although the mechanism underlying cisplatin nephrotoxicity is not yet clear, the available evidence suggests that mitochondrial dysfunction plays a key role in renal tubular cell injury and death. Ultrastructural analysis of cisplatin-treated renal tubular cells of mouse kidney demonstrates the decrease in mitochondrial mass, disruption of cristae, and extensive mitochondrial swelling [66], supporting the involvement of mitochondria in cisplatin-induced nephrotoxicity. Cisplatin decreases manganese superoxide dismutase and complex II activity in rodents' kidney [67]. The GSH-reductase activity and the levels of GSH are markedly diminished in porcine proximal tubular cells [68]. These observations suggest that cisplatin strongly reduces the antioxidant defenses and favors ROS formation. However, agents that are able to prevent ROS formation, do not prevent cell death, suggesting that ROS formation is not the direct cause of cell death [68]. Furthermore, cisplatin significantly impairs kidney mitochondrial bioenergetic functions. In porcine proximal tubular cells, cisplatin inhibits complexes I to IV and decreases intracellular ATP [68]. In fact, the kidney of animals treated with cisplatin presents decreased mtDNA content and reduced complex I, III and IV protein expression [67].

Cisplatin is a rare cause of hepatotoxicity (steatosis and cholestasis) at standard doses, but high doses may lead to liver damage, revealed by abnormal liver tests, especially aspartate aminotransferase (AST) and alanine aminotransferase (ALT) [69]. Light microscopic observations confirmed that high doses of cisplatin cause massive hepatotoxicity; alterations at the ultrastructural level, including atrophied mitochondria, were also found [70]. Cisplatin induces MPT in rat liver mitochondria [71]. Moreover, cisplatin stimulates state 4 respiration, but does not affect FCCP-uncoupled respiration, suggesting that cisplatin affects mitochondrial bioenergetics by increasing the IMM permeability to protons and not by interfering with respiratory chain complexes activity [71]. Both the induction of MPT and the effects on liver mitochondrial bioenergetics are prevented by thiol group protecting agents, suggesting that changes on the redox-status of thiol groups affect membrane permeability to cations and underlie liver mitochondrial dysfunction [71]. Accordingly, it was proposed that the mechanism of cisplatin-induced hepatotoxicity involves membrane rigidification, lipid peroxidation, oxidative damage of cardiolipin and protein sulfhydryl groups, as well as decreased GSH/GSSG ratio, ATP, GSH and NADPH [72].

#### *4.3.2. Nitrogen mustards*

Cyclophosphamide is an alkylating agent used in the treatment of lymphomas, multiple myeloma, and certain types of leukemia, retinoblastoma, neuroblastoma, ovarian cancer, and breast cancer. Generally, cyclophosphamide does not cause relevant cardiotoxicity, but when it occurs, it appears to be related to a single dose, unlike the anthracyclines [3]. Patients who were previously medicated with anthracyclines or that underwent chest irradiation are more prone to suffer from cyclophosphamide-induced cardiotoxicity [3]. Liver damage was also reported [73, 74].

Cyclophosphamide compromises calcium accumulation by heart or liver mitochondria, which can almost be restored by CyA [75]. As the increases in the levels of serum AST, serum ALT, glucose-6-phosphate dehydrogenase and creatine phosphokinase induced by cyclophosphamide can also be attenuated by the simultaneous administration of CyA, the induction of MPT is closely related to the hepatotoxicity and cardiotoxicity promoted by cyclophosphamide (Fig.1) [75].

Ifosfamide, another nitrogen mustard, is one of the most commonly implicated drugs in kidney injury [76]. Using mitochondria isolated from the kidney of rats treated with ifosfamide, it was shown that this alkylating agent significantly inhibits complex I, resulting in NADH elevation and $NAD^+$depletion, and Krebs cycle impairment (Fig.1) [77]. Among the ifosfamide metabolites, only chloroacetaldehyde, which reaches high concentrations in the renal cortex, inhibits complex I, suggesting that this metabolite is responsible for the ifosfamide-induced nephrotoxicity [77].

#### *4.3.3. Alkyl sulfonates*

Busulfan is an alkylating drug, which forms DNA intrastrand crosslinks, used in the clinical management of chronic myelogenous leukemia. Although in standard doses busulfan rarely causes liver dysfunction, some cases of hepatotoxicity during busulfan treatment were reported [78-80].

The toxicity of busulfan is thought to involve oxidative stress mechanisms as it promotes decreases in GSH in hepatocytes both *in vivo* and *in vitro* [81]. Considering that glutathione S-transferase inhibitors and antioxidants prevent busulfan toxicity *in vitro*, it is likely that busulfan toxicity requires glutathione conjugation [81] Moreover, the effects of busulfan are strongly exacerbated on GSH-depleted hepatoctyes [81], which may provide a basis to explain the enhanced sensitivity to the liver damaging effects of busulfan under certain circumstances.

### 4.4. Enzyme inhibitors

#### *4.4.1. Anthracyclines*

Doxorubicin is used in the clinical management of a wide range of cancers, and particularly in breast cancer treatment. The anticancer activity of doxorubicin involves its intercalation into DNA and disruption of topoisomerase-II-mediated DNA repair, as well as the generation of ROS that lead to lipid peroxidation, as well as membrane and DNA damage [82]. However, its therapeutic use is limited by its side-effects, mainly the dose-dependent myelosuppression and the cumulative and irreversible cardiotoxicity, which in the most severe forms may lead to patient death [83].

Acute cardiotoxicity occurs in less than 1 % of the patients immediately after infusion and is usually reversible; the early-onset chronic progressive form affects 1.6–2.1 % of patients, during therapy or within the first year after treatment; the late-onset chronic progressive form occurs after one year of completion of therapy in 1.6–5 % of patients, supporting the need of long-term follow-up [3]. Doxorubicin causes myocardial damage as shown by the increase in serum levels of AST, ALT, LDH isoenzyme and creatine phosphokinase isoenzyme [84]. Doxorubicin-induced cardiotoxicity etiology seems complex, and several effects may be involved, triggering a domino effect [83]. Among the several mechanisms postulated, the induction of oxidative stress is the most widely accepted. The univalent reduction of the tetracyclic ring of anthracycline by complex I generates a semiquinone free radical; the unpaired electron of this semiquinone is transferred to oxygen, forming the superoxide radical, while the tetracyclic ring returns to the parent quinone [85]. The free radicals generated are thought to be related to the interference with calcium homeostasis and bioenergetic functions, lipid peroxidation, and mtDNA damage, which play a key role in the pathogenesis of doxorubicin cardiotoxicity (Fig.1).

Heart mitochondria isolated from rats treated with doxorubicin present decreased state 3 respiration and respiratory control ratio (RCR), whereas the state 4 respiration is not affected [86-88]; complex I activity is also inhibited [87]. Besides affecting nuclear DNA, doxorubicin damages mtDNA [89-91] and decreases its content in human hearts [90]. Accordingly, doxorubicin-exposed human hearts show low activity of complex I and IV (encoded by mtDNA) but not of complex II (exclusively encoded by nuclear DNA) [90]. The higher levels of superoxide in doxorubicin-exposed hearts correlate negatively with mtDNA content and with the activities of respiratory chain complexes encoded by mtDNA [90]. The damage leading to mtDNA adducts, as well as the higher rate of ROS formation and depression of GSH in heart tissue, persist for several weeks after cessation of doxorubicin treatment [92, 93].

Furthermore, mitochondria isolated from the heart of rats treated with doxorubicin present diminished ability to accumulate calcium [84, 86, 87, 94]. Similar effects were reported in mitochondria isolated from doxorubicin-treated human atrial trabeculae, and were shown to be reversed by CyA [95]. Considering that the decrease in left ventricular fractional survival promoted by doxorubicin is improved by the simultaneous administration of CyA, it seems that doxorubicin-induced heart damage is closely related to the induction of MPT pore opening [84, 96]. As discussed in section 3.3, oxidative stress is a major factor regulating MPT and doxorubicin leads to the oxidation of mitochondrial glutathione and to the accumulation of membrane disulfides, which may contribute to MPT induction. On the other hand, it has been proposed that the ANT is a key target for doxorubicin, as following doxorubicin treatment the amount of ANT protein and its active content are reduced in rats [94, 97]. The effects of doxorubicin on the ANT explain both the MPT induction and the effects on mitochondrial respiration [97]. Indeed, the decrease in state 3 respiration observed in heart mitochondria isolated from doxorubicin-treated rats is partially reversed by CyA or dithiothreitol, but not by trolox, suggesting that the toxic effects of doxorubicin on mitochondrial bioenergetics are at least in part a consequence of MPT induction and involve changes in the redox state of thiol groups [88]. Noteworthy, among several agents, including antioxidants, CyA was the only agent that was able to reverse the doxorubicin-induced alterations in the calcium accumulation capacity when added *ex vivo* [94]. Although the triggering of MPT by doxorubicin may initially involve the oxidation of regulatory components of the MPT pore megacomplex, once it occurs thiol protecting agents are unable to restore the pore to its original closed state [94, 98]. Therefore, antioxidants may be useful in the preventive setting, as discussed in section 5. Moreover, by increasing the generation of free radicals, doxorubicin also significantly enhances lipid peroxidation, as well as alterations in proteins and biomolecules that act as signaling molecules [99-101].

Altogether, the results obtained so far suggest that the persistent nature of doxorubicin cardiotoxicity reflects a self-perpetuating mechanism, where mtDNA alterations accumulate, leading to a damaged respiratory chain and decreased calcium loading ability; the defective respiratory chain further enhances ROS generation and mtDNA insult (Fig.1) [83, 98].

The heart is the main target of doxorubicin toxicity, due to the abundance of mitochondria in heart tissue, the elevated rate of oxygen consumption and the lower antioxidant defenses [83]. However, mitochondrial dysfunction has also been observed in other tissues. Indeed, in isolated mitochondrial fractions from the brain of rats treated with doxorubicin, the thiobarbituric acid-reactive substances and the vitamin E levels are increased, whereas the reduced glutathione content is diminished [102]. In addition, doxorubicin increases the sensibility of brain mitochondria to MTP pore opening [102]. The use of doxorubicin was also associated with a higher risk for developing hepatotoxicity among breast cancer patients [103]. Liver mitochondria isolated from doxorubicin-treated rats present decreased RCR and the activity of complex IV is inhibited [107]. In addition, light microscopic observations confirmed that doxorubicin at high doses caused massive liver injury; alterations at the ultrastructural level, such as atrophied mitochondria, were shown [70].

*4.4.2. Topoisomerase inhibitors*

Etoposide is a podophyllotoxin derivative used in the treatment of several cancers that acts as a topoisomerase II inhibitor. Cases of hepatic injury were reported using either standard doses [104] or high-dose regimens [105]. Etoposide induces calcium-dependent MPT in rat liver mitochondria [106]. Since the etoposide-induced MPT is prevented by several antioxidants, it was proposed that etoposide triggers MPT pore opening through the generation of oxidant species, which is further corroborated by the ability of antioxidants to prevent the apoptosis promoted by etoposide (Fig.1) [107]. Therefore, the generation of oxidant species that are able to induce mitochondrial dysfunction may contribute to hepatic injury.

### 4.5. Antimicrotubules — Taxanes

Paclitaxel is a taxane-derived drug used in monotherapy or in combination with other agents, for the treatment of ovarian, breast and advanced non-small cell lung cancers, and AIDS-related Kaposi's sarcoma.

Painful peripheral neuropathy is the major dose-limiting side-effect of paclitaxel therapy, with the major drawback that the pain and sensory abnormalities can persist for months or years. Moreover, it may turn the patients unable to complete optimal chemotherapy schedules thus potentially compromising the treatment efficacy [108].

The involvement of mitochondrial dysfunction in paclitaxel-induced pain is suggested by the presence of swollen and vacuolated neuronal mitochondria [109]. Earlier investigations demonstrated that paclitaxel promotes a CyA-sensitive swelling in liver, kidney, heart, and brain mitochondria; the highest degree and slope of the swelling are observed in liver mitochondria, whereas the lowest are detected in brain mitochondria [110].

Using a rat model of paclitaxel-induced pain, it was shown that the non-specific ROS scavenger N-tert-butyl-α-phenylnitrone significantly decreases paclitaxel-induced mechanical hypersensitivity, whereas the superoxide selective scavenger 4-hydroxy-2, 2, 6, 6-tetramethylpiperidine-1-oxyl (TEMPOL) does not present significant effects [108]. Therefore, the authors suggest that ROS are involved in the development and maintenance of paclitaxel-induced pain, although such effects cannot be attributed to superoxide radicals alone [108]. Moreover, rat sciatic nerve samples taken after induction of painful peripheral neuropathy with paclitaxel exhibit significant impairment of both complex I- and complex II-mediated respiration and deficits in ATP synthesis; the mitochondrial dysfunction promoted by paclitaxel is abrogated by acetyl-l-carnitine, again supporting that paclitaxel promotes oxidative damage [65].

Paclitaxel is extensively excreted by the liver, and therefore its administration to patients with liver impairment should be handled with care [69]. Alterations of liver functions are seen in 4-17 % of patients treated with doses up to 190 $mg/m^2$, but they can occur in 16-37 % of patients taking higher doses [69].

In isolated liver mitochondria, paclitaxel induces large amplitude swelling, the dissipation of mitochondrial membrane potential and the release of cytochrome c; these effects are inhibited by CyA, suggesting that paclitaxel induces MPT pore opening [110]. Paclitaxel also significantly increases complex IV-mediated ROS production (Fig.1) [110]. Paclitaxel does not inhibit mitochondrial respiration, but ROS formation is abolished by complex IV inhibitors, suggesting that paclitaxel promotes ROS production not by inhibiting the respiratory complexes, but through an effect on complex IV [110]. The abrogation of ROS formation does not prevent paclitaxel-induced MPT, suggesting that the induction of MPT is not secondary to enhanced ROS generation [110]. The combination with doxorubicin enhances the induction of oxidative stress [111].

The cardiotoxicity promoted by paclitaxel is usually represented by subclinical sinus bradycardia (approximately 30 % of patients), but more severe conditions were also reported [3]. A recent study suggests that microtubule disorganization in cardiac myocytes promoted by paclitaxel leads to MTP pore opening [112]. However, when isolated mitochondria are exposed to paclitaxel, no significant effects are detected; the authors suggested that paclitaxel does not promote MPT due to a direct effect on mitochondria [112]. However, it must be noted that lower concentrations were used in the latter study in comparison with previous work using liver mitochondria [110, 112].

Therefore, both the induction of MPT and mitochondrial ROS production can contribute to paclitaxel side effects in the nerve, liver, kidney and heart.

### 4.6. Antimetabolites

#### *4.6.1. Folate antagonists*

Methotrexate is a folic acid antagonist widely used in the treatment of leukemia and other malignancies. Gastrointestinal toxicity and liver function abnormalities are common in patients taking methotrexate and the use of methotrexate in patients with history of liver disease is not advisable [113].

In liver mitochondria, methotrexate promotes a significant rise in superoxide radical formation, as well as in lipid peroxidation, whereas the GSH levels are decreased [114]. Likewise, methotrexate significantly impairs the function of isolated heart mitochondria by promoting lipid peroxidation, mitochondrial swelling and by inhibiting complex I, II and IV activities [115].

Methotrexate administration also leads to small intestinal injury and damages in enterocyte mitochondria, as shown by the decrease in the RCR, an indicator of mitochondrial function [116]. Moreover, the activities of complexes II and IV are markedly decreased in enterocyte mitochondria, suggesting that the deleterious effects promoted by methotrexate on enterocyte mitochondria can compromise ATP synthesis (Fig.1) [116], thereby leading to the gastrointestinal toxicity seen in patients.

http://dx.doi.org/10.5772/59488

#### *4.6.2. Purine analogs*

6-Mercaptopurine is an orally administered immunosuppressive drug used to treat acute lymphocytic leukemia. 6-Mercaptopurine is converted to its active metabolites, the 6-thioguinine nucleotides, or inactivated by xanthine oxidase or by thiopurine methyltransferase to 6-thiouric acid or 6-methylmercaptopurine, respectively [117]. Liver injury is an important adverse effect of 6-mercaptopurine, with an estimated frequency of liver test abnormalities within 1-9 % range [118]. Clinically relevant concentrations of 6-mercaptopurine are toxic to rat hepatocyte cultures by a mechanism that involves oxidative stress and ATP depletion (Fig. 1) [119]. The decreased rat hepatocytes viability promoted by 6-mercaptopurine is nearly prevented by allopurinol (xanthine oxidase inhibitor) together with trolox (vitamin E analog), implying xanthine oxidase-mediated metabolism of the thiopurines and oxidative stress in the hepatotoxicity promoted by 6-mercaptopurine [119].

### 4.7. Retinoids

All-*trans*-retinoic acid was approved in 1995 by the Food and Drug Administration for the treatment of acute promyelocytic leukemia, changing the outcome of this disease, which was associated with a significant mortality until then. Retinoids induce hepatotoxicity, either during dietary supplementation [120] or treatment of acute promyelocytic leukemia patients [121], and hypertriglyceridemia [122]. Moreover, vitamin A supplementation in rats induces slight enlargement of mitochondria [123], hepatic oxidative insult and mitochondrial dysfunction [124], supporting the view that mitochondria are a target of retinoid toxicity.

All-*trans*-retinoic acid is a known inducer of MPT pore opening [125-127], which is thought to reflect its ability to modulate ANT activity in both liver and heart mitochondria [126]. All-*trans*-retinoic acid depresses the phosphorylation efficiency of mitochondria and, at higher concentrations, induces uncoupling of mitochondria [127]. Whereas earlier studies attribute the uncoupling promoted by retinoids to an increase in the IMM permeability [128], a more recent study suggests that the leak of protons through the Fo fraction of complex V is the underlying mechanism [127]. Thus, is seems likely that the liver injury promoted by all-*trans*-retinoic acid reflects its effects on mitochondria (Fig.1).

### 4.8. Targeted therapy

#### *4.8.1. Monoclonal antibodies*

Trastuzumab is a recombinant humanized monoclonal antibody against the human epidermal growth factor receptor 2 (HER2), which is overexpressed by many adenocarcinomas. Trastuzumab improves cancer patient survival, but it also causes cardiotoxicity in a significant number of patients, ranging from 2-7 % when used as monotherapy, 2-13 % when used combined with paclitaxel, and up to 27 % when trastuzumab is used with both anthracyclines and cyclophosphamide [3]. In contrast to the cardiomyopathy promoted by doxorubicin, the cardiac dysfunction induced by trastuzumab does not appear to be dose dependent and is often reversible [123]. Neonatal rat cardiomyocytes treated with an inhibitory HER2 antibody exhibit an increased ROS production and cell death, which are reversed by N-acetylcysteine and by CyA, suggesting that the toxic effects of trastuzumab on the heart involve mitochondrial damage and enhanced ROS production (Fig.1) [129].

#### *4.8.2. Tyrosine kinase inhibitors*

Sorafenib is effective against renal-cell carcinoma and hepatocellular carcinoma, whereas sunitinib is used in the management of advanced kidney cancer, gastrointestinal stromal tumor, and pancreatic neuroendocrine tumors. In phase I–II trials, 11 % of patients taking sunitinib experienced cardiovascular events and approximately half of the patients developed hypertension [130]. The incidence of sorafenib-associated heart toxicity is lower than that of sunitinib, and hypertension occurred in about 17 % of patients in clinical trials [131].

Sorafenib compromises mitochondrial function at clinically relevant concentrations in a myoblastic cell line grown under conditions where cells are either glycolytically or aerobically poised; the other tyrosine kinase inhibitors investigated (imatinib, dasatinib, sunitinib) do not affect the mitochondria [132]. Sorafenib uncouples heart mitochondria and inhibits complex V and complex II+III; at much higher concentrations the complex I and IV are also inhibited (Fig.1) [132].

Using neonatal rat cardiomyocyte cultures, it was shown that sunitinib decreases the mitochondrial membrane potential, and that both sunitinib and sorafenib reduce the intracellular ATP levels [133]. Echocardiographic abnormalities are apparent in sorafenib, but not in sunitinib or pazopanib treated animals; the analysis of ventricular cardiomyocytes revealed that sunitinib promotes mitochondrial swelling, dense deposits, and matrix cavitation, whereas sorafenib disrupted mitochondrial cristae [133].

#### *4.8.3. Proteasome inhibitors*

Bortezomib is a proteasome-inhibitor approved for the treatment of multiple myeloma and mantle cell lymphoma and its use in other types of cancer is currently under investigation. However, bortezomib induces dose-limiting peripheral neuropathy and compromises complex I- and complex II-mediated respiration, as well as ATP production in peripheral nerve axons, suggesting that mitochondrial dysfunction plays a key role in bortezomib-induced peripheral neuropathy (Fig.1) [134].

| **Mechanism** | **Drug class** | **Target organ** | **References** |
|---|---|---|---|
| **MPT** | | | |
| *MPT induction* | | | |
| All-*trans*-retinoic acid | Miscellaneous agents | Heart and liver | [125-127] |
| Paclitaxel | Antimicrotubules | Heart, liver, kidney | [110] |
| Doxorubicin | Enzyme inhibitors | Heart and brain | [84, 86, 87, 94, 95, 102] |
| Etoposide | Enzyme inhibitors | Liver | [106] |
| Cisplatin | Alkylating agents | Liver | [71] |

| Mechanism | Drug class | Target organ | References |
|---|---|---|---|
| Cyclophosphamide | Alkylating agents | Heart and liver | [75] |
| *MPT inhibition* | | | |
| Tamoxifen | SERMs | Liver | [51-55] |
| **Mitochondrial bioenergetics** | | | |
| Tamoxifen | SERMs | Liver | [40, 41, 159] |
| Flutamide | Antiandrogens | Liver | [59, 60] |
| All-*trans*-retinoic acid | Miscellaneous agents | Liver | [127] |
| Cisplatin | Alkylating agents | Liver and kidney | [67, 68, 71] |
| Oxaliplatin | Alkylating agents | Nerve | [65] |
| 6-Mercaptopurine | Antimetabolite | Liver | [119] |
| Ifosfamide | Alkylating agents | Kidney | [77] |
| Methotrexate | Antimetabolites | Heart and GI | [115, 116] |
| Paclitaxel | Antimicrotubules | Nerve | [65] |
| Doxorubicin | Enzyme inhibitors | Heart and liver | [86-88] |
| Sorafenib | Targeted Therapy | Heart | [132, 133] |
| Sunitinib | Targeted Therapy | Heart | [133] |
| Bortezomib | Targeted therapy | Nerve | [134] |
| **mtDNA damage** | | | |
| Tamoxifen | SERMs | Liver | [47] |
| Cisplatin | Alkylating agents | Neurons and kidney | [63, 67] |
| Doxorubicin | Enzyme inhibitors | Heart | [89-91] |
| **Oxidative stress** | | | |
| Flutamide | Antiandrogens | Liver | [59, 60] |
| Doxorubicin | Enzyme inhibitors | Heart and brain | [85, 102] |
| Paclitaxel | Antimicrotubules | Liver and nerve | [108, 110] |
| 6-Mercaptopurine | Antimetabolites | Liver | [119] |
| Busulfan | Alkylating agents | Liver | [81] |
| Cisplatin | Alkylating agents | Kidney and liver | [67, 68, 72] |
| Methotrexate | Antimetabolites | Heart and liver | [114, 115] |
| Trastuzumab | Targeted therapy | Heart | [129] |

**Table 1.** Summary of the mechanisms of mitochondrial dysfunction promoted by anticancer agents (GI, gastrointestinal tract; MPT, mitochondrial permeability transition; mtDNA, mitochondrial DNA; SERMs, selective estrogen receptors modulators).

## 5. A mitochondrial basis for anticancer drugs combinations: a promising approach to therapy

The severe toxicity promoted by anticancer agents represents a substantial health care burden that may seriously affect the treatment outcome. Based on the previous sections, mitochondria take center stage within the toxicity mechanisms, and are in the first line for protection by pharmacological strategies aiming to avoid alterations that may prove deleterious both in the short and in the long term. Considering that some of these effects are irreversible or cumulative, it is desirable to prevent these events when planning the therapy of cancer patients.

As discussed in the previous section, oxidative stress has been established as one of the primary cause of mitochondrial dysfunction and toxicity induced by anticancer agents and, therefore, several antioxidants have been tested *in vitro* and *in vivo* as a prophylactic measure. In particular, naturally occurring antioxidants have been investigated as therapeutic adjuvants, as they are considered safe and well-tolerated, and may afford protection against cancer treatment-related toxicity by improving mitochondrial functions.

Alpha-lipoic acid affords protection against the neurotoxic effects promoted by cisplatin and paclitaxel through its antioxidant and mitochondrial regulatory functions [135]. The toxic effects promoted by cisplatin on rat liver mitochondria are also prevented by thiol group protecting agents [71]. Curcumin, which has anti-inflammatory and anticancerous properties, counteracts the mitochondrial lipid peroxidation and GSH levels alterations in mitochondria isolated from the brain and liver of rats treated with cisplatin, suggesting that it can abrogate the toxic effects of cisplatin on brain and liver [136]. Likewise, epicatechin prevents the renal damage and mitochondrial dysfunction promoted by cisplatin by decreasing oxidative stress; noteworthy, epicatechin does not compromise the antitumor actions of cisplatin in HeLa cells [67].

The etoposide-induced MPT is prevented by ascorbate, the primary reductant of the phenoxyl radicals generated by etoposide, and by thiol protecting agents [107].

An *in vitro* study demonstrated that Vitamin E decreases the oxidative stress induced by methotrexate in rat heart mitochondria and thereby minimizes mitochondrial dysfunction [115]. Likewise, the administration of lipoic acid decreases oxidative stress induced by methotrexate, which affects liver mitochondrial function [114].

Acetyl-L-carnitine completely blocks the effects of bortezomib on mitochondria and pain [134].

Strategies to prevent doxorubicin-induced cardiotoxicity are probably the best studied, given the significant number of patients affected and the impact on the overall success of the treatment. Many studies reported that antioxidants could afford cardioprotection against doxorubicin therapy. The broad antioxidant resveratrol markedly ameliorates the cardiac dysfunction promoted by doxorubicin, while the ROS generation is decreased, and glutathione, superoxide dismutase and catalase activities are improved [137]. Also, flavonoids, and particularly 7-monohydroxyethylrutoside, protect against the cardiac toxic effects promoted by doxorubicin both *in vitro* and *in vivo* [138]. In addition, 7-monohydroxyethylrutoside does not compromise the antitumor activity of doxorubicin in human ovarian cell lines and in the corresponding mouse xenograft models, and even inhibits the overexpression of adhesion molecules promoted by doxorubicin on vascular endothelial cells [138]. The combination of doxorubicin and vitamin E-succinate cooperates to induce apoptosis in human gastric cancer cells, by promoting doxorubicin influx and suppressing its efflux [139]. On the other hand, vitamin E also aggravates the heart damage promoted by doxorubicin in P388 tumor-bearing mice [140].

Studies in animals demonstrated that the inhibition of mitochondrial respiration and the decrease in mitochondrial calcium accumulation capacity promoted by doxorubicin are prevented by the coadministration of the beta-adrenergic receptor antagonist carvedilol [87]. The prophylactic use of carvedilol in patients receiving doxorubicin contributes to maintain left ventricle diameters constant and to preserve diastolic function [141]. Interestingly, the toxic effects promoted by doxorubicin on heart mitochondria and cardiac cell apoptosis are prevented by carvedilol, but not by atenolol, another beta-adrenergic receptor antagonist with no antioxidant action, suggesting that the antioxidant properties and not the beta-adrenergic receptor antagonism are responsible for the cardioprotective effects of carvedilol [142]. Likewise, metoprolol, which also has no antioxidative properties, failes to afford cardioprotection in lymphoma patients treated with doxorubicin [143].

Dexrazoxane, a well-studied therapeutic adjuvant for doxorubicin chemotherapy, is a free radical scavenger that was found to have cardioprotective effects by preventing the functional damage of cardiac mitochondria initiated by ROS [83, 144]. Dexrazoxane prevents or reduces cardiac injury in doxorubicin-treated children with acute lymphoblastic leukemia without affecting the antitumor activity of doxorubicin [145]. In contrast, other iron chelators have failed to afford the same degree of cardioprotection, suggesting that iron does not play a crucial role in the oxidative stress-mediated toxicity of doxorubicin [138, 146, 147].

Promising results were obtained when the potent phosphodiesterase-5 inhibitor sildenafil is combined with doxorubicin. Prophylactic treatment with sildenafil prevents cardiomyocyte apoptosis and left ventricular dysfunction in a mouse chronic model of doxorubicin-induced cardiotoxicity [148]. On the other hand, in breast cancer cells, sildenafil enhances sensitivity to doxorubicin without enhancing its toxicity in bone marrow cells or macrophages [149]. Furthermore, cotreatment with sildenafil enhances doxorubicin-induced apoptosis in prostate cancer cells and inhibits tumor growth in mice bearing prostate tumor xenografts, while attenuating left ventricular dysfunction promoted by doxorubicin [150].

Interesting results were also observed when retinoids and antiestrogens are combined. Antiestrogenic compounds inhibit the MPT-induced by retinoids in isolated liver mitochondria [127, 151, 152]. Noteworthy, the prevention of MPT by antiestrogens does not compromise the antitumor efficacy of all-*trans*-retinoic acid, as an additive/synergistic action was demonstrated in breast cancer [153-156] and melanoma [157] cell lines. Therefore, we propose that studies *in vivo* with combined therapies are now required to confirm that these results obtained *in vitro* will translate into more therapeutic benefits in humans while attenuate mitochondrial dysfunctions promoted by drugs used individually.

## 6. Concluding remarks

Considering the key role played by mitochondria in cell survival and death, the pharmacological modulation of mitochondrial activity has been investigated in cancer therapy [13, 158]. It is thought that this strategy may overcome the resistance mechanisms related with conventional chemotherapy that do not target mitochondria directly, but interfere with signaling pathways which lie upstream of mitochondria and that are frequently deregulated in cancer [158]. However, the targeting of mitochondria as a therapeutic strategy is often compromised by the absence of significant pathophysiological differences between mitochondria in normal and malignant cells, leading to reduced selectivity of drugs targeting mitochondria. Therefore, the actions that are beneficial in cancer cells may, in contrast, underlie some of the severe toxic effects promoted by these agents.

Indeed, the induction of mitochondrial damage is an important contributor for some of the most well-known toxic effects of anticancer agents, namely the liver injury promoted by tamoxifen [159], the cardiotoxicity of doxorubicin or the cisplatin-induced neuropathy and nephrotoxicity. Organ dysfunction has a significant impact on the treatment outcomes and, therefore, the better understanding of the mechanisms of toxicity may unveil strategies to limit, or preferably to prevent, the incidence of these events and thereby improve the overall clinical success.

The recognition that mitochondrial dysfunction plays a key role in drug-induced toxicity may contribute to identify the drugs that are more likely to lead to such effects at an early stage. In this context, the use of isolated mitochondria fractions is a valuable tool to predict drug safety, since it provides relevant information while allowing to reduce the number of laboratory animals and the costs of preclinical studies [8].

On the other hand, our current knowledge does not allow to predict the idiosyncratic injury related with drug-induced mitochondrial dysfunction. It seems that genetic, metabolic and environmental factors that impair mitochondrial function can add their effects to those of anticancer drugs, compromising mitochondrial function to an extent where manifestations start to occur [17]. Therefore, therapeutic drug monitoring is mandatory. Furthermore, as organ damage may become apparent months or even years after the completion of the treatment (e.g. late-onset doxorubicin toxicity) the need of long-term follow-up is reinforced.

Finally, future studies should aim to develop strategies which are able to afford protection against both the short-term and long-term effects of anticancer drugs and without compromising their antitumor activity. Although antioxidants showed promise in *in vitro* studies, inconsistent results and failure in clinical trials turn the use of antioxidants as adjuvants in cancer therapy hardly consensual [7, 83]. However, in this context, we need to take into consideration that antioxidants may present different intracellular localization patterns and interfere with normal redox signaling pathways in specific cell compartments; an approach involving the targeted delivery of antioxidants to mitochondria can possibly provide better outcomes [7, 83]. Moreover, there are important differences between *in vitro* and *in vivo* toxicities and between animal models and humans. The different drug metabolism and clearance, as well as the asymmetries in redox regulation may account for the difficulty in translating these strategies into human subjects [83].

In conclusion, studies in suitable animal models are vital for a better understanding of the mechanisms underlying drug toxicity and the benefits of strategies aiming to prevent mitochondrial damage. So far most studies have used animal models devoid of tumors, which add an extra physiological burden that may influence the effects of drugs [83]. Moreover, as

http://dx.doi.org/10.5772/59488

described in the previous section, some of the toxic effects on mitochondria are observed in several organs, including the liver and kidneys, which may compromise both the pharmacokinetics and the efficacy of the anticancer drugs, but also the benefit of therapeutic adjuvants aiming to protect the mitochondria. These observations emphasize the importance of performing *in vivo* studies in relevant models, as well as the crucial importance of the clinical control and therapeutic drug monitoring of patients treated with anticancer drugs.

## Author details

Mariana Ponte Cardoso Ribeiro, Armanda Emanuela Castro e Santos and José Barata Antunes Custódio*

*Address all correspondence to: custodio@ci.uc.pt

Center for Neuroscience and Cell Biology, Faculty of Pharmacy, University of Coimbra, Coimbra, Portugal

## References

[1] Bray F, Jemal A, Grey N, Ferlay J, Forman D. Global cancer transitions according to the Human Development Index (2008-2030): a population-based study. The Lancet Oncology 2012;13(8): 790-801. http://www.ncbi.nlm.nih.gov/pubmed/22658655 (accessed 28 June 2014).

[2] Senior JR. Unintended hepatic adverse events associated with cancer chemotherapy. Toxicologic Pathology 2010;38(1): 142-7. http://www.ncbi.nlm.nih.gov/pubmed/19858501 (accessed 14 June 2014).

[3] Berardi R, Caramanti M, Savini A, Chiorrini S, Pierantoni C, Onofri A, Ballatore Z, De Lisa M, Mazzanti P, Cascinu S. State of the art for cardiotoxicity due to chemotherapy and to targeted therapies: a literature review. Critical Reviews in Oncology/Hematology 2013;88(1): 75-86. http://www.ncbi.nlm.nih.gov/pubmed/23522920 (accessed 8 July 2014).

[4] Bahirwani R, Reddy KR. Drug-Induced Liver Injury due to Cancer Chemotherapeutic Agents. Seminars in Liver Disease 2014;34(2): 162-71. http://www.ncbi.nlm.nih.gov/pubmed/24879981 (accessed 21 June 2014).

[5] Humphreys BD, Soiffer RJ, Magee CC. Renal failure associated with cancer and its treatment: an update. Journal of the American Society of Nephrology 2005;16(1): 151-61. http://www.ncbi.nlm.nih.gov/pubmed/15574506 (accessed 12 July 2014).

[6] Skinner R, Kaplan R, Nathan PC. Renal and pulmonary late effects of cancer therapy. Seminars in Oncology 2013;40(6): 757-73. http://www.ncbi.nlm.nih.gov/pubmed/24331195 (accessed 27 July 2014).

[7] Areti A, Yerra VG, Naidu V, Kumar A. Oxidative stress and nerve damage: Role in chemotherapy induced peripheral neuropathy. Redox Biology 2014;2: 289-95. http://www.ncbi.nlm.nih.gov/pubmed/24494204 (accessed 29 June 2014).

[8] Pereira SP, Pereira GC, Moreno AJ, Oliveira PJ. Can drug safety be predicted and animal experiments reduced by using isolated mitochondrial fractions? Alternatives to Laboratory Animals: ATLA 2009;37(4): 355-65. http://www.ncbi.nlm.nih.gov/pubmed/19807208 (accessed 12 June 2014).

[9] Cohen BH. Pharmacologic effects on mitochondrial function. Developmental Disabilities Research Reviews 2010;16(2): 189-99. http://www.ncbi.nlm.nih.gov/pubmed/20818734 (accessed 13 July 2014).

[10] Nadanaciva S, Will Y. Investigating mitochondrial dysfunction to increase drug safety in the pharmaceutical industry. Current Drug Targets 2011;12(6): 774-782. http://www.ncbi.nlm.nih.gov/pubmed/21275886 (accessed 2 August 2014).

[11] Nadanaciva S, Will Y. New insights in drug-induced mitochondrial toxicity. Current Pharmaceutical Design 2011;17(20): 2100-2112. http://www.ncbi.nlm.nih.gov/pubmed/21718246 (accessed 8 June 2014).

[12] Nadanaciva S, Will Y. Current concepts in drug-induced mitochondrial toxicity. In: Maines MD. (ed.) Current Protocols in Toxicology. Hoboken, NJ: John Wiley & Sons, Inc; 2009. p2.15.1-2.15.9. Available from http://www.ncbi.nlm.nih.gov/pubmed/20941696 (accessed 8 June 2014).

[13] Scatena R, Bottoni P, Botta G, Martorana GE, Giardina B. The role of mitochondria in pharmacotoxicology: a reevaluation of an old, newly emerging topic. American Journal of Physiology. Cell Physiology 2007;293(1): C12-C21. http://www.ncbi.nlm.nih.gov/pubmed/17475665 (accessed 5 July 2014).

[14] Wallace KB, Starkov AA. Mitochondrial targets of drug toxicity. Annual Review of Pharmacology and Toxicology 2000;40: 353-88. http://www.ncbi.nlm.nih.gov/pubmed/10836141 (accessed 29 July 2014).

[15] Begriche K, Igoudjil A, Pessayre D, Fromenty B. Mitochondrial dysfunction in NASH: causes, consequences and possible means to prevent it. Mitochondrion 2006;6(1): 1-28. http://www.ncbi.nlm.nih.gov/pubmed/16406828 (accessed 29 June 2014).

[16] Rolo AP, Teodoro JS, Palmeira CM. Role of oxidative stress in the pathogenesis of nonalcoholic steatohepatitis. Free Radical Biology & Medicine 2012;52(1): 59-69. http://www.ncbi.nlm.nih.gov/pubmed/22064361 (accessed 14 July 2014).

[17] Labbe G, Pessayre D, Fromenty B. Drug-induced liver injury through mitochondrial dysfunction: mechanisms and detection during preclinical safety studies. Fundamen-

tal & Clinical Pharmacology 2008;22(4): 335-53. http://www.ncbi.nlm.nih.gov/pubmed/18705745 (accessed 5 August 2014).

[18] Rasola A, Bernardi P. The mitochondrial permeability transition pore and its involvement in cell death and in disease pathogenesis. Apoptosis 2007;12(5): 815-33. http://www.ncbi.nlm.nih.gov/pubmed/17294078 (accessed 19 July 2014).

[19] Siemen D, Ziemer M. What is the nature of the mitochondrial permeability transition pore and what is it not? IUBMB Life 2013;65(3): 255-62. http://www.ncbi.nlm.nih.gov/pubmed/23341030 (accessed 25 June 2014).

[20] Baines CP, Kaiser RA, Purcell NH, Blair NS, Osinska H, Hambleton MA, Brunskill EW, Sayen MR, Gottlieb RA, Dorn GW, Robbins J, Molkentin JD. Loss of cyclophilin D reveals a critical role for mitochondrial permeability transition in cell death. Nature 2005;434(7033): 658-62. http://www.ncbi.nlm.nih.gov/pubmed/15800627 (accessed 17 June 2014).

[21] Nakagawa T, Shimizu S, Watanabe T, Yamaguchi O, Otsu K, Yamagata H, Inohara H, Kubo T, Tsujimoto Y. Cyclophilin D-dependent mitochondrial permeability transition regulates some necrotic but not apoptotic cell death. Nature 2005;434(7033): 652-8. http://www.ncbi.nlm.nih.gov/pubmed/15800626 (accessed 11 July 2014).

[22] Basso E, Fante L, Fowlkes J, Petronilli V, Forte MA, Bernardi P. Properties of the permeability transition pore in mitochondria devoid of Cyclophilin D. The Journal of Biological Chemistry 2005;280(19): 18558-61. http://www.ncbi.nlm.nih.gov/pubmed/15792954 (accessed 5 June 2014).

[23] Kokoszka JE, Waymire KG, Levy SE, Sligh JE, Cai J, Jones DP, MacGregor GR, Wallace DC. The ADP/ATP translocator is not essential for the mitochondrial permeability transition pore. Nature 2004;427(6973): 461-5. http://www.ncbi.nlm.nih.gov/pubmed/14749836 (accessed 24 July 2014).

[24] Baines CP, Kaiser RA, Sheiko T, Craigen WJ, Molkentin JD. Voltage-dependent anion channels are dispensable for mitochondrial-dependent cell death. Nature Cell Biology 2007;9(5): 550-5. http://www.ncbi.nlm.nih.gov/pubmed/17417626 (accessed 17 July 2014).

[25] Leung AW, Varanyuwatana P, Halestrap AP. The mitochondrial phosphate carrier interacts with cyclophilin D and may play a key role in the permeability transition. The Journal of Biological Chemistry 2008;283(39): 26312-23. http://www.ncbi.nlm.nih.gov/pubmed/18667415 (accessed 19 June 2014).

[26] Varanyuwatana P, Halestrap AP. The roles of phosphate and the phosphate carrier in the mitochondrial permeability transition pore. Mitochondrion 2012;12(1): 120-5. http://www.ncbi.nlm.nih.gov/pubmed/21586347 (accessed 1 July 2014).

[27] Giorgio V, von Stockum S, Antoniel M, Fabbro A, Fogolari F, Forte M, Glick GD, Petronilli V, Zoratti M, Szabó I, Lippe G, Bernardi P. Dimers of mitochondrial ATP synthase form the permeability transition pore. Proceedings of the National Academy of

Sciences of the United States of America 2013;110(15): 5887-92. http://www.ncbi.nlm.nih.gov/pubmed/23530243 (accessed 20 June 2014).

[28] McStay GP, Clarke SJ, Halestrap AP. Role of critical thiol groups on the matrix surface of the adenine nucleotide translocase in the mechanism of the mitochondrial permeability transition pore. Biochemical Journal 2002;367(Pt 2): 541-8. http://www.ncbi.nlm.nih.gov/pubmed/12149099 (accessed 30 June 2014).

[29] Sánchez G, Fernández C, Montecinos L, Domenech RJ, Donoso P. Preconditioning tachycardia decreases the activity of the mitochondrial permeability transition pore in the dog heart. Biochemical and Biophysical Research Communications 2011;410(4): 916-21. http://www.ncbi.nlm.nih.gov/pubmed/21708132 (accessed 23 June 2014).

[30] Halestrap AP. What is the mitochondrial permeability transition pore? Journal of Molecular and Cellular Cardiology 2009;46(6): 821-31. http://www.ncbi.nlm.nih.gov/pubmed/19017630 (accessed 21 June 2014).

[31] Kinnally KW, Peixoto PM, Ryu SY, Dejean LM. Is mPTP the gatekeeper for necrosis, apoptosis, or both? Biochimica et Biophysica Acta 2011;1813(4): 616-22. http://www.ncbi.nlm.nih.gov/pubmed/20888866 (accessed 22 July 2014).

[32] Baines CP. The mitochondrial permeability transition pore and ischemia-reperfusion injury. Basic Research in Cardiology 2009;104(2): 181-8. http://www.ncbi.nlm.nih.gov/pubmed/19242640 (accessed 25 June 2014).

[33] Mailloux RJ, Jin X, Willmore WG. Redox regulation of mitochondrial function with emphasis on cysteine oxidation reactions. Redox Biology 2014;2: 123-39. http://www.ncbi.nlm.nih.gov/pubmed/24455476 (accessed 11 June 2014).

[34] Dalla Via L, García-Argáez AN, Martínez-Vázquez M, Grancara S, Martinis P, Toninello A. Mitochondrial permeability transition as target of anticancer drugs. Current Pharmaceutical Design 2014;20(2): 223-44. http://www.ncbi.nlm.nih.gov/pubmed/23701547 (accessed 12 July 2014).

[35] Günel N, Coşkun U, Toruner FB, Sancak B, Yilmaz E, Cengiz O, Elbeg S, Uner A, Ozkan S. Serum leptin levels are associated with tamoxifen-induced hepatic steatosis. Current Medical Research and Opinion 2003;19:47-50. http://www.ncbi.nlm.nih.gov/pubmed/12661780 (accessed 17 August 2014).

[36] Liu CL, Huang JK, Cheng SP, Chang YC, Lee JJ, Liu TP. Fatty liver and transaminase changes with adjuvant tamoxifen therapy. Anticancer Drugs 2006;17(6):709-13. http://www.ncbi.nlm.nih.gov/pubmed/16917217 (accessed 17 August 2014).

[37] Oien KA, Moffat D, Curry GW, Dickson J, Habeshaw T, Mills PR, MacSween RN. Cirrhosis with steatohepatitis after adjuvant tamoxifen. Lancet 1999;353(9146): 36-7. http://www.ncbi.nlm.nih.gov/pubmed/10023952 (accessed 25 July 2014).

[38] Farrell GC. Drugs and steatohepatitis. Seminars in Liver Disease 2002;22(2): 185-94. http://www.ncbi.nlm.nih.gov/pubmed/12016549 (accessed 23 July 2014).

[39] Saphner T, Triest-Robertson S, Li H, Holzman P. The association of nonalcoholic steatohepatitis and tamoxifen in patients with breast cancer. Cancer 2009;115(14): 3189-95. http://www.ncbi.nlm.nih.gov/pubmed/19484789 (accessed 30 July 2014).

[40] Cardoso CMP, Custódio JBA, Almeida LM, Moreno AJM. Mechanisms of tamoxifen deleterious effects on the respiration rate and phosphorylation efficiency of mitochondria. Toxicology and Applied Pharmacology 2001;176(3): 145-52. http://www.ncbi.nlm.nih.gov/pubmed/11714246 (accessed 11 June 2014).

[41] Cardoso CM, Moreno AJ, Almeida LM, Custódio JB. Comparison of the changes in adenine nucleotides of rat liver mitochondria induced by tamoxifen and 4-hydroxytamoxifen. Toxicology In Vitro 2003;17(5-6): 663-70. http://www.ncbi.nlm.nih.gov/pubmed/15276871 (accessed 6 July 2014).

[42] Tuquet C, Dupont J, Mesneau A, Roussaux J. Effects of tamoxifen on the electron transport chain of isolated rat liver mitochondria. Cell Biology and Toxicology 2000;16(4): 207-19. http://www.ncbi.nlm.nih.gov/pubmed/11101003 (accessed 9 July 2014).

[43] Custódio JB, Almeida LM, Madeira VM. The effect of the anticancer drugs tamoxifen and hydroxytamoxifen on the calcium pump of isolated sarcoplasmic reticulum vesicles. Toxicology In Vitro 1996;10(5): 523-31. http://www.ncbi.nlm.nih.gov/pubmed/20650233 (accessed 16 July 2014).

[44] Chen Y, Schindler M, Simon SM. A mechanism for tamoxifen-mediated inhibition of acidification. The Journal of Biological Chemistry 1999;274(26): 18364-73. http://www.ncbi.nlm.nih.gov/pubmed/10373441 (accessed 17 June 2014).

[45] Moreira PI, Custódio J, Moreno A, Oliveira CR, Santos MS. Tamoxifen and estradiol interact with the flavin mononucleotide site of complex I leading to mitochondrial failure. The Journal of Biological Chemistry 2006;281(15): 10143-52. http://www.ncbi.nlm.nih.gov/pubmed/16410252 (accessed 30 July 2014).

[46] Custódio JB, Almeida LM, Madeira VM. The anticancer drug tamoxifen induces changes in the physical properties of model and native membranes. Biochimica et Biophysica Acta 1993;1150(2): 123-9. http://www.ncbi.nlm.nih.gov/pubmed/8347666 (accessed 8 June 2014).

[47] Larosche I, Lettéron P, Fromenty B, Vadrot N, Abbey-Toby A, Feldmann G, Pessayre D, Mansouri A. Tamoxifen inhibits topoisomerases, depletes mitochondrial DNA, and triggers steatosis in mouse liver. The Journal of Pharmacology and Experimental Therapeutics 2007;321(2): 526-35. http://www.ncbi.nlm.nih.gov/pubmed/17277197 (accessed 23 June 2014).

[48] Lim YC, Desta Z, Flockhart DA, Skaar TC. Endoxifen (4-hydroxy-N-desmethyl-tamoxifen) has anti-estrogenic effects in breast cancer cells with potency similar to 4-hydroxy-tamoxifen. Cancer Chemotherapy and Pharmacology 2005;55(5): 471-8. http://www.ncbi.nlm.nih.gov/pubmed/15685451 (accessed 17 August 2014).

[49] Cardoso CM, Moreno AJ, Almeida LM, Custódio JB. 4-Hydroxytamoxifen induces slight uncoupling of mitochondrial oxidative phosphorylation system in relation to the deleterious effects of tamoxifen. Toxicology 2002;179(3): 221-32. http://www.ncbi.nlm.nih.gov/pubmed/12270594 (accessed 27 June 2014).

[50] Ribeiro MP, Silva FS, Santos AE, Santos MS, Custódio JB. The antiestrogen endoxifen protects rat liver mitochondria from permeability transition pore opening and oxidative stress at concentrations that do not affect the phosphorylation efficiency. Toxicology and Applied Pharmacology 2013;267(1): 104-12. http://www.ncbi.nlm.nih.gov/pubmed/23274567 (accessed 8 June 2014).

[51] Custódio JBA, Moreno AJM, Wallace KB. Tamoxifen inhibits induction of the mitochondrial permeability transition by $Ca^{2+}$and inorganic phosphate. Toxicology and Applied Pharmacology 1998;152(1): 10-7. http://www.ncbi.nlm.nih.gov/pubmed/9772195 (accessed 9 July 2014).

[52] Cardoso CM, Almeida LM, Custódio JB. Protection of tamoxifen against oxidation of mitochondrial thiols and NAD(P)H underlying the permeability transition induced by prooxidants. Chemico-Biological Interactions 2004;148(3): 149-61. http://www.ncbi.nlm.nih.gov/pubmed/15276871 (accessed 5 June 2014).

[53] Moreira PI, Custódio JB, Nunes E, Moreno A, Seiça R, Oliveira CR, Santos MS. Estradiol affects liver mitochondrial function in ovariectomized and tamoxifen-treated ovariectomized female rats. Toxicology and Applied Pharmacology 2007;221(1): 102-10. http://www.ncbi.nlm.nih.gov/pubmed/17397887 (accessed 15 June 2014).

[54] Hernández-Esquivel L, Natalia-Pavón, Zazueta C, García N, Correa F, Chávez E. Protective action of tamoxifen on carboxyatractyloside-induced mitochondrial permeability transition. Life Sciences 2011;88(15-16): 681-7. http://www.ncbi.nlm.nih.gov/pubmed/21324322 (accessed 23 June 2014).

[55] Hernández-Esquivel L, Zazueta C, Buelna-Chontal M, Hernández-Reséndiz S, Pavón N, Chávez E. Protective behavior of tamoxifen against Hg2+-induced toxicity on kidney mitochondria: in vitro and in vivo experiments. The Journal of Steroid Biochemistry and Molecular Biology 2011;127(3-5): 345-50. http://www.ncbi.nlm.nih.gov/pubmed/21821123 (accessed 6 July 2014).

[56] Cardoso CM, Almeida LM, Custódio JB. 4-Hydroxytamoxifen is a potent inhibitor of the mitochondrial permeability transition. Mitochondrion 2002;1(6): 485-95. http://www.ncbi.nlm.nih.gov/pubmed/16120301 (accessed 22 June 2014).

[57] Ribeiro MP, Santos AE, Custódio JB. Mitochondria: the gateway for tamoxifen-induced liver injury. Toxicology 2014;323C: 10-8. http://www.ncbi.nlm.nih.gov/pubmed/24881593 (accessed 4 August 2014).

[58] Bruni V, Peruzzi E, Dei M, Nannini S, Seravalli V, Sisti G, Fambrini M. Hepatotoxicity with low-and ultralow-dose flutamide: a surveillance study on 203 hyperandro-

genic young females. Fertility and Sterility 2012;98(4): 1047-52. http://www.ncbi.nlm.nih.gov/pubmed/22795685 (accessed 1 July 2014).

[59] Kashimshetty R, Desai VG, Kale VM, Lee T, Moland CL, Branham WS, New LS, Chan EC, Younis H, Boelsterli UA. Underlying mitochondrial dysfunction triggers flutamide-induced oxidative liver injury in a mouse model of idiosyncratic drug toxicity. Toxicology and Applied Pharmacology 2009;238(2): 150-9. http://www.ncbi.nlm.nih.gov/pubmed/19442681 (accessed 14 June 2014).

[60] Fau D, Eugene D, Berson A, Letteron P, Fromenty B, Fisch C, Pessayre D. Toxicity of the antiandrogen flutamide in isolated rat hepatocytes. Journal of Pharmacology and Experimental Therapeutics 1994;269(3): 954-62. http://www.ncbi.nlm.nih.gov/pubmed/8014883 (accessed 12 June 2014).

[61] Yang Y, Liu H, Liu F, Dong Z. Mitochondrial dysregulation and protection in cisplatin nephrotoxicity. Archives of Toxicology 2014;88(6): 1249-56. http://www.ncbi.nlm.nih.gov/pubmed/24859930 (accessed 23 July 2014).

[62] McWhinney SR, Goldberg RM, McLeod HL. Platinum neurotoxicity pharmacogenetics. Molecular Cancer Therapeutics 2009;8(1): 10-6. http://www.ncbi.nlm.nih.gov/pubmed/19139108 (accessed 24 June 2014).

[63] Podratz JL, Knight AM, Ta LE, Staff NP, Gass JM, Genelin K, Schlattau A, Lathroum L, Windebank AJ. Cisplatin induced mitochondrial DNA damage in dorsal root ganglion neurons. Neurobiology of Disease 2011;41(3): 661-8. http://www.ncbi.nlm.nih.gov/pubmed/21145397 (accessed 14 August 2014).

[64] Ta LE, Espeset L, Podratz J, Windebank AJ. Neurotoxicity of oxaliplatin and cisplatin for dorsal root ganglion neurons correlates with platinum-DNA binding. Neurotoxicology 2006;27(6): 992-1002. http://www.ncbi.nlm.nih.gov/pubmed/16797073 (accessed 12 June 2014).

[65] Zheng H, Xiao WH, Bennett GJ. Functional deficits in peripheral nerve mitochondria in rats with paclitaxel-and oxaliplatin-evoked painful peripheral neuropathy. Experimental Neurology 2011;232(2): 154-61. http://www.ncbi.nlm.nih.gov/pubmed/21907196 (accessed 3 July 2014).

[66] Zsengellér ZK, Ellezian L, Brown D, Horváth B, Mukhopadhyay P, Kalyanaraman B, Parikh SM, Karumanchi SA, Stillman IE, Pacher P. Cisplatin nephrotoxicity involves mitochondrial injury with impaired tubular mitochondrial enzyme activity. The Journal of Histochemistry & Cytochemistry 2012;60(7): 521-9. http://www.ncbi.nlm.nih.gov/pubmed/22511597 (accessed 19 June 2014).

[67] Tanabe K, Tamura Y, Lanaspa MA, Miyazaki M, Suzuki N, Sato W, Maeshima Y, Schreiner GF, Villarreal FJ, Johnson RJ, Nakagawa T. Epicatechin limits renal injury by mitochondrial protection in cisplatin nephropathy. American Journal of Physiology. Renal Physiology 2012;303(9): F1264-74. http://www.ncbi.nlm.nih.gov/pubmed/22933302 (accessed 13 July 2014).

[68] Kruidering M, Van de Water B, de Heer E, Mulder GJ, Nagelkerke JF. Cisplatin-induced nephrotoxicity in porcine proximal tubular cells: mitochondrial dysfunction by inhibition of complexes I to IV of the respiratory chain. The Journal of Pharmacology and Experimental Therapeutics 1997;280(2): 638-49. http://www.ncbi.nlm.nih.gov/pubmed/9023274 (accessed 2 July 2014).

[69] King PD, Perry MC. Hepatotoxicity of chemotherapy. Oncologist 2001;6(2): 162-76. http://www.ncbi.nlm.nih.gov/pubmed/11306728 (accessed 17 July 2014).

[70] El-Sayyad HI, Ismail MF, Shalaby FM, Abou-El-Magd RF, Gaur RL, Fernando A, Raj MH, Ouhtit A. Histopathological effects of cisplatin, doxorubicin and 5-flurouracil (5-FU) on the liver of male albino rats. International Journal of Biological Sciences 2009;5(5): 466-73. http://www.ncbi.nlm.nih.gov/pubmed/19584954 (accessed 6 July 2014).

[71] Custódio JB, Cardoso CM, Santos MS, Almeida LM, Vicente JA, Fernandes MA. Cisplatin impairs rat liver mitochondrial functions by inducing changes on membrane ion permeability: prevention by thiol group protecting agents. Toxicology 2009;259(1-2): 18-24. http://www.ncbi.nlm.nih.gov/pubmed/19428939 (accessed 27 June 2014).

[72] Martins NM, Santos NA, Curti C, Bianchi ML, Santos AC. Cisplatin induces mitochondrial oxidative stress with resultant energetic metabolism impairment, membrane rigidification and apoptosis in rat liver. Journal of Applied Toxicology 2008;28(3): 337-44. http://www.ncbi.nlm.nih.gov/pubmed/17604343 (accessed 3 August 2014).

[73] Mok CC, Wong WM, Shek TW, Ho CT, Lau CS, Lai CL. Cumulative hepatotoxicity induced by continuous low-dose cyclophosphamide therapy. The American Journal of Gastroenterology 2000;95(3): 845-6. http://www.ncbi.nlm.nih.gov/pubmed/10710110 (accessed 19 June 2014).

[74] Subramaniam SR, Cader RA, Mohd R, Yen KW, Ghafor HA. Low-dose cyclophosphamide-induced acute hepatotoxicity. The American Journal of Case Reports 2013;14: 345-9. http://www.ncbi.nlm.nih.gov/pubmed/24023976 (accessed 16 July 2014).

[75] Al-Nasser IA. In vivo prevention of cyclophosphamide-induced Ca2+dependent damage of rat heart and liver mitochondria by cyclosporin A. Comparative Biochemistry and Physiology Part A: Molecular & Integrative Physiology. 1998;121(3): 209-14. http://www.ncbi.nlm.nih.gov/pubmed/9972318 (accessed 18 June 2014).

[76] Airy M, Raghavan R, Truong LD, Eknoyan G. Tubulointerstitial nephritis and cancer chemotherapy: update on a neglected clinical entity. Nephrology Dialysis Transplantation 2013;28(10): 2502-9. http://www.ncbi.nlm.nih.gov/pubmed/24009289 (accessed 14 June 2014).

[77] Nissim I, Horyn O, Daikhin Y, Nissim I, Luhovyy B, Phillips PC, Yudkoff M. Ifosfamide-induced nephrotoxicity: mechanism and prevention. Cancer Research

2006;66(15): 7824-31. http://www.ncbi.nlm.nih.gov/pubmed/16885387 (accessed 30 June 2014).

[78] Underwood JC, Shahani RT, Blackburn EK. Cholestatic jaundice following treatment of chronic granulocytic leukemia with busulphan. Journal of Clinical Pathology 1970;23(9): 827. http://www.ncbi.nlm.nih.gov/pubmed/5278972 (accessed 16 June 2014).

[79] Morris LE, Guthrie TH Jr. Busulfan-induced hepatitis. The American Journal of Gastroenterology 1988;83(6): 682-683. http://www.ncbi.nlm.nih.gov/pubmed/3376924 (accessed 19 June 2014).

[80] Adang RP, Breed WP. Liver damage during use of busulfan. Nederlands Tijdschrift voor Geneeskunde 1989;133(30): 1515-8. http://www.ncbi.nlm.nih.gov/pubmed/2797253 (accessed 23 June 2014).

[81] DeLeve LD, Wang X. Role of oxidative stress and glutathione in busulfan toxicity in cultured murine hepatocytes. Pharmacology 2000;60(3): 143-54. http://www.ncbi.nlm.nih.gov/pubmed/10754451 (accessed 1 July 2014).

[82] Thorn CF, Oshiro C, Marsh S, Hernandez-Boussard T, McLeod H, Klein TE, Altman RB. Doxorubicin pathways: pharmacodynamics and adverse effects. Pharmacogenetics and Genomics 2011;21(7): 440-6. http://www.ncbi.nlm.nih.gov/pubmed/21048526 (accessed 23 June 2014).

[83] Carvalho FS, Burgeiro A, Garcia R, Moreno AJ, Carvalho RA, Oliveira PJ. Doxorubicin-induced cardiotoxicity: from bioenergetic failure and cell death to cardiomyopathy. Medical Research Reviews 2014;34(1): 106-35. http://www.ncbi.nlm.nih.gov/pubmed/23494977 (accessed 14 July 2014).

[84] Al-Nasser IA. In vivo prevention of adriamycin cardiotoxicity by cyclosporin A or FK506. Toxicology 1998;131(2-3): 175-81. http://www.ncbi.nlm.nih.gov/pubmed/9928632 (accessed 1 July 2014).

[85] Doroshow JH. Effect of anthracycline antibiotics on oxygen radical formation in rat heart. Cancer Research 1983;43(2): 460-72. http://www.ncbi.nlm.nih.gov/pubmed/6293697 (accessed 2 July 2014).

[86] Solem LE, Henry TR, Wallace KB. Disruption of mitochondrial calcium homeostasis following chronic doxorubicin administration. Toxicology and Applied Pharmacology 1994;129(2): 214-22. http://www.ncbi.nlm.nih.gov/pubmed/7527602 (accessed 19 June 2014).

[87] Santos DL, Moreno AJ, Leino RL, Froberg MK, Wallace KB. Carvedilol protects against doxorubicin-induced mitochondrial cardiomyopathy. Toxicology and Applied Pharmacology 2002;185(3): 218-27. http://www.ncbi.nlm.nih.gov/pubmed/12498738 (accessed 11 August 2014).

[88] Oliveira PJ, Santos MS, Wallace KB. Doxorubicin-induced thiol-dependent alteration of cardiac mitochondrial permeability transition and respiration. Biochemistry (Mos-

cow) 2006;71(2):194-99. http://www.ncbi.nlm.nih.gov/pubmed/16489925 (accessed 27 June 2014).

[89] Ellis CN, Ellis MB, Blakemore WS. Effect of adriamycin on heart mitochondrial DNA. The Biochemical Journal 1987;245(1): 309-12. http://www.ncbi.nlm.nih.gov/pubmed/3663157 (accessed 2 August 2014).

[90] Lebrecht D, Kokkori A, Ketelsen UP, Setzer B, Walker UA. Tissue-specific mtDNA lesions and radical-associated mitochondrial dysfunction in human hearts exposed to doxorubicin. Journal of Pathology 2005;207(4): 436-44. http://www.ncbi.nlm.nih.gov/pubmed/16278810 (accessed 8 July 2014).

[91] Ashley N, Poulton J. Mitochondrial DNA is a direct target of anti-cancer anthracycline drugs. Biochemical and Biophysical Research Communications 2009;378(3): 450-5. http://www.ncbi.nlm.nih.gov/pubmed/19032935 (accessed 7 July 2014).

[92] Zhou S, Palmeira CM, Wallace KB. Doxorubicin-induced persistent oxidative stress to cardiac myocytes. Toxicology Letters 2001;121(3): 151-7. http://www.ncbi.nlm.nih.gov/pubmed/11369469 (accessed 27 July 2014).

[93] Lebrecht D, Setzer B, Ketelsen UP, Haberstroh J, Walker UA. Time-dependent and tissue-specific accumulation of mtDNA and respiratory chain defects in chronic doxorubicin cardiomyopathy. Circulation 2003;108(19): 2423-9. http://www.ncbi.nlm.nih.gov/pubmed/14568902 (accessed 17 June 2014).

[94] Zhou S, Starkov A, Froberg MK, Leino RL, Wallace KB. Cumulative and irreversible cardiac mitochondrial dysfunction induced by doxorubicin. Cancer Research 2001;61(2): 771-7. http://www.ncbi.nlm.nih.gov/pubmed/11212281 (accessed 15 June 2014).

[95] Montaigne D, Marechal X, Preau S, Baccouch R, Modine T, Fayad G, Lancel S, Neviere R. Doxorubicin induces mitochondrial permeability transition and contractile dysfunction in the human myocardium. Mitochondrion 2011;11(1): 22-6. http://www.ncbi.nlm.nih.gov/pubmed/20599629 (accessed 13 July 2014).

[96] Marechal X, Montaigne D, Marciniak C, Marchetti P, Hassoun SM, Beauvillain JC, Lancel S, Neviere R. Doxorubicin-induced cardiac dysfunction is attenuated by ciclosporin treatment in mice through improvements in mitochondrial bioenergetics. Clinical Science 2011;121(9): 405-13. http://www.ncbi.nlm.nih.gov/pubmed/21605084 (accessed 2 July 2014).

[97] Oliveira PJ, Wallace KB. Depletion of adenine nucleotide translocator protein in heart mitochondria from doxorubicin-treated rats – relevance for mitochondrial dysfunction. Toxicology 2006;220(2-3): 160-8. http://www.ncbi.nlm.nih.gov/pubmed/16427179 (accessed 5 August 2014).

[98] Wallace KB. Adriamycin-induced interference with cardiac mitochondrial calcium homeostasis. Cardiovascular Toxicology 2007;7(2): 101-7. http://www.ncbi.nlm.nih.gov/pubmed/17652813 (accessed 18 June 2014).

[99] Meredith MJ, Reed DJ. Depletion in vitro of mitochondrial glutathione in rat hepatocytes and enhancement of lipid peroxidation by adriamycin and 1, 3-bis(2-chloroethyl)-1-nitrosourea (BCNU). Biochemical Pharmacology 1983;32(8): 1383-8. http://www.ncbi.nlm.nih.gov/pubmed/6860357 (accessed 12 August 2014).

[100] Mimnaugh EG, Trush MA, Bhatnagar M, Gram TE. Enhancement of reactive oxygen-dependent mitochondrial membrane lipid peroxidation by the anticancer drug adriamycin. Biochemical Pharmacology 1985;34(6): 847-56. http://www.ncbi.nlm.nih.gov/pubmed/3977958 (accessed 7 July 2014).

[101] Berthiaume JM, Wallace KB. Adriamycin-induced oxidative mitochondrial cardiotoxicity. Cell Biology and Toxicology 2007;23(1): 15-25. http://www.ncbi.nlm.nih.gov/pubmed/17009097 (accessed 3 June 2014).

[102] Cardoso S, Santos RX, Carvalho C, Correia S, Pereira GC, Pereira SS, Oliveira PJ, Santos MS, Proença T, Moreira PI. Doxorubicin increases the susceptibility of brain mitochondria to Ca(2+)-induced permeability transition and oxidative damage. Free Radical Biology & Medicine 2008;45(10):1395-402. http://www.ncbi.nlm.nih.gov/pubmed/18775776 (accessed 21 June 2014).

[103] Damodar G, Smitha T, Gopinath S, Vijayakumar S, Rao Y. An evaluation of hepatotoxicity in breast cancer patients receiving injection Doxorubicin. Annals of Medical and Health Sciences Research 2014;4(1): 74-9. http://www.ncbi.nlm.nih.gov/pubmed/24669335 (accessed 19 June 2014).

[104] Tran A, Housset C, Boboc B, Tourani JM, Carnot F, Berthelot P. Etoposide (VP 16-213) induced hepatitis. Report of three cases following standard-dose treatments. Journal of Hepatology 1991;12(1): 36-9. http://www.ncbi.nlm.nih.gov/pubmed/2007774 (accessed 22 July 2014).

[105] Johnson DH, Greco FA, Wolff SN. Etoposide-induced hepatic injury: a potential complication of high-dose therapy. Cancer Treatment Reports 1983;67(11): 1023-4. http://www.ncbi.nlm.nih.gov/pubmed/6315228 (accessed 10 August 2014).

[106] Custódio JB, Cardoso CM, Madeira VM, Almeida LM. Mitochondrial permeability transition induced by the anticancer drug etoposide. Toxicology In Vitro 2001;15(4-5): 265-70. http://www.ncbi.nlm.nih.gov/pubmed/11566547 (accessed 23 July 2014).

[107] Custódio JB, Cardoso CM, Almeida LM. Thiol protecting agents and antioxidants inhibit the mitochondrial permeability transition promoted by etoposide: implications in the prevention of etoposide-induced apoptosis. Chemico-Biological Interactions 2002;140(2): 169-84. http://www.ncbi.nlm.nih.gov/pubmed/12076523 (accessed 14 June 2014).

[108] Fidanboylu M, Griffiths LA, Flatters SJ. Global inhibition of reactive oxygen species (ROS) inhibits paclitaxel-induced painful peripheral neuropathy. PLoS One 2011;6(9): e25212. http://www.ncbi.nlm.nih.gov/pubmed/21966458 (accessed 14 July 2014).

[109] Flatters SJ, Bennett GJ. Studies of peripheral sensory nerves in paclitaxel-induced painful peripheral neuropathy: evidence for mitochondrial dysfunction. Pain 2006;122(3): 245-57. http://www.ncbi.nlm.nih.gov/pubmed/12016549 (accessed 1 August 2014).

[110] Varbiro G, Veres B, Gallyas F Jr, Sumegi B. Direct effect of Taxol on free radical formation and mitochondrial permeability transition. Free Radical Biology & Medicine 2001;31(4):548-58. http://www.ncbi.nlm.nih.gov/pubmed/11498288 (accessed 3 August 2014).

[111] Pieniążek A, Czepas J, Piasecka-Zelga J, Gwoździński K, Koceva-Chyła A. Oxidative stress induced in rat liver by anticancer drugs doxorubicin, paclitaxel and docetaxel. Advances in Medical Sciences 2013;58(1): 104-11. http://www.ncbi.nlm.nih.gov/pubmed/23612702 (accessed 17 August 2014).

[112] Kumazawa A, Katoh H, Nonaka D, Watanabe T, Saotome M, Urushida T, Satoh H, Hayashi H. Microtubule disorganization affects the mitochondrial permeability transition pore in cardiac myocytes. Circulation Journal 2014;78(5): 1206-15. http://www.ncbi.nlm.nih.gov/pubmed/24614510 (accessed 13 July 2014).

[113] Cronstein BN. Low-dose methotrexate: a mainstay in the treatment of rheumatoid arthritis. Pharmacological Reviews 2005;57(2): 163-72. http://www.ncbi.nlm.nih.gov/pubmed/15914465 (accessed 4 July 2014).

[114] Tabassum H, Parvez S, Pasha ST, Banerjee BD, Raisuddin S. Protective effect of lipoic acid against methotrexate-induced oxidative stress in liver mitochondria. Food and Chemical Toxicology 2010;48(7): 1973-9. http://www.ncbi.nlm.nih.gov/pubmed/20451574 (accessed 4 August 2014).

[115] Singh K, Malviya A, Bhori M, Marar T. An in vitro study of the ameliorative role of $\alpha$-tocopherol on methotrexate-induced oxidative stress in rat heart mitochondria. Journal of Basic and Clinical Physiology and Pharmacology 2012;23(4): 163-8. http://www.ncbi.nlm.nih.gov/pubmed/23072846 (accessed 6 June 2014).

[116] Kolli V, Natarajan K, Isaac B, Selvakumar D, Abraham P. Mitochondrial dysfunction and respiratory chain defects in a rodent model of methotrexate-induced enteritis. Human & Experimental Toxicology 2013. http://www.ncbi.nlm.nih.gov/pubmed/24347301 (accessed 13 August 2014).

[117] Sandborn WJ. State-of-the-art: Immunosuppression and biologic therapy. Digestive Diseases 2010;28(3): 536-42. http://www.ncbi.nlm.nih.gov/pubmed/20926883 (accessed 3 July 2014).

[118] King PD, Perry MC. Hepatotoxicity of chemotherapeutic and oncologic agents. Gastroenterology Clinics if North America 1995;24(4): 969-90. http://www.ncbi.nlm.nih.gov/pubmed/8749907 (accessed 18 August 2014).

[119] Tapner MJ, Jones BE, Wu WM, Farrell GC. Toxicity of low dose azathioprine and 6-mercaptopurine in rat hepatocytes. Roles of xanthine oxidase and mitochondrial injury. Journal of Hepatology 2004;40(3): 454-63. http://www.ncbi.nlm.nih.gov/pubmed/15123360 (accessed 7 August 2014).

[120] Stickel F, Kessebohm K, Weimann R, Seitz HK. Review of liver injury associated with dietary supplements. Liver International 2011;31(5):595-605. http://www.ncbi.nlm.nih.gov/pubmed/21457433 (accessed 12 July 2014).

[121] de-Medeiros BC, Strapasson E, Pasquini R, de-Medeiros CR. Effect of all-trans retinoic acid on newly diagnosed acute promyelocytic leukemia patients: results of a Brazilian center. Brazilian Journal of Medical and Biological Research 1998;31(12): 1537-43. http://www.ncbi.nlm.nih.gov/pubmed/9951549 (accessed 15 June 2014).

[122] Standeven AM, Beard RL, Johnson AT, Boehm MF, Escobar M, Heyman RA, Chandraratna RA. Retinoid-induced hypertriglyceridemia in rats is mediated by retinoic acid receptors. Fundamental and Applied Toxicology 1996;33(2): 264-71. http://www.ncbi.nlm.nih.gov/pubmed/8921345 (accessed 23 July 2014).

[123] Leo MA, Arai M, Sato M, Lieber CS. Hepatotoxicity of vitamin A and ethanol in the rat. Gastroenterology 1982;82(2): 194-205. http://www.ncbi.nlm.nih.gov/pubmed/6274729 (accessed 5 July 2014).

[124] de Oliveira MR, Oliveira MW, Lorenzi R, Fagundes da Rocha R, Fonseca Moreira JC. Short-term vitamin A supplementation at therapeutic doses induces a pro-oxidative state in the hepatic environment and facilitates calcium-ion-induced oxidative stress in rat liver mitochondria independently from permeability transition pore formation: detrimental effects of vitamin A supplementation on rat liver redox and bioenergetic states homeostasis. Cell Biology and Toxicology 2009;25(6): 545-60. http://www.ncbi.nlm.nih.gov/pubmed/19043787 (accessed 9 June 2014).

[125] Rigobello MP, Scutari G, Friso A, Barzon E, Artusi S, Bindoli A. Mitochondrial permeability transition and release of cytochrome c induced by retinoic acids. Biochemical Pharmacology 1999;58(4): 665-70. http://www.ncbi.nlm.nih.gov/pubmed/10413304 (accessed 19 July 2014).

[126] Notario B, Zamora M, Viñas O, Mampel T. All-trans-retinoic acid binds to and inhibits adenine nucleotide translocase and induces mitochondrial permeability transition. Molecular Pharmacology 2003;63(1): 224-31. http://www.ncbi.nlm.nih.gov/pubmed/12488555 (accessed 5 July 2014).

[127] Ribeiro MP, Santos AE, Santos MS, Custódio JB. Effects of all-*trans*-retinoic acid on the permeability transition and bioenergetic functions of rat liver mitochondria in

combination with endoxifen. Life Sciences 2013;93(2-3): 96-107. http://www.ncbi.nlm.nih.gov/pubmed/23764110 (accessed 7 July 2014).

[128] Stillwell W, Nahmias S. Effect of retinol and retinoic acid on P/O ratios of coupled mitochondria. Biochemistry International 1983;6(3): 385-92. http://www.ncbi.nlm.nih.gov/pubmed/6679330 (accessed 7 June 2014).

[129] Gordon LI, Burke MA, Singh AT, Prachand S, Lieberman ED, Sun L, Naik TJ, Prasad SV, Ardehali H. Blockade of the erbB2 receptor induces cardiomyocyte death through mitochondrial and reactive oxygen species-dependent pathways. The Journal of Biological Chemistry 2009;284(4): 2080-7. http://www.ncbi.nlm.nih.gov/pubmed/19017630 (accessed 1 July 2014).

[130] Chu TF, Rupnick MA, Kerkela R, Dallabrida SM, Zurakowski D, Nguyen L, Woulfe K, Pravda E, Cassiola F, Desai J, George S, Morgan JA, Harris DM, Ismail NS, Chen JH, Schoen FJ, Van den Abbeele AD, Demetri GD, Force T, Chen MH. Cardiotoxicity associated with tyrosine kinase inhibitor sunitinib. Lancet 2007;370(9604): 2011-9. http://www.ncbi.nlm.nih.gov/pubmed/18083403 (accessed 19 June 2014).

[131] Escudier B, Eisen T, Stadler WM, Szczylik C, Oudard S, Siebels M, Negrier S, Chevreau C, Solska E, Desai AA, Rolland F, Demkow T, Hutson TE, Gore M, Freeman S, Schwartz B, Shan M, Simantov R, Bukowski RM; TARGET Study Group. Sorafenib in advanced clear-cell renal-cell carcinoma. The New England Journal of Medicine 2007;356(2): 125-34. http://www.ncbi.nlm.nih.gov/pubmed/17215530 (accessed 11 June 2014).

[132] Will Y, Dykens JA, Nadanaciva S, Hirakawa B, Jamieson J, Marroquin LD, Hynes J, Patyna S, Jessen BA. Effect of the multitargeted tyrosine kinase inhibitors imatinib, dasatinib, sunitinib, and sorafenib on mitochondrial function in isolated rat heart mitochondria and H9c2 cells. Toxicological Sciences 2008;106(1): 153-61. http://www.ncbi.nlm.nih.gov/pubmed/18664550 (accessed 14 July 2014).

[133] French KJ, Coatney RW, Renninger JP, Hu CX, Gales TL, Zhao S, Storck LM, Davis CB, McSurdy-Freed J, Chen E, Frazier KS. Differences in effects on myocardium and mitochondria by angiogenic inhibitors suggest separate mechanisms of cardiotoxicity. Toxicologic Pathology 2010;38(5): 691-702. http://www.ncbi.nlm.nih.gov/pubmed/20616376 (accessed 6 July 2014).

[134] Zheng H, Xiao WH, Bennett GJ. Mitotoxicity and bortezomib-induced chronic painful peripheral neuropathy. Experimental Neurology 2012;238(2): 225-34. http://www.ncbi.nlm.nih.gov/pubmed/11212281 (accessed 3 August 2014).

[135] Melli G, Taiana M, Camozzi F, Triolo D, Podini P, Quattrini A, Taroni F, Lauria G. Alpha-lipoic acid prevents mitochondrial damage and neurotoxicity in experimental chemotherapy neuropathy. Experimental Neurology 2008;214(2): 276-84. http://www.ncbi.nlm.nih.gov/pubmed/18809400 (accessed 31 July 2014).

[136] Waseem M, Parvez S. Mitochondrial dysfunction mediated cisplatin induced toxicity: modulatory role of curcumin. Food and Chemical Toxicology 2013;53: 334-42. http://www.ncbi.nlm.nih.gov/pubmed/23246825 (accessed 25 July 2014).

[137] Tatlidede E, Sehirli O, Velioğlu-Oğünc A, Cetinel S, Yeğen BC, Yarat A, Süleymanoğlu S, Sener G. Resveratrol treatment protects against doxorubicin-induced cardiotoxicity by alleviating oxidative damage. Free Radical Research 2009;43(3):195-205. http://www.ncbi.nlm.nih.gov/pubmed/19169920 (accessed 21 June 2014).

[138] Bast A, Kaiserová H, den Hartog GJ, Haenen GR, van der Vijgh WJ. Protectors against doxorubicin-induced cardiotoxicity: flavonoids. Cell Biology and Toxicology 2007;23(1): 39-47. http://www.ncbi.nlm.nih.gov/pubmed/17063376 (accessed 4 June 2014).

[139] Zhang X, Peng X, Yu W, Hou S, Zhao Y, Zhang Z, Huang X, Wu K. Alpha-tocopheryl succinate enhances doxorubicin-induced apoptosis in human gastric cancer cells via promotion of doxorubicin influx and suppression of doxorubicin efflux. Cancer Letters 2011;307(2): 174-81. http://www.ncbi.nlm.nih.gov/pubmed/21536373 (accessed 6 June 2014).

[140] Liu QY, Tan BK. Dietary fish oil and vitamin E enhance doxorubicin effects in P388 tumor-bearing mice. Lipids 2002;37(6): 549-56. http://www.ncbi.nlm.nih.gov/pubmed/12120952 (accessed 31 July 2014).

[141] Kalay N, Basar E, Ozdogru I, Er O, Cetinkaya Y, Dogan A, Inanc T, Oguzhan A, Eryol NK, Topsakal R, Ergin A. Protective effects of carvedilol against anthracycline-induced cardiomyopathy. Journal of the American College of Cardiology 2006;48(11): 2258-62. http://www.ncbi.nlm.nih.gov/pubmed/17161256 (accessed 12 June 2014).

[142] Oliveira PJ, Bjork JA, Santos MS, Leino RL, Froberg MK, Moreno AJ, Wallace KB. Carvedilol-mediated antioxidant protection against doxorubicin-induced cardiac mitochondrial toxicity. Toxicology Applied Pharmacology 2004;200(2):159-68. http://www.ncbi.nlm.nih.gov/pubmed/15476868 (accessed 18 August 2014).

[143] Georgakopoulos P, Roussou P, Matsakas E, Karavidas A, Anagnostopoulos N, Marinakis T, Galanopoulos A, Georgiakodis F Zimeras S, Kyriakidis M, Ahimastos A. Cardioprotective effect of metoprolol and enalapril in doxorubicin-treated lymphoma patients: a prospective, parallel-group, randomized, controlled study with 36-month follow-up. American Journal of Hematology 2010;85(11): 894-6. http://www.ncbi.nlm.nih.gov/pubmed/20872550 (accessed 7 August 2014).

[144] Swain SM, Whaley FS, Gerber MC, Ewer MS, Bianchine JR, Gams RA. Delayed administration of dexrazoxane provides cardioprotection for patients with advanced breast cancer treated with doxorubicin-containing therapy. Journal of Clinical Oncology 1997;15(4): 1333-40. http://www.ncbi.nlm.nih.gov/pubmed/9193324 (accessed 1 July 2014).

[145] Lipshultz SE, Rifai N, Dalton VM, Levy DE, Silverman LB, Lipsitz SR, Colan SD, Asselin BL, Barr RD, Clavell LA, Hurwitz CA, Moghrabi A, Samson Y, Schorin MA,

Gelber RD, Sallan SE. The effect of dexrazoxane on myocardial injury in doxorubicin-treated children with acute lymphoblastic leukemia. The New England Journal of Medicine 2004;351(2): 145-53. http://www.ncbi.nlm.nih.gov/pubmed/15247354 (accessed 21 July 2014).

[146] Voest EE, van Acker SA, van der Vijgh WJ, van Asbeck BS, Bast A. Comparison of different iron chelators as protective agents against acute doxorubicin-induced cardiotoxicity. Journal of Molecular and Cellular Cardiology 1994;26(9): 1179-85. http://www.ncbi.nlm.nih.gov/pubmed/7815460 (accessed 12 July 2014).

[147] Hasinoff BB, Patel D, Wu X. The oral iron chelator ICL670A (deferasirox) does not protect myocytes against doxorubicin. Free Radical Biology & Medicine 2003;35(11): 1469-79. http://www.ncbi.nlm.nih.gov/pubmed/14642395 (accessed 9 August 2014).

[148] Fisher PW, Salloum F, Das A, Hyder H, Kukreja RC. Phosphodiesterase-5 inhibition with sildenafil attenuates cardiomyocyte apoptosis and left ventricular dysfunction in a chronic model of doxorubicin cardiotoxicity. Circulation 2005;111(13): 1601-10. http://www.ncbi.nlm.nih.gov/pubmed/15811867 (accessed 29 June 2014).

[149] Di X, Gennings C, Bear HD, Graham LJ, Sheth CM, White KL Jr, Gewirtz DA. Influence of the phosphodiesterase-5 inhibitor, sildenafil, on sensitivity to chemotherapy in breast tumor cells. Breast Cancer Research and Treatment 2010;124(2): 349-60. http://www.ncbi.nlm.nih.gov/pubmed/20155316 (accessed 6 July 2014).

[150] Das A, Durrant D, Mitchell C, Mayton E, Hoke NN, Salloum FN, Park MA, Qureshi I, Lee R, Dent P, Kukreja RC. Sildenafil increases chemotherapeutic efficacy of doxorubicin in prostate cancer and ameliorates cardiac dysfunction. Proceedings of the National Academy of Sciences of the United States of America 2010;107(42): 18202-7. http://www.ncbi.nlm.nih.gov/pubmed/20884855 (accessed 14 June 2014).

[151] Silva FS, Ribeiro MP, Santos MS, Rocha-Pereira P, Santos-Silva A, Custódio JB. The antiestrogen 4-hydroxytamoxifen protects against isotretinoin-induced permeability transition and bioenergetic dysfunction of liver mitochondria: comparison with tamoxifen. Journal of Bioenergetics and Biomembranes 2013;45(4): 383-96. http://www.ncbi.nlm.nih.gov/pubmed/23779226 (accessed 2 August 2014).

[152] Silva FS, Ribeiro MP, Santos MS, Rocha-Pereira P, Santos-Silva A, Custódio JB. Acitretin affects bioenergetics of liver mitochondria and promotes mitochondrial permeability transition: potential mechanisms of hepatotoxicity. Toxicology 2013;306: 93-100. http://www.ncbi.nlm.nih.gov/pubmed/23384448 (accessed 15 July 2014).

[153] Wetherall NT, Taylor CM. The effects of retinoid treatment and antiestrogens on the growth of T47D human breast cancer cells. European Journal of Cancer & Clinical Oncology 1986;22(1): 53-9. http://www.ncbi.nlm.nih.gov/pubmed/3007157 (accessed 1 August 2014).

[154] Danforth DNJr. All trans-retinoic acid acts synergistically with hydroxytamoxifen and transforming-growth factor beta to stimulate apoptosis in MCF-7 breast cancer

cells. The Journal of Endocrinology 2004; 183(2): 395-404. http://www.ncbi.nlm.nih.gov/pubmed/15531727 (accessed 21 June 2014).

[155] Wang Y, He QY, Chen H, Chiu JF. Synergistic effects of retinoic acid and tamoxifen on human breast cancer cells: proteomic characterization. Experimental Cell Research 2007;313(2): 357-68. http://www.ncbi.nlm.nih.gov/pubmed/17098229 (accessed 21 July 2014).

[156] Koay DC, Zerillo C, Narayan M, Harris LN, DiGiovanna MP. Anti-tumor effects of retinoids combined with trastuzumab or tamoxifen in breast cancer cells: induction of apoptosis by retinoid/trastuzumab combinations. Breast Cancer Research 2010;12(4): R62. http://www.ncbi.nlm.nih.gov/pubmed/20696059 (accessed 1 August 2014).

[157] Ribeiro MP, Silva FS, Paixão J, Santos AE, Custódio JB. The combination of the anti-estrogen endoxifen with all-*trans*-retinoic acid has anti-proliferative and anti-migration effects on melanoma cells without inducing significant toxicity in non-neoplasic cells. European Journal of Pharmacology 2013;715(1-3): 354-62. http://www.ncbi.nlm.nih.gov/pubmed/23712006 (accessed 25 June 2014).

[158] Fulda S, Galluzzi L, Kroemer G. Targeting mitochondria for cancer therapy. Nature Reviews Drug Discovery 2010;9(6): 447-64. http://www.ncbi.nlm.nih.gov/pubmed/20467424 (accessed 10 August 2014).

[159] Moreira PI, Custódio JB, Nunes E, Oliveira PJ, Moreno A, Seiça R, Oliveira CR, Santos MS. Mitochondria from distinct tissues are differently affected by 17β-estradiol and tamoxifen. The Journal of Steroid Biochemistry and Molecular Biology 2011;123(1-2): 8-16. http://www.ncbi.nlm.nih.gov/pubmed/20932907 (accessed 27 July 2014).

Chapter 3

# Mitochondrial Targeting for Drug Development

Jalal Pourahmad, Ahmad Salimi and
Enayatollah Seydi

Additional information is available at the end of the chapter

http://dx.doi.org/10.5772/59719

## 1. Introduction

What is the reason that mitochondrion is so attractive target for pharmacotherapy? The problem raised is a bit complex. Although the appearance of mitochondria in animal cells started more than one million years ago, when the proteobacteria (in particular, Rickettsiales or close relatives) entered and practiced coexistence inside eukaryotic cells via endocymbiosis, But the biological science started to pay attention on mitochondria in the middle of $19^{th}$ century, the time that mitochondria were discovered in tissue section of liver and flight muscle. The earliest definition of this organelle in cells was written by Richard Altmann on 1890, when he named them as "bioblasts" and hypothesized that they were "elementary organisms" living inside cells with "vital functions" [1]. After 1890, the progress in understanding the structure and function of mitochondria was quite steady, but we can single out major milestones in every decade. In the 1950s, investigators analyzed mitochondria by electron microscopy and characterized that they are the sites of respiration, Oxidative Phosphorylation (OXPHOS) and fatty acid oxidation. In the 1960s, investigators found out mitochondrial DNA (mtDNA) and described chemiosmotic theory. In the 1980s, the first consummate sequence of mammalian mtDNA and the first molecular identification of a cause of mitochondrial diseases were reported. A great incrementation in interest on mitochondria occurred in 1996, when researchers demonstrated that the organelles are associated with programming cell death or apoptosis [2]. After this manifestation, mitochondrial study commenced growing as a biomedical field. Owing to the unique structure and function of mitochondria, several clinically used drugs can improve or damage their bioenergetics. These drugs can act via the regulation of: (a) permeability transition pores (PTPs), (b) fatty acid uptake or oxidation, (c) the electron transport chain (ETC), (d) cardiolipin (CL) content (e) ion channels and transporters, (f) Adenosine triphosphate (ase) (ATPase) and (g) mtDNA and protein synthesis [3]. Mitochondria are subcellular organelles that play pivotal roles essential for energy (ATP) production, metabolism, and homeostasis. In addition, mitochondria orchestrate some survival and cell death signaling. The reason why the mitochondria is considered as a potential drug target for the treatment of hyperproliferative and metabolic disorders. Unsimilarities in the reduction/oxidation condition of tumor versus non-tumor cells may be beneficial to get selective cytotoxic and anti-colonygenic effect on tumor cell populations. It was shown that pro-oxidant drugs, including Elesclomol and Trisenox have therapeutic benefits in the treatment of cancer. Findings obtained with Bz-423 in mouse demonstrate the potential for mitochondria-targeted drugs to control disorders of immune function. Investigation associating an elevated oxidant state with mitochondrial damage, aging dictates, and degenerative disease the need for a better understanding of how and when pharmacological manipulation of mitochondrial function prepares most therapeutic benefit [4].

Mitochondria carry out vital biochemical functions essential for cells such as homeostasis calcium, cell death and survival, in addition to ATP production. They represent a convergence point for death signals triggered by both intracellular and extracellular cues. Not surprisingly it's incoherent, therefore, mitochondria additionally offer targets for xenobiotics to exert either detrimental or therapeutic effects on cell survival and function. Efforts to harness mitochondrial targets for therapeutic benefit have focused largely on cancer, although treatments for ischemia, metabolic diseases and neurodegenerative diseases also are being explored. This chapter will describe current thinking and recent advances in the discovery of small molecule drugs acting on targets in the mitochondrion [5].

## 2. Why we choose mitochondria for drug targeting

The mitochondrion is as a respiratory organelle exists in almost all eukaryotic nucleated cells. Its unique structure is consisted of four distinct sub-structures with different specific functions: the mitochondrial matrix, the inner mitochondrial membrane (IMM), the outer mitochondrial membrane (OMM) and the intermembrane space (IMS). The structure of the inner mitochondrial membrane (IMM), is extensively folded and compartmentalized. The numerous invaginations of the membrane are called cristae, which house the 4 complexes of the mitochondrial respiratory chain and ATP synthase, controlling the vital levels of cellular bioenergetics. This primary function of the mitochondrion is responsible for supplying cellular energy, the reason why we call it power plant of the cell.'' However, it is not the only important function of mitochondria in the cell [6]. Adenosine triphosphate (ATP) production through the oxidative phosphorylation (OXPHOS) process requires a continuous flow of electrons. As such, mitochondria are the major so are the major source of reactive oxygen species (ROS, i.e. superoxide and $H_2O_2$), generated as byproducts of the ETC. ROS reflect the level of cellular oxidative stress, causing severe damage to macromolecules when overproduced. Consequently, according to the Harman's oxidative stress theory, they have been linked to aging, age-related pathologies, and death. However, when produced in a controlled amount, ROS may also play important signaling roles in various redox-dependent processes, including apoptosis, cell proliferation and hypoxia. Furthermore, mitochondria are active players in cellular calcium homeostasis. Mitochondrial $Ca^{2+}$ accumulation regulates functions as diverse as aerobic metabolism and induction of cell death. Finally, mutations in mitochondrial DNA (mtDNA) are responsible

http://dx.doi.org/10.5772/59719

for many mitochondrial metabolic disorders, and are thought to contribute to aging by promoting apoptosis. Thus, because of their pivotal role in regulating cell life and death, mitochondria represent an attractive target for mitochondrial gene therapy as well as drugs treating either degenerative or hyper proliferative diseases (figure 1) [7].

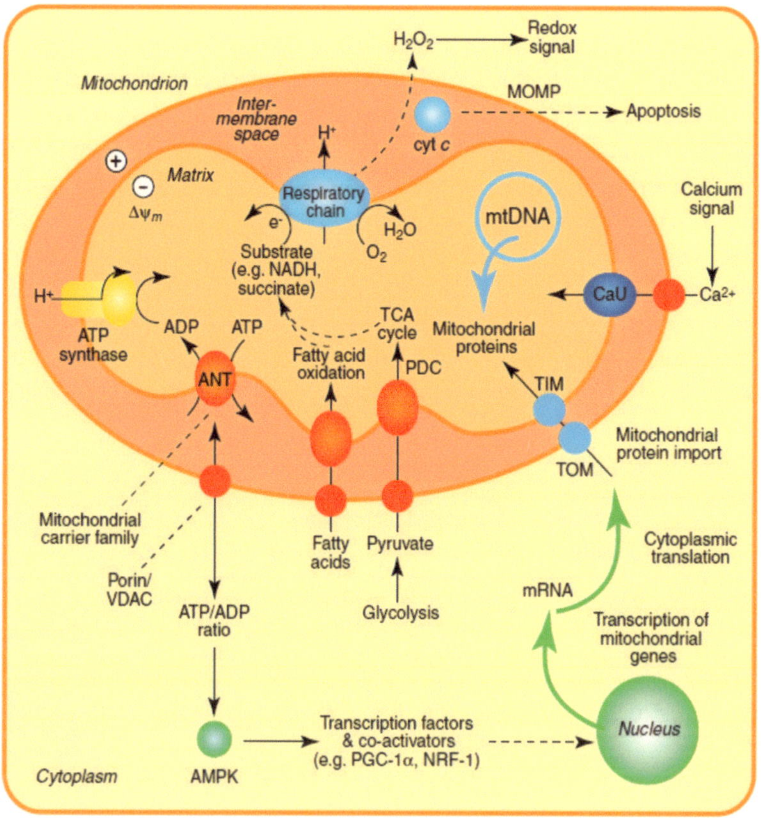


Some aspects of mitochondrial biogenesis and some important roles of mitochondria in cell function are illustrated. One major function of mitochondria is the production of energy (ATP) via aerobic metabolism of glucose which is called oxidative phosphorylation. Initially, glucose is metabolized to pyruvate through cytosolic glycolysis (anaerobic metabolism). Voltage-dependent anion channels (VDACs), also called porin channels, allow low molecular weight molecules to enter the mitochondrial inter membrane space. Following the activation of AMPK (AMP-dependent kinase), cell responds to the decreased ATP/ADP ratio in the cytosol through alterations in AMP, and affects several targets. Mitochondrial mtDNA encodes 37 genes that are involved in the synthesis of the respiratory chain and the ATP production. Additional proteins are imported through TIM (transporter inner membrane) and TOM (transporter outer membrane), translocases of the inner and outer membranes that transport nuclear-encoded proteins into mitochondria. The adenine nucleotide translocase (ANT) enables the mitochondrion to import ADP and export ATP. Mitochondria also contribute to calcium homeostasis by taking up calcium into the mitochondrial matrix through the calcium uniporter in response to changes in cytosolic calcium. In addition, mitochondria play a crucial role in cell death such as apoptosis and necrosis. When apoptotic signals occur, the outer membrane becomes compromised and the mitochondrion experiences mitochondrial outer membrane permeabilization (MOMP), leading to the release of cytochrome c (cyt c) and many other pro-apoptotic proteins from the intermembrane space into the cytosol where they activate apoptotic cell death [6].

**Figure 1.** Mitochondrial biogenesis and function.

## 3. Mitochondrial diseases

Mitochondrial dysfunction triggers the cell death signaling cascade and results in organ failure and disease. Therapeutic intervention at the mitochondrial level can be envisioned for general cell-degenerative as well as hyper proliferative diseases, i.e. cancers. Hyper proliferative cells are sensitive to pro-oxidant that induced apoptosis through increasing of their oxidative stress level. The redox status of many tumors is significantly changed compared with normal tissue, and pro-oxidant drugs can use this difference for treatment of proliferative disorder. Conversely, degenerative and aging diseases are associated with an elevated oxidant state that may associate mitochondrial damage. In these cases, antioxidants targeting mitochondria are hoped to exert a justifying effect. Several studies are found in this category, all sharing the common features of disturbances of mitochondrial ROS, ATP or $Ca^{2+}$ metabolism. They contain cardiovascular diseases (for example atherosclerosis, ischemia/reperfusion injury, heart failure, stroke); aging and neurodegenerative diseases (for example Alzheimer's disease (AD), Parkinson's disease (PD), Huntington's disease (HD), amyotrophic lateral sclerosis (ALS) and Friedreich's ataxia (FRDA)); chronic autoimmune inflammatory diseases (for example rheumatoid arthritis (RA)) ; metabolic diseases(for example diabetes and obesity) ; as well as ionizing radiation injury (Table 1) [6].

| Cardiovascular diseases | Neurodegenerative diseases | Chronic autoimmune inflammatory diseases | Metabolic diseases | Cancer |
|---|---|---|---|---|
| **Atherosclerosis** | Alzheimer's disease (AD) | rheumatoid arthritis (RA) | diabetes | Hepatocellular carcinoma |
| **Ischemia/reperfusion injury** | Parkinson's disease (PD) | | obesity | Adenocarcinoma |
| **Heart failure** | Huntington's disease (HD) | | | Breast cancer |
| **Stroke** | amyotrophic lateral sclerosis (ALS) | | | Prostate cancer |
| **Congestive heart failure** | Friedreich's ataxia (FRDA) | | | |

**Table 1.** The table above contains some disease that role of mitochondria in these diseases has been demonstrated. Which are divided into five categories.

## 4. Strategies to target mitochondria

Small molecule drugs or biologics can act on mitochondria through various pathways. Many of these mechanisms will be argued in more detail in the below sections, and a detailed discussion would immensely encroach the purpose of this chapter, but attractive current approaches include OXPHOS uncoupling, mitochondrial $Ca^{2+}$ modulation, ETC inhibition and control of oxidative stress through increase or decrease of mitochondrial ROS accumulation. The inhibition of the ETC can happen through direct inhibition of a protein subunit of one or more of the enzyme complexes or via reception of electrons current across the ETC instead of the natural receiver cytochrome c or ubiquinone. In the Oxidative Phosphorylation (OXPHOS) uncoupling occurrence, protons are shifted from the mitochondrial matrix to the intermembrane space (IMS) and do not avert across the F1F0-ATPase and back to the matrix, but instead migrate directly across the inner mitochondrial membrane (IMM). This bypass results in lack of ATP formation but heat production. Typical instances for agents that elevate OXPHOS uncoupling are weak bases and weak acids, which can be protonated in the IMS and carry protons across the IMM. Interestingly, compounds affecting the activity of inner membrane uncoupling proteins (UCPs) can inhibit cell death. An important occurrence starting the apoptotic cascade is the mitochondrial membrane permeabilization (MMP), which begins the collapse of the mitochondrial potential ($\Delta\Psi$), the release of cyt c and other protease and nuclease activators. The inhibition of this process can be attained with inhibitors of the mitochondrial permeability transition pore (mPTP) complex, openers of the mitochondrial ATP-regulated (mitoKATP) or inhibitors of the mitochondrial $Na^+$-$Ca^{2+}$ exchange or $Ca^{2+}$activated (mitoKCa) potassium channels. Modulation of mitochondrial $Ca^{2+}$ can also be envisioned by interference with mitochondria-specific $Ca^{2+}$ transporters. Additional strategies for drug-induced perturbation of mitochondrial biochemistry include the inhibition of the cyt c-catalyzed peroxidation of the mitochondria-specific phospholipid CL, and the targeting of other specific mitochondrial proteins via inhibition of kinases, F1F0-ATPase, enzymes of the Krebs cycle, or members of the anti-apoptotic Bcl-2 family. It has been known for a while that inhibition of the oxidative cellular damage through a decrease of mitochondrial ROS accumulation can be attained by the delivery of antioxidants acting as radical and/or electron scavengers. Many compounds are able to inhibit the β-oxidation of unsaturated fatty acids, causing cellular accumulation of fat. Alternatively, anti-apoptotic agents could be designed via inhibition of the cyt c-catalyzed peroxidation of CL. Finally, the mitochondrial biochemistry is also severely derailed by mtDNA binding/oxidation or inhibition of mtDNA synthesis, or modulation of mitochondrial fission/fusion. Chemical agents that bind to mtDNA often result in inhibition of DNA synthesis. If adequate selectivity in the binding process can be acceded, this mechanism f action may display an attractive strategy to block the expression of mutated mtDNA accountable for genetic mitochondrial disarrays. Lately, compounds that modulate mitochondrial fission/fusion have been suggested as a valuable replacement in treatment of neurodegenerative diseases (figure 2) [6]. While the OMM is relatively permeable due to the abundance of the VDAC protein, the IMM is extremely impermeable and acts as a stiff barrier to the passive propagation of all types of molecules. It is also wealthy in the unusual phospholipid cardiolipin (CL), and keeps a strong negative internal potential of −180 mV needed for the ETC function. A widely used strategy for targeting mitochondria takes benefit of this considerable biophysical membrane nature, since cationic molecules are attracted to and accumulate preferentially within the negatively charged mitochondrial matrix. Another strategy is based on the access of an agent to mitochondrial membrane components, particularly to the phospholipid cardiolipin CL which is particularly found in the IMM. Moreover the former more specific properties, adequate lipophilicity is also needed to achieve an adequate enrichment in mitochondrial compartments. A rising approach to the selective delivery of bioactive cargo molecule into mitochondria uses a carrier of short peptide sequences with specific physicochemical properties. For example, Horton *et al.* newly reported such mitochondria-penetrating peptides with changing cationic and hydrophobic residues. Other variants have been based on an oligomeric carbohydrate scaffold, always attaching key guanidinium moieties due to their delocalized cationic form. Finally, the tethering of active molecules to mitochondrial targeting sequences (MTSs) has also been successively utilized. Mitochondrial targeting sequences (MTSs) are peptides applied by cells for the delivery of nuclear-encoded mitochondrial proteins, comprising structural motifs recognized by the mitochondrial import machinery. Another class of mitochondrial delivery vectors, appropriate for the import of impermeable or big molecules, is the vesicle-based transporter system. The targeted agent is encapsulated in a cationic liposome, which undergoes cellular internalization and subsequent fusion with the OMM. In summary, by the utilization of a wide range of various delivery systems, the targeting of mitochondria for therapeutic advantages can be employed to enrich both pro-oxidants as well as antioxidants in mitochondrial compartments. Antioxidants are of preliminary interest for their antiaging properties, with some of the main applications centered neurodegenerative and cardioprotection diseases, while cytotoxic and pro-oxidant agents are under research for cancer therapy [6].

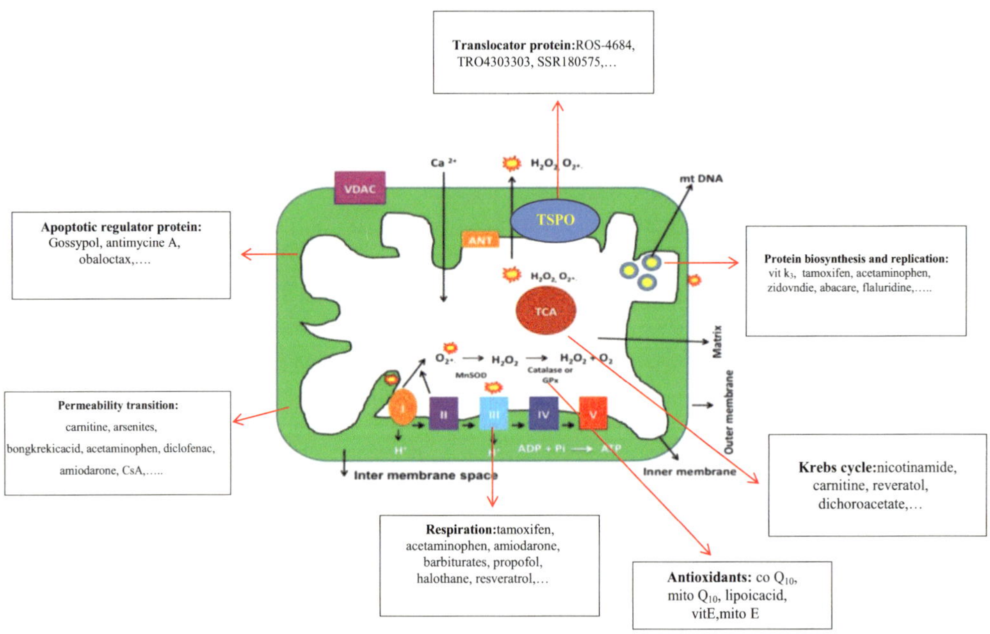


**Figure 2.** Pharmacological targeting of mitochondria of possible sites of drug action.

### 4.1. Targeting the mitochondrial electron transport chain

Mitochondria are unusual organelles. They act as the power plants of the cell, are surrounded by two membranes, and have their own genome. The mitochondrion consists a matrix encircled by two membranes, the MOM and the MIM. The MIM comprises several invaginations called cristae and is very impermeable to ions and small molecules, which need specific transport proteins to exit or enter the mitochondrial matrix. Under aerobic statuses, the proteins of the ETC, placed in the MIM, reduce oxygen to water through a series of steps along the electron transport chain that use NADH and FADH2 derived from the glycolysis and tricarboxylic acid cycle. These reductions effectively efflux protons ($H^+$) through the MIM such that they accumulate in the IMS creating a pH gradient across the MIM that contribute to an overall electrochemical gradient (DC). This gradient as a source of energy to drive the synthesis of ATP from ADP and phosphate is applied by the mitochondrial F1F0-ATPase. This succession of chemical stages is collectively known as OXPHOS.

Small amounts of ROS are generated as a result of incomplete oxygen reduction in during normal OXPHOS. ROS comprise superoxide, the result of partial oxygen reduction, hydroxyl radicals and the subsequently formed hydrogen peroxide, each of which displays different chemistry. A high NADH: $NAD^+$ ratio (as may arise owing to high rates of glycolysis) can increase ROS production, as does state 4 respiration in which electron transport occurs in the loss of ATP synthesis, for instance, when ADP levels are low [8]. Inhibitors of the ETC and of the F1F0- ATPase can also enhance mitochondrial ROS production. ROS act as secondary messengers with important signaling roles, but in addition ROS contribute to oxidative damage of cellular macromolecules. It is also remarkable that the production of ROS has been recognized as a widespread mechanism for the bactericidal effect of many widely used antibiotics including drugs targeting DNA, the cell wall and protein synthesis [9]. Thus, ROS perform both a destructive role and necessary role in cells. Inhibitors of the electron transport chain are useful tools for furthering our understanding of this essential bioenergetics process [10]. Inhibitors of complex I (NADH ubiquinone oxidoreductase) include the photochemical Annonaceousacet ogenins that have been attributed with antimicrobial and anticancer properties and rotenone used as a rodenticide. The widely used diabetes drug metformin inhibits complex I and has been shown to induce AMP-activated protein kinase-dependent and p53 increase in glycolysis to countervail for modulation of the respiratory chain, which effectively increases glucose utilization. Succinate–ubiquinone oxidoreductase (Complex II) is one proposed target of redox-silent vitamin E analogs such as $\alpha$-tocopheryl succinate. Cytochrome c oxidoreductase (complex III) is inhibited by the natural product myxothiazole and by antimycin A (the active constituent of the piscicide Fintrol).Cytochrome c oxidase (complex IV) is a target of cyanide. Complex I and complex III are the main sources of mitochondria derived ROS in vitro, although the synthesis of superoxide by complex III is considered to be more physiologically related. The electron transport chain provides the $H^+$ gradient that is necessary for the mitochondrial F1F0- ATPase to function. The related macrolide apoptolidin and Oligomycin, a natural product that blocks the proton channel are both inhibitors of the F1F0-ATPase.Apoptolidins display remarkably selective cytotoxicity toward a subset of tumor cell lines in vitro, suggesting that inhibition of the ATPase is not exactly cytotoxic. Other compounds reported to bind to the F1F0-ATPase include aurovertin, resveratrol, PK1119, Bz-423, and diindolyl methane (DIM) [11]. The benzodiazepine derivative Bz-423 was identified as a lead for the treatment of autoimmune diseases.Bz-423 reduces disease in murine models of lupus, psoriasis, and arthritis and has cytotoxic and anti-proliferative effects on tumor cells in vitro. Bz-423 is an uncompetitive inhibitor of the F1F0-ATPase, deceleration the ATPase without causing a significant drop in cellular ATP levels. The therapeutic effects of this compound are moderated by the induction of superoxide $O_2^-$. Resveratrol, a constituent of grape skins, increases longevity in rodents and has been attributed with beneficial effects against inflammation, heart disease, and cancer. Notwithstanding the existence of a crystal structure of resveratrol bound to the F1F0-ATPase, this protein is one of several reported targets for resveratrol and related compounds, including the protein deacetylase, sirtuin [5].

The ETC and the F1F0-ATPase proteins can be decoupled by uncoupling proteins that promote the leakage of protons back through the MIM. The resulting drop in membrane potential reduces ROS production and represents a natural protective mechanism against inhibition of respiration. This is a natural process that results in thermogenesis. F1F0-ATPase inhibitors, without affecting ATP synthesis, specifically block ATP hydrolysis have been described: such compounds should be effective under ischemic conditions when the ATPase can operate in the reverse of its normal direction leading to a catastrophic drop in ATP levels that causes cell death [12]. This premise has not been tested clinically. Mammalian and bacterial ATP synthases exhibit substantial differences in structure and intracellular location presenting the opportunity for species selective ATP synthase modulation [5]. The mycobacterial ATP synthase inhibitor, R207910, is currently in Phase III trials for the treatment of tuberculosis [13].

### 4.2. Targeting transporters and channels in mitochondria

It is well recognized that the totality of the mitochondrial membrane is crucial for mitochondrial function. Not only are the inner and outer membranes targeted by drugs, but, in addition, many of the ion channels, proteins, and transporters embedded within the lipid membrane are also targeted. Among the main drug targets are: 1) lipophilic cations targeting the IMM (e.g., rhodamine-123) 2)cardiolipin(CL) (e.g., 10-N-alkyl-arcine orange), 3) carnitine palmitoyltransferase- 1 (CPT-1) inhibitors (e.g., oxfenicine, perhexiline, and etomoxir), 4) $Na^+$/ $Ca^{+2}$ exchanger regulators, 5) B-cell lymphoma 2 (Bcl-2) protein inhibitors (e.g., gossypol) 6) IMM potassium channel regulators (e.g., glibencamide and diazoxide), and 7) MPT pore complex regulators (e.g., CsA).We can activate permeabilization of the mitochondrial membrane or can protect membrane integrity. Among the best mitochondrial protein targets for many drugs are a group of proteins that form the PTP complex across the OMM and IMM. This complex is responsible for mitochondrial permeability transition and plays a crucial role in both survival and death signaling pathways. Depending on the pharmacological strategy, MPT pore activation stimulates apoptosis and prevents the differentiation of many tumor cells. Strategies to induce this effect typically involve direct action against the MPT pore protein complex or indirect action via depleting endogenous inhibitors of MPT pore or increasing ROS and calcium ions in the cytoplasm. Various MPT pore complex inhibitors, in anticancer therapeutic approaches, are used, including: 1) hexokinase modulators such as glucose-6-phosphate and glucose 2)creatine kinase modulators such as cyclocreatine and creatine; 3) cyclophilin D (CypD) -affecting drugs such as sanglipherin A and CsA; 4) voltage dependent ion channel modulators such as arsenic trioxide; 5) benzodiazepine receptor modulators such as Ro-54846 and PK11195; and 6) adeninenucleotide translocase modulators such as CD437, PENAO (4-(N

(Spenicillaminylacetyl) amino) phenylarsonous acid), lonidamide, betulinic acid, clotrane, and bongkrekic acid, GSAO (4-[N-[S-glutathionylacetylamino] phenylarsenoxide)[14], GSAO and PENAO are tumor-metabolism inhibitors that target ANT of the inner-mitochondrial membrane. Both the compounds are currently being appraised in trials in patients with solid tumors. The trivalent arsenical moiety reacts with the two matrix-facing cysteine residues of ANT, inactivating the transporter. This leads to tumor-supporting cells and death and proliferation arrest of tumor cells [14].Above-mentioned drugs grouping although useful appears to be synthetic, and surely will be modified. According to some authors MPT pore may consist of quite different proteins. Recent investigation on MPT pore molecular identity has to redefine a new context on described interaction.CL, a negatively charged phospholipid, is almost exclusively localized in the mitochondrial inner membrane. CL maintains architecture and membrane potential. A loss of CL content has been associated with mitochondrial damage in multiple tissues in a variety of pathological conditions, including aging, heart failure, and ischemia. It was reported that preadministration of NAO (10-N-alkyl-arcine orange), that is a dye associated specifically with CL, decreased the release of cytochrome c, a component of the ETC in mitochondria, released in response to pro-apoptotic stimuli [15]. Another drug target example is CPT-1, an enzyme located in the OMM and responsible for the transport of long-chain fatty acids across the membrane by binding them to carnitine. Perhexiline and etomoxir (antianginal agents) act by inhibiting CPT-1 and protect heart from fatty acid-induced ischemic injury [16].

In contrast to the MIM, the mitochondrial outer membrane is more permeable to small molecules so that the IMS resembles cytosol in its small molecule composition. In addition, however, the IMS sequesters proteins such as apoptosis inducing factor (AIF), smac/ Diablo (second mitochondria derived activator of caspases), and cyt c that when released into the cytosol activate caspases and induce apoptosis. One process for the release of these death inducing protein factors involves swelling of the mitochondrion so that the outer membrane ruptures producing MPT. These events are mediated by the MPT, a channel that comprises multiple proteins including the VDAC located in the MOM, ANT located in the MIM, as well as the peripheral benzodiazepine receptor (PBR), CypD, hexokinase, and possibly also Bax.andBcl-2 Inhibitors of the MPTP have been reviewed elsewhere as have inhibitors of Bcl-family proteins. High affinity ligands of the PBR have been associated with immunotherapeutic and anticancer properties. The relationship of these effects to physiological functions of the PBR requires more study. Newly, VDAC ligands identified in cell-based screens were shown to be cytotoxic toward cells bearing oncogenic Ras protein [4].

#### *4.2.1. Targeting mitochondrial Adenine nucleotide translocator (ANT)*

Adenine nucleotide transporter interacts with Voltage dependent anion channel (VDAC) and cyclophilin D *and* other proteins to make the mitochondrial permeability transition pore (mPTP) at locations where IM contacts OM [17]. Adenine nucleotide transporter (ANT), the key IM protein of mPTP, exchanges ATP and ADP. ANT can form mitochondrial permeability transition pores (mPTP) which induces other membrane leakiness of mitochondria and subsequent swelling of matrix. This event happens following the surface area of the IM (with its folded cristae) exceeds that of the OM. Quite in contrast, the conformation of ANT is modulated by ANT ligands [18] and sensitive interaction of cyclosporine A with cyclophilin D, indirectly blocks VDAC activity. When reconstructed into planar lipid bilayers or into liposomes or into planar lipid bilayers, ANT can form nonspecific channels in response to proapoptotic agents such as the HIV-1 viral protein R (Vpr), $Ca^{2+}$, lonidamine and atractyloside. Moreover, ANT channel formation is inhibited by Bcl-2 and enhanced by Bax. However, mouse knockout studies led to the conclusion that ANT would not (always) be required for apoptotic MPT. Recent evidence suggests that some ANT isoforms (ANT1, ANT3) are apoptogenic while others are not (ANT2)[19]. In 2005, a fourth ANT isoform (ANT4) has been identified in mouse and man by means of two independent experimental approaches. ANT2, which are over expressed in cancer cells, help to stabilize mitochondrial membranes and survival cell. Indeed, it was suggested that in cancer cells, small interfering RNA (siRNA) that down regulate ANT2 may constitute a valid strategy for the selective induction of tumor cell apoptosis [20].

#### *4.2.2. Targeting mitochondrial cyclophilin D*

CypD is a nuclear-encoded mitochondrial isoform of cyclophilin, with a molecular mass of 18 kDa. It enters mitochondria using a targeting sequence that is cleaved following translocation into the matrix. At present, extensive data have been obtained in favor of Cyclophilin D as an essential component and key regulator of MPT pore using various pharmacological inhibitors and genetic manipulations. The first evidence for the involvement of Cyclophilin D in MPT pore formation came from studies showing an inhibitory effect of CsA, extensively used in tissue and organ transplantation, as an immunosuppressant, on pore opening. Other document for the essential role of Cyp D in MPT pore formation has been reported by several independent groups in reports with Cyp D knockout mice in which mitochondria isolated from these animals displayed a low sensitivity to $Ca^{2+}$and, as a result, a delayed MPT pore opening. The inhibitory effect of CsA and its analogs involves interaction with Cyp D that reduces sensitivity of pore opening to $Ca^{2+}$. Cyp D favors MPT pore opening by facilitating the $Ca^{2+}$triggered conformational change. Most probable, interaction of CypD and $Ca^{2+}$, P and the pore is a multifaceted process that also includes enhancement of susceptibility of the MPT pore proteins to oxidative stress [21].

Several studies have shown that Cyp D is up-regulated in many human tumors and can function as an apoptosis repressor. Growing number of evidence demonstrated that the anti-apoptotic regulation of Cyp D might be associated with the stabilization of hexokinase II binding to mitochondria. Inactivation of CypD with cyclosporine A or knock- down of the expression using siRNA was shown to release hexokinase II from mitochondria. Because Cyp D is a mitochondrial matrix protein, an intermediate in the IMM between the OMM and matrix is necessary for its modulation of hexokinase II binding to VDAC. ANT in the IMM could play this intermediation role.However, study showed the opposing pro-apoptotic role of Cyclophilin D in apoptosis. They demonstrated that hexokinase II detachment-triggering apoptosis might be associated with a disruption of the interaction of Cyp D with ANT. Furthermore, inhibition of CyP-D was shown to prevent the onset of the MPT pore [22].

The MPT pore, a critical mediator of cell death, has appeared as a serious therapeutic target for limiting acute ischemia reperfusion injury. The genetic amputation and pharmacological inhibition of mitochondrial Cyp D, a key mediator of apoptosis signaling, has emerged as an important therapeutic target for minimizing acute hypoxic/ischemic injury. The genetic ablation and biological inhibition of mitochondrial cyclophilin-D (CypD), a regulatory component of the mitochondrial permeability transition pore (mPTP), has been reported to decrease myocardial infarction progression in in vivo studies. However, it is note worthy that CypD-deficient hearts are still susceptible to mPTP opening and cell death signaling occurred through mechanisms which are not dependent on CypD. Very recently, cyclosporin-A (CsA), an immunosuppressive therapeutic agent and biological inhibitor of CypD has been shown to reduce myocardial infarction progression and improve left ventricular function in ST-elevated MI patients undergoing primary percutaneous coronary surgery, given at reperfusion [23].

Animals lacking CypD display increased resistance to ischemic insults, muscular dystrophies, multiple sclerosis (MS), ALS, and AD, and the CypD inhibitor CsA and its analogs have displayed neuroprotective effects in several animal models of acute neurological damage and chronic neurodegenerative disease. Preserving the integrity of mitochondrial membranes through inhibition of mPT has been put forward as the central mechanism for the neuroprotective and cardioprotective effects of CsA, even though the drug has several pharmacological targets. It has also been suggested that CypD is downregulated in neurons during development, which would decrease the sensitivity of the MPT pore to calcium, and prohibit the use of CypD as a pharmacological target in disorders of the adult central nervous system (CNS) [24].

#### *4.2.3. Targeting mitochondrial peripheral benzodiazepine receptor (PBR)*

The elaborate structure of mitochondria is important for the normal performance of the organelle and as a potential therapeutic target. Two specialized membranes embed each mitochondrion, dividing the organelle into an arrow IMS restricted by the OMM and the inner IMM. The OMM comprises many channels formed by the protein porin that makes the membrane relatively permeable. One of the membrane proteins is the peripheral benzodiazepine receptor (PBR). PBR is a small evolutionarily conserved protein involved in steroid synthesis and cholesterol transport; it is also a regulator of apoptosis. The PBR is also involved in OMM permeabilization by interaction with the pro-apoptotic Bcl family of proteins. However, OMM permeability maybe independent of MPT pore opening because blocking PBR with 4′-chlorodiazepam (CDZ) prevents against ischemia-induced cytochrome c release independent of damage to the IMM;4′-chlorodiazepam (CDZ)also reduces ischemia-induced arrhythmias. PBR is found in close association with the VDAC and additional components of the mitochondrial contact site. This close association also suggests that PBR-VDAC may serve as a target for modulating apoptosis and may have implications for drug design to treat such disorders as cancer and neurodegenerative diseases [20].

#### *4.2.4. Voltage-dependent anion channel (VDAC)*

VDACs, also known as mitochondrial porins that show 68% similarity between mice and humans. Among three VDAC isoforms, VDAC1 is the most widely expressed in mammals followed by VDAC2 and then VDAC3. Studies have found that VDACs are highly conserved.

Three isoforms of VDAC: VDAC1, VDAC2 and VDAC3 are reported. The additional exon in VDAC2 is believed to encode part of the 5′-UTR region. VDAC1 and VDAC2 are expressed in the skeletal muscles, heart, liver, and brain. There is also very low level expression of VDAC1 but only in the testes. VDAC3 is expressed in the spleen, lung, adrenal, ovary, liver, testicular tissue and kidney muscles. Voltage dependent anion channel (VDAC) function functions in the cell, including regulating mitochondrial shape and structural changes, regulating ATP transport, regulating calcium transport, regulating apoptosis signaling, regulating hexokinase interactions with mitochondria, regulating cell survival, growth, and fertility and maintaining synaptic plasticity through mitochondrial permeability in the transition pore. These functions have been found to be altered in cells from patients with mitochondrial and neurodegenerative diseases, leading to mitochondrial dysfunction. As well as, increasing evidence suggests that VDAC interacts with several cytoplasmic proteins, changes channel activity and VDAC closure and reduces VDAC channel conductance. It is believed that VDAC is constantly open in metabolic state. However, recent evidence suggests that VDAC closes intelligibly during apoptosis in unhealthy neurons. As a result, with its pores closed, mitochondria may not be able to uptake ADP, inorganic phosphate and respiratory substrates from the cytoplasm and to release ATP into the cytoplasm. The pro-apoptotic protein tBid has been found to promote the pore closure whereas anti-apoptotic proteinBcl2-XL has been found to prevent VDAC closure. VDAC displays to be involved in both anti - and pro – apoptosis aspects of mitochondria. VDAC channel conductance may be impaired in a couple different ways. (1)Phosphorylated VDAC may also interact with cytoplasmic proteins, leading to the blockade of mitochondrial pores. Recently, in a study of brain tissue from postmortem brains of patients with AD, Reddy and Manczak found that VDAC interacted with mutant AD proteins, which in turn blocked mitochondrial pores and interrupted the flow of ADP, ATP, respiratory substrates and inorganic phosphate substrates between mitochondria and the cytoplasm, ultimately leading to mitochondrial dysfunction. (2) In neurons from mitochondrial diseases, VDAC may interact with cytoskeletal and mutant proteins that may have accumulated during disease progression and may have blocked the mitochondrial pores [25].

A lot of literature testes the role of VDAC in the regulation of cell death. VDAC is being studied as a cancer-specific target because tumor cells have increased VDAC expression and glycolysis. The role of VDAC1, VDAC2 and VDAC3, in cell death is intricate, but importantly, in vivo evidence shows that in cancer cells, the association of VDAC1with HK prevents against mitochondrial-mediated apoptosis. Therefore, disruption of the VDAC1-hexokinase (HK) complex exhibits an attractive therapeutic cancer target. Over expression of HK1, 2 and their connection with VDAC are notable characteristics of glycolytic cancer cells. It was found that the VDACs expression has been elevated in cancerous cells compared with normal cells and could be altered with chemotherapy. Increased VDAC concentration is an unfavorable prognostic factor; moreover, RNA interference induced VDAC down regulation inhibits cancer growth. This evidence seems in contrast with the finding that over expression of VDAC induces apoptosis, but it illustrates how the context may influence the functional meaning of a biological parameter. In cancer up regulation of VDAC goes hand in with HK2 up-regulation and can be considered a component of glycolytic up-regulation. HK2 binding to VDAC, which allows for ATP transport out of mitochondria, leads to a cancer cell metabolic advantage (termed the Warburg effect), and it antagonizes cell death through the inhibition of Bax-induced cytochrome c release and/or inhibition of the MPT pore [26].

#### *4.2.5. Changes in the configuration of MPT pore as a target in treatment*

Cellular redox potential can be changed by function of OXPHOS proteins as well as by the proliferative state. Elevations in intracellular oxidant potential can have discrete chemical consequences: for example, a pair of cysteine thiols in the ANT becomes oxidized to a disulfide linkage that results in opening of the MPT pore. Thus, manipulating cellular redox represents an approach to altering mitochondrial function. Arsenic trioxide is currently marketed for the treatment of acute promyelocytic leukemia. Its mechanism of action is undoubtedly multifactorial but is understood to involve the formation of disulfide linkages in mitochondrial proteins, including members of the MPT pore leading to their inhibition and the production of ROS [27]. Elesclomol (STA-4783), an injectable drug currently undergoing Phase III clinical evaluation for the treatment of metastatic melanoma, selectively kills cancer cells through apoptosis as a result of an increase in their already raised oxidant level [28].

### **4.3. Superoxide dismutase (SOD) as a target in mitochondria**

Superoxide dismutase (SOD) represents a group of enzymes that use as cofactor zinc and copper, or nickel, iron, or manganese ions. There are three major families of superoxide dismutase, depending on the metal cofactor: The Ni type, which binds nickel (only in prokaryotes) and Cu/Zn (which binds both copper and zinc), Fe and Mn types (which bind either iron or manganese). SOD1 is located in the cytoplasm, SOD2 in the mitochondria, and SOD3 is extracellular. The first is a dimer, whereas the others are tetramers (four subunits).SOD2, the mitochondrial enzyme, has manganese in its reactive site whereas SOD1 and SOD3 contain copper and zinc. [28]

A key role in oxidative stress protection is played by the manganese containing SOD2 in mitochondria. This enzyme is also critical for fetus growth and viability n many eukaryotic organisms, since complete loss of the enzyme results in neonatal lethality in mice. In addition to oxidative tress nitrosative stress can completely inactivate mitochondrial Mn-SOD as well, possibly through nitration of a single tyrosine residue (Tyr-34). Consequently, this favors peroxynitrite generation in mitochondrion. Tyrosine nitration induced Mn-SOD inactivation being identified in more than 50 human diseases including ischemia/reperfusion, inflammation, human kidney allograft rejection and human pancreatic ductal adenocarcinoma [29].

The renal ischemia-reperfusion injury is one of the most important clinical xamples in which Mn-SOD represents the main antioxidant protective mechanism. A significant increase in superoxide production is usually associated with Ischemia/reperfusion conditions which leads to a rapid depletion of SOD. Therefore, any external therapeutic involvement needs the sufficient amount of SOD to overcome the superoxide radical byproduct of ischemia-reperfusion conditions. Any therapeutic administration of exogenous SOD fails due to short half-life of the enzyme in plasma. A way to ensure a continuous production of SOD is entering SOD gene in renal tissue which guarantees protection from renal ischemia-reperfusion injury. The effective gene delivery without toxic side effects was established by intravenous injection of the gene vectors during experiments on animal models before the ischemic insult. A significant progress in the area of kidney biology, especially in hereditary kidney disease and inflammatory and fibrotic diseases was achieved by the use of adenovirus as a vector for kidney-directed gene therapy [30]. Although some advantages make adenoviral vectors suitable for gene transfer into complex organs such as the kidney. But in contrast some disadvantages downgrade these vectors. For instance, the expression of the transfected gene is limited to weeks or months in this technique, because adenovirus does not integrate into the host genome. Secondly, the adenovirus can elicit immunological responses, therefore vector cannot be administered repeatedly. During emergency situations in other inflammatory renal disease states, the SOD gene therapy with adenoviral vector is recommended, however, occurrence of harmful effects maximum within a week is expected (e.g., post-transplant acute renal failure) [29].

ALS a neurodegenerative disease leads to paralysis, muscle wasting, and death, usually within 2 - 3 years of symptom onset due to death of motor neurons. The central mechanism by which motor neuron death occurs in familial ALS is oxidative stress which is due to the mutations in the antioxidant enzyme SOD1gene. Many hypotheses studied so far using ALS mouse models. Some of these studies showed that SOD1 mutants have very low benefits (3, 35). One of the most important pharmacological outcomes obtained in ALS mouse models was increasing expression of either growth factors such glial cell-derived neurotrophic factor, IGF-1, and VEGF (11–13) or RNAi molecules by the delivery of viral vectors (14–16) to silence SOD1 mutant gene expression. In gene therapy the primary cause of toxicity (i.e. mutant SOD1 proteins) is targeted, unlike drug therapy which usually acts on cell survival or deleterious pathways [29].

Reduction of myocardial reperfusion injury through an effective immunization with SOD and catalase has also been hypothesised. Indeed, the cardioprotective effect of intracoronary infusion of SOD may further increase with coadministration of catalase. It is proven that calcium antagonists, rennin-angiotensin system antagonists, Na+/H+ exchanger inhibitors, nitric oxide donors and adenosine induce cardioprotective effects during primary angioplasty for the management of acute myocardial infarction. When these reagents were administrated using intracoronary infusion, their efficiency has increased. Another way to attenuate myocardial ischemia-reperfusion injury is anterograde intracoronary and intravenous administration of anti- P-selectin and anti- ICAM-1 antibodies. The ideal injection route for these antibodies is retrograde intracoronary infusion, which has direct access to postcapillary venules [29].

Application of inhibitors of cellular redox maintaining proteins which reduce intracellular ROS is complementary to the use of pro-oxidant molecules, for example, administeration of catalase or SOD in association with various peroxidases. 2-Methoxyestradiol by increasing cellular ROS formation due to its inhibition of SOD, enhances the cytotoxic effects of apoptotic agents and displays anti-leukemic activity in culture. On the other hand it has been hypothesized, continuous mitochondrial ROS formation leading to oxidative stress and mitochondrial damage has link to degenerative diseases and aging. Based on the ROS etiology of aging the

ROS inhibition should have therapeutic benefit. Administration of antioxidants manganese (III) tetrakis (4-benzoic acid) porphyrin (MnTBAP) or N-acetylcysteine also improved glucose homoeostasis and insulin sensitivity in obese insulin-resistant mice [31]. MitoQ, a coenzyme Q analog is currently in trial for the treatment of Parkinson's Disease due to its potential mitochondrial ROS inhibition. Knowing the beneficial effects of ROS shouldn't underscore the importance of a detailed knowledge of pathological conditions under which ROS formation is happening, as well as the identity and biological half-life of the ROS produced.

Free radicals are generally involved in many pathological processes. The injuring mechanism of reactive radical species is concentration dependent, which finally damages all cellular constituents. Any insufficiency or functional failure in the body antioxidant systems results in the shortening of the lifespan. Therefore, the first therapeutic approach is restoring the normal function of the antioxidant enzymes like SOD.

### 4.4. Mitochondrial $K_{ATP}$ channels target for therapy

Potassium channel openers (KCOs) are agents, discovered in the early 1980s, that act by stimulating ion flux through $K^+$ channels. Many drugs such as, diazoxide, nicorandil, and cromakalim have been identified as KCOs. KCOs act on two types of ion channels: $Ca^{2+}$ activated $K^+$ channels (BK channels) and ATP-regulated $K^+$ channels ($K_{ATP}$ channels). KCOs were first identified by their antihypertensive or antianginal mode of action. Now, they are at various stages of development as and cardioprotective agents. Preclinical and clinical evidence also supports the therapeutic role of KCOs in vascular and pulmonary hypertension, and the treatment of overactive bladder. Until recently, it was believed that the effects of KCOs were entirely attributed to the modulation of K+ channels in cell plasma membranes. However, it is now proven, that new targets for KCOs exist in intracellular membranes including those of mitochondria, zymogen granules, and sarcoplasmic reticulum. It seems that Mitochondria are particularly very important targets for KCOs, because the interaction of these compounds with mitochondria appears to mediate the cardioprotection of KCOs. The protective role of mitochondrial ion channels was recently summarized and mitochondrial targets for anti-ischemic drugs were recently described [32].

#### *4.4.1. Potassium channel openers and mitochondrial $K^+$ channels*

A small-conductance potassium channel, with properties similar to those of the $K_{ATP}$ channel from the plasma membrane, in the inner membrane of rat heart and liver mitochondria and designated the mito$K_{ATP}$. The mito$K_{ATP}$ channel was blocked not only by ATP, but also, similarly to the plasma membrane $K_{ATP}$ channel, by antidiabetic sulfonylureas. These observations raised the question whether the mito$K_{ATP}$ channel could be activated by KCOs. In fact, an increased influx of $K^+$ and depolarization of liver mitochondria in the presence of KCOs was observed. Also, other KCOs were shown to activate potassium ion transport into mitochondria. KCOs such as levcromakalim, cromakalim, and pinacidil have been shown to depolarize cardiac mitochondria. KCO-induced membrane depolarization was associated with an increase in the rate of mitochondrial respiration and decreased ATP synthesis.Moreover, KCOs released cytochrome *c*and calcium ions from cardiac mitochondria. Despite the effect on $K^+$ transport, diazoxide also exhibits a direct effect on mitochondrial energy metabolism by inhibition of respiratory chain complex II in liver mitochondria. Recently, mito$K_{ATP}$ channel opener BMS-191095 with no peripheral vasodilator activity was described.Using isolated mitochondria or proteoliposomes reconstituted with partly purified mito$K_{ATP}$ channel and measuring potassium flux demonstrated that heart and liver liver mitochondrial $K_{ATP}$ channels have some pharmacological similarities with the cell membrane $K_{ATP}$ channel, i.e., both channels are activated by KCOs. Mitochondrial $K_{ATP}$ channels are 1000 times more sensitive to diazoxide than that of cell membrane $K_{ATP}$ channels. This document concluded that the interaction of mitochondrial $K_{ATP}$ channels with KCOs plays a key role in cardioprotection [32].

#### *4.4.2. Mitochondrial $K_{ATP}$ channel: A novel target for cardioprotection*

Mitochondrial $K_{ATP}$ channel: A Novel target for Cardioprotection. KCOs mimic hypoxic/ ischemic preconditioning in the absence of ischemia in the heart myocardial cells, the reason why antagonists of $K_{ATP}$ channel, like 5-hydroxydecanoic acid and glibenclamide, ameliorate the positive effects of short time hypoxic/ischemic conditions on the heart myocardium. The primary postulation to justify these events includes cell membrane $K_{ATP}$ channels. Newly, it was shown that in fact KCOs including diazoxide affect the mito$K_{ATP}$ channel in mitochondria. In a complementary approach, it was shown that diazoxide did not activate plasma membrane $K_{ATP}$ channels, but induced oxidation of mitochondrial flavoproteins, due to the activation of mito$K_{ATP}$ channel. These findings established the fact that the target for the diazoxide protective effects in heart myocytes is the mitochondrial $K_{ATP}$ channel rather than the cell membrane $K_{ATP}$ channel. It is also note worthy that evidence for mitochondrial $K_{ATP}$ channels as effectors of cardiac myocardial preconditioning has also been proven in human subjects. The initial observations on the cardioprotective action of KCOs on mitochondria were further confirmed and developed in a series of reports. It has been shown that other KCOs such as nicorandil, cromakalim, and pinacidil modulate mitochondrial $Ca^{2+}$ uptake, respiration, mitochondrial membrane potential, ATP generation, and mitochondrial $Ca^{2+}$ uptake. The main question remains how the opening of the mito$K_{ATP}$ channel could protect cells against ischemic damage. 1) Opening of the mito$K_{ATP}$ channel followed by mitochondrial swelling could improve mitochondrial $_{ATP}$ handling and/or production. 2) The protective effect of mito$K_{ATP}$ activation could be mediated by lowering $Ca^{2+}$ overloading of mitochondria. In fact, it was found that diazoxid preserves mitochondrial function in ischaemic rat cardiomyocyte. It is now proven that hypoxia approximately decreases mitochondrial oxygen consumption rate to 40% of the normal value, and administration of diazoxide maintains the prehypoxic mitochondrial oxygen consumption rate during hypoxia/ischemia. Cardiac ATP concentration was significantly raised following diazoxide treatment. Secondly, by lowering Ca2+ overloading of mitochondria the protective effect of mitochondrial KATP activation could be induced. It was shown that the opening of the mitochondrial KATP channel may increase mitochondrial reactive oxygen species (ROS) formation. This increase could lead to protein kinase C activation, which is known to be necessary for the cardioprotection. Besides, it seems that mitochondrial KATP channel is enrolled in delayed preconditioning because of an alteration in expression of "protective" proteins (3). It was that pretreatment of hippocampal neurons with cromakalim and diazoxide increases the expression level of Bcl-2 and Bcl-XL which are involved in the control of apoptosisBcl-2 [32].

## 5. Mitochondria as a biosensor for drug development

Extensive study over the last 50 years indicates that many medications can induce mitochondrial damage [33]. Medication- induced dysfunctions include the alteration of mitochondrial components and metabolic pathways. These dysfunctions are a major challenge and problem for drug development. There is mounting evidence of the mitotoxicity (table 2).

Interestingly knowledge of the mechanisms that trigger drug-induced mitochondrial damage will be helpful in the development of strategies to decrease the potentially toxic effects of medications. Additional, these issues affect the most aerobically poised organs such as heart and kidneys or organs exposed to higher concentrations of the drug for example liver. Recently using mitochondria as a biosensor for determination safety of drug development has increased. The reasons are as follows: A) in general, mitochondria control many of the pro-death and anti-death cell signals; B) a number of reports describe an association between patients receiving medication and effects on mitochondrial metabolism 3) drug safety has become a priority of many pharmaceutical companies [4].

It is quite obvious that mitochondria are key elements of cell life which several well known drugs induce toxic effects on them in several non-target and target organs. As soon as possible by improvement of preliminary drug safety assessment the possibility of drug toxic reactions during clinical practice will be avoided. Depending on the targeted organ, severe in vitro mitochondrial impairment may be sufficient to ban an efficient drug in the market or preventing a promising drug candidate from further clinical trials. Drug companies now have a new dilemma, which is to realize how much of the evaluated mitochondrial toxicity is a key predictor of the drug pharmacological or adverse effects. Pharmaceutical suppliers have also now a difficult problem which is to know how much of the supposedly mitochondrial impairment is a component of the therapeutic effect. On the other hand, it may be a tough choice to remove dispensing drugs showing a certain degree of mitochondrial toxicity *in vitro* evaluations but with a very unique significant therapeutic effect. Despite showing mitochondrial toxicity, sometimes pharmaceutical companies may decide to push the lead candidate molecule forward for further in *vivo* assays in order to also clarify ways of reducing adverse mitochondrial toxicity [3]. Some pharmacological strategies could be used to decrease mitochondrial toxicity. For example in the cardiac toxicity of doxorubicin (DOX), One possibility is to improve drug targeting, decreasing the amount of drug that reach non-target organs. One successful example of this strategy is the use of pegylated liposomal DOX, which has a quite different pharmacokinetic profile including an increased circulation time and a decreased volume of distribution [34]. Another strategy is the co-administration of protective agents, one example of which being the preventive role of the beta-blocker carvedilol on DOX induced cardiac mitochondrial impairment.

| Hepatic Toxicity | Renal Toxicity | Cardiovascular Toxicity |
|---|---|---|
| - Metformin | - Cysplatin | - Lidocaine |
| - Valproic acid | - Gentamicin | - Doxorubicin (DOX) |
| - Ketoconazole | - Doxorubicin (DOX) | - Celecoxib |
| - Isoniazid | - Cyclosporin A | - Sorafenib |
| - Nefazodone | - Statins | - Bupivacaine |
| - Lamivudine | - Ifosfamide | - Diclofenac |
| - Divalproex Sodium | - Tenofovi | - Daunorubicin |
| - Tenofovir | | - Ibuprofen |
| - Didanosine | | - Piroxicam |
| - Tamoxifen | | - Thiazolidinediones |
| - Nevirapine | | - Indomethacin |
| - Zidovudine (AZT) | | - Rosiglitazone |
| - Stavudine | | - Atenolol |
| - Flutamide | | -Nucleoside reverse transcriptase inhibitors (NRTIs) |
| - Abacavir | | - Meloxicam |
| - Phenoformin | | - Pioglitazone |
| - Zalcitabine | | - Sulindac |
| | | - Zidovudine (AZT) |
| | | - Idarubicin |
| | | - Piroxicam |
| | | - Mefenamic acid |
| | | - Daunorubicin |

**Table 2.** Examples of Drugs with Black Box Warnings for Mitochondrial Toxicity

Refining of the different methodologies results into higher achievement in the isolation of functional mitochondria from different organs, which can be used in further mechanistic studies to identify tissue-specific drug-induced mitochondrial toxicity. Nevertheless, studies with isolated mitochondria lack the complexity associated with experiments in intact cells, isolated organs or even in vivo studies. But the use of isolated mitochondrial fractions helps determining precise sites of action of the molecule on mitochondria. If everything works OK, the accurate drug safety assessment would correlate data in isolated mitochondria with data collected in intact cells and *in vivo* (figure 3).One important issue in this discussion includes what can be gained by using mitochondria as a biosensor to search drug safety. One particular example was nefazodone, an anti-depressant. This drug was withdrawn from the market in 2004, following several clinical reports of serious liver toxicity [35]. Would the use of mitochondria as cost effective accelerated biosensors of drug safety helped in avoiding the entry of the drug in the market? The answer is, maybe so. Dykens*et al.* demonstrated that nefazodone is highly toxic to isolated liver mitochondria, human hepatocytes and HepG2 cells, showing an obvious cytotoxicity even when cell lines were used. [36] If an initial assessment of mitochondrial toxicity for nefazodone had been done, it is very unlikely that the drug would have been pushed forward for further clinical trials.

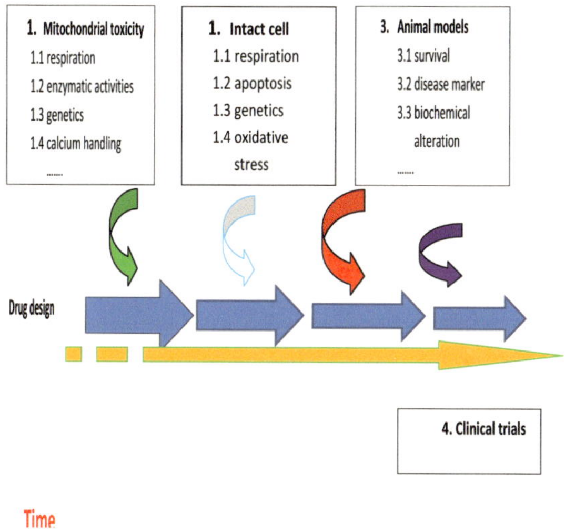


**Figure 3.** Basic scheme of the drug development process involving mitochondria as an important marker for drug-induced toxicity. The thickness of each arrow exemplifies the number of different molecules in each evaluation stage. Drug toxicity on mitochondria is proposed as the bottleneck step in decision-making [3].

It is now apparent that mitochondrial toxicology has become an area of interest to the industry, since a primary assessment of mitochondrial toxicity of a range of compounds can be performed in a fast and relatively inexpensive way, avoiding some later human toxicity problems that may arise during subsequent testing stages or even during clinical use. Some companies will focus more on investigating direct drug-induced mitochondrial dysfunction, others will rather measure drug-induced alterations in mitochondrial-relevant genes. Whatever the chosen strategy is, the final outcome is the prediction of drug safety based on a mitochondrial end-point.

## Author details

Jalal Pourahmad*, Ahmad Salimi and Enayatollah Seydi

*Address all correspondence to: j.pourahmadjaktaji@utoronto.ca

Faculty of Pharmacy, Shahid Beheshti University of Medical Sciences, Tehran, Iran

## References

[1] O'Rourke B: From bioblasts to mitochondria. ever expanding roles of mitochondria in cell physiology. Frontiers in physiology 2010; 1.

[2] Liu X, Kim CN, Yang J, Jemmerson R, Wang X. Induction of apoptotic program in cell-free extracts: requirement for dATP and cytochrome c. Cell 1996; 86(1):147-157.

[3] Pereira CV, Moreira AC, Pereira SP, Machado NG, Carvalho FS, Sardão VA, Oliveira PJ. Investigating drug-induced mitochondrial toxicity: a biosensor to increase drug safety? Current Drug Safety 2009; 4(1):34-54.

[4] Olszewska A, Szewczyk A. Mitochondria as a pharmacological target: magnum overview. IUBMB life 2013; 65(3):273-281.

[5] Toogood PL. Mitochondrial drugs. Current opinion in chemical biology 2008; 12(4): 457-463.

[6] Smith RA, Hartley RC, Cocheme HM, Murphy MP. Mitochondrial pharmacology. Trends in pharmacological sciences 2012; 33(6):341-352.

[7] Frantz MC, Wipf P. Mitochondria as a target in treatment. Environmental and molecular mutagenesis 2010; 51(5):462-475.

[8] Adam-Vizi V, Chinopoulos C. Bioenergetics and the formation of mitochondrial reactive oxygen species. Trends in pharmacological sciences 2006;27(12):639-645.

[9] Kohanski MA, Dwyer DJ, Hayete B, Lawrence CA, Collins JJ. A common mechanism of cellular death induced by bactericidal antibiotics. Cell 2007; 130(5):797-810.

[10] Dias N, Bailly C. Drugs targeting mitochondrial functions to control tumor cell growth. Biochemical pharmacology 2005; 70(1):1-12.

[11] Cleary J, Johnson KM, Opipari AW, Glick GD. Inhibition of the mitochondrial F 1 F 0-ATPase by ligands of the peripheral benzodiazepine receptor. Bioorganic & medicinal chemistry letters 2007; 17(6):1667-1670.

[12] Atwal KS, Wang P, Rogers WL, Sleph P, Monshizadegan H, Ferrara FN, Traeger S, Green DW, Grover GJ. Small molecule mitochondrial F1F0 ATPase hydrolase inhibitors as cardioprotective agents. Identification of 4-(N-arylimidazole)-substituted benzopyran derivatives as selective hydrolase inhibitors. Journal of medicinal chemistry 2004; 47(5):1081-1084.

[13] Koul A, Dendouga N, Vergauwen K, Molenberghs B, Vranckx L, Willebrords R, Ristic Z, Lill H, Dorange I, Guillemont J. Diarylquinolines target subunit c of mycobacterial ATP synthase. Nature chemical biology 2007; 3(6):323-324.

[14] Neuzil J, Dong L-F, Rohlena J, Truksa J, Ralph SJ. Classification of mitocans, anti-cancer drugs acting on mitochondria. Mitochondrion 2013;13(3):199-208.

[15] Biasutto L, Dong L-F, Zoratti M, Neuzil J. Mitochondrially targeted anti-cancer agents. Mitochondrion 2010;10(6):670-681.

[16] Hamann LG, Ding CZ, Miller AV, Madsen CS, Wang P, Stein PD, Pudzianowski AT, Green DW, Monshizadegan H, Atwal KS.Benzodiazepine-based selective inhibitors

of mitochondrial F 1 F 0 ATP hydrolase. Bioorganic & medicinal chemistry letters 2004; 14(4):1031-1034.

[17] Marzo I, Brenner C, Zamzami N, Susin SA, Beutner G, Brdiczka D, Rémy R, Xie Z-H, Reed JC, Kroemer G. The permeability transition pore complex: a target for apoptosis regulation by caspases and Bcl-2–related proteins. The Journal of experimental medicine 1998;187(8):1261-1271.

[18] Brustovetsky N, Brustovetsky T, Jemmerson R, Dubinsky JM. Calcium-induced Cytochrome c release from CNS mitochondria is associated with the permeability transition and rupture of the outer membrane. Journal of neurochemistry 2002; 80(2): 207-218.

[19] Galluzzi L, Larochette N, Zamzami N, Kroemer G. Mitochondria as therapeutic targets for cancer chemotherapy. Oncogene 2006;25(34):4812-4830.

[20] Camara AK, Lesnefsky EJ, Stowe DF. Potential therapeutic benefits of strategies directed to mitochondria. Antioxidants & redox signaling 2010; 13(3):279-347.

[21] Javadov S, Karmazyn M, Escobales N. Mitochondrial permeability transition pore opening as a promising therapeutic target in cardiac diseases. Journal of Pharmacology and Experimental Therapeutics 2009; 330(3):670-678.

[22] Suh DH, Kim M-K, Kim HS, Chung HH, Song YS. Mitochondrial permeability transition pore as a selective target for anti-cancer therapy. Frontiers in oncology 2013; 3.

[23] Lim SY, Hausenloy DJ, Arjun S, Price AN, Davidson SM, Lythgoe MF, Yellon DM. Mitochondrial cyclophilin-D as a potential therapeutic target for post-myocardial infarction heart failure. Journal of cellular and molecular medicine 2011; 15(11): 2443-2451.

[24] Hansson MJ, Morota S, Chen L, Matsuyama N, Suzuki Y, Nakajima S, Tanoue T, Omi A, Shibasaki F, Shimazu M. Cyclophilin D-sensitive mitochondrial permeability transition in adult human brain and liver mitochondria. Journal of neurotrauma 2011; 28(1):143-153.

[25] Reddy PH. Is the mitochondrial outermembrane protein VDAC1 therapeutic target for Alzheimer's disease? Biochimica et Biophysica Acta (BBA)-Molecular Basis of Disease 2013; 1832(1):67-75.

[26] Leanza L, Venturini E, Kadow S, Carpinteiro A, Gulbins E, Becker KA.Targeting a mitochondrial potassium channel to fight cancer. Cell calcium 2014.

[27] Dilda PJ, Hogg PJ. Arsenical-based cancer drugs. Cancer treatment reviews 2007; 33(6):542-564.

[28] Berkenblit A, Eder JP, Ryan DP, Seiden MV, Tatsuta N, Sherman ML, Dahl TA, Dezube BJ, Supko JG. Phase I clinical trial of STA-4783 in combination with paclitaxel in patients with refractory solid tumors. Clinical cancer research 2007; 13(2):584-590.

[29] Cristiana F, Elena A, Nina Z: Superoxide Dismutase. Therapeutic Targets in SOD Related Pathology. Health 2014; 2014.

[30] Yin M, Wheeler MD, Connor HD, Zhong Z, Bunzendahl H, Dikalova A, Samulski RJ, Schoonhoven R, Mason RP, Swenberg JA. Cu/Zn-superoxide dismutase gene attenuates ischemia-reperfusion injury in the rat kidney. Journal of the American Society of Nephrology 2001; 12(12):2691-2700.

[31] Houstis N, Rosen ED, Lander ES. Reactive oxygen species have a causal role in multiple forms of insulin resistance. Nature 2006; 440(7086):944-948.

[32] Szewczyk A, Wojtczak L. Mitochondria as a pharmacological target. Pharmacological reviews 2002; 54(1):101-127.

[33] Neustadt J, Pieczenik SR. Medication-induced mitochondrial damage and disease. Molecular nutrition & food research 2008; 52(7):780-788.

[34] Solomon R, Gabizon AA. Clinical pharmacology of liposomal anthracyclines: focus on pegylated liposomal Doxorubicin. Clinical Lymphoma and Myeloma 2008; 8(1): 21-32.

[35] Lucena MI, Carvajal A, Andrade RJ, Velasco A. Antidepressant-induced hepatotoxicity. Expert opinion on drug safety 2003; 2(3):249-262.

Section 2

# Drug Toxicology

Chapter 4

# Forensic Toxicology

Donata Favretto, Massimo Montisci and
Rossella Snenghi

Additional information is available at the end of the chapter

http://dx.doi.org/10.5772/60445

## 1. Introduction

Forensic toxicology can be defined as the discipline of studiying under a forensic profile the pathologies induced by xenobiotics. This term comprehends all substances of exogenous origin that do not have a physiological role in the biochemical processes of the organism. Xenobiotics are poisons, drugs, drugs of abuse, toxins, pesticides, chemicals and agrochemicals, doping substances and, in part, food supplements.

The following application areas will be discussed: poisoning; alcohol, drugs and driving; workplace drug testing (WDT); doping-antidoping.

## 2. Poisoning

In the field of forensic toxicology, concepts of poisoning and adverse reaction are encompassed in the concept of intoxication according to a unitary criteriological vision; always oriented at resolving a fundamental query concerning the nexus between the action of one or more xenobiotics and the functional and/or morphological harm on the organism until its death. Substances considered *poisons* are those capable of causing damage even in low doses. Even drugs, and in any case all xenobiotics, can exert a poisonous action for an absolute overdose, for pharmacokinetic-pharmacodynamic synergies or for endogenous or exogenous factors.

The classification of poisons in Forensic Toxicology is traditionally dependent on the basis of chemico-physical characteristics of substances and on the consequent possibility of extractions from biological fluids with a method specific for classes. Therefore they have six groups: 1) *poisons in a gaseous or vaporous state* that when inhaled cause intoxication (carbon monoxide, hydrogen sulphide, ethylic ether, chloroform, etc.); 2) *poisons in a liquid state prone to volatility* (benzene and derivatives, glycols, aldehydes, essential oils of some plants, etc); 3) *acids and strong bases* (hydrochloric, sulphuric and nitric acids, sodium or potassium hydrate, etc.); 4) *inorganic anions* (permanganates, chromates); 5) *metals* o salts of metals (arsenic, thallium, mercury, lead); 6) non volatile *organic compounds* of acidic, neutral or basic nature (the most of drugs of synthesis, alkaloids, narcotics, insecticides, agrochemicals etc.). It must be considered, however, that some toxins and many drugs, with a polypeptidic (for example insulin) or protein structure (for example erythropoietin), have physical and analytical chemical peculiarities that do render their extraction and analysis and also their classification more complex.

In many cases, poisoning represents an unknown event that can be demonstrated only through a balanced criteriology for obtaining a differential diagnoses, often inopportunely overlooked in the number of tests to be executed in cases of unexpected death. All of this leads to an underestimation of poisoning incidence in the field of so-called *medico-legal pathologies*. Included in this field are *drug related deaths (DRD)*, a widely investigated and delineated phenomenon in terms of incidence, prevalence and social impact. The multiplicity of pathological factors that contribute to its cause is demonstrated by a complex definition elaborated by a German study group [1], according to which DRD term groups deaths due to *"accidental or intentional overdoses, long term drug abuse, suicide associated to toxic dependency, lethal accidents influenced by the use of drugs"*. DRD is a pathological epiphenomenon reductively denominated an "overdose" or "adverse reaction", originating from variable physiopathological pharmacotoxicological and immunological mechanisms, whose genesis has not found and cannot find a comprehensive explanation in a morphological or chemical-toxicological cause, considered in isolation.

The phenomenon also assumes particular connotations in relation to the quali-quantitative heterogeneity of active drugs, the peculiarity of pre-existent psychophysical conditions, the unpredictability of pharmacotoxicological interactions from poly-drug abuse, capable of inducing a sometimes exponential increase of the risk of lethal *adverse reactions*.

Post-mortem diagnosis of acute and/or chronic intoxication is a paradigmatic example of the necessity to correlate circumstantial, clinical (documentary, anamnestic, objective), necroscopic (autoptic, histologic, immunohistochemical, microbiological, thanatochemical) and chemical toxicological data, obtained following an accurate methodological approach; the gathered data must successively be the object of an evaluative forensic toxicological criteriology. In this view the existence of standardised methodological protocols finds its reason, applied to the resolution of cases where an acute or chronic intoxication of forensic concern is suspected. The necessity of uniform autoptic procedures has been expressed in Recommendation N. 99 of the Committee of Ministers of the Council of Europe, relative to the harmonisation of the rules concerning the legal medical autopsy [2].

The circumstantial data draw on the spatio-temporal circumstances of the presumed "contact" with the toxicant; they can derive from police investigations, testimonial depositions, technical inspections, site inspection reports, etc., and are for example the insurgence of pathological phenomenon or of death following the ingestion of foods or beverages, or contact with chemical substances, or the retrieval of pharmaceutical provisions or paraphernalia in the location where a corpse is discovered.

http://dx.doi.org/10.5772/60445

The clinical data refer to sanitary documentation that is examined to evidence any general or local disorder, in order to outline the objective symptoms characterizing an intoxication. In this view an appropriate toxicological evaluation needs a profound knowledge of the spectrum of biological effects of a specific chemical substance, of the intensity of individual effects dependent on the dose (*dose-effect relationship*) and on the frequency or probability of the appearance of a dose-dependent effect in a determined population (*dose-response relationship*).

The anatomopathological data are intended to reveal morphological modifications, pathognomonic and not, of the organs and systems of the deceased for suspected (acute or chronic) intoxication. In this field the medico-legal literature is lacking thorough studies, extended to all the organs and to the diverse modes of poisoning. In some cases, a macro and microscopic observation can enable identification of toxic-related harmfulness, also non-specific, apt to explain the death or direct the chemical-toxicological investigation. The examinations must include observance of cadaveric phenomena to capture changes in the normal coloration of hypostatic stains, detection of changes in rigidity and evolution of putrefactive phenomena, external examination (presence of jaundice, alterations in cutaneous appendages) and autopsy. A complete evaluation of macroscopic investigations, integrated by the optic and electronic microscope analyses, as well as by specific immunohistochemical techniques, may enable comprehension of the ethiopathogenesis and physiopathogenesis of the intoxication. In particular, it is important to examine the whole encephalon and the heart [3], as well as anatomical organs and structures sometimes undervalued, such as the carotid body, bone tissue and sexual organs. Examination of the *carotid body* provides indications as to possible alterations resulting from chronic hypoxic states and abuse of opiates [4]; *bone tissue*, as to alterations of bone marrow due to toxic or neoplastic diseases; *sexual organs*, as to testicular atrophy attributable to chronic exposure to steroid hormones; the *lymphonodal stations* to distinguish hypertrophy of an infective, inflammatory or neoplastic origin.

The anatomo-pathological findings allow, therefore, to address investigations in two directions:

**a.** To exclude acute intoxication as the principal cause of death when a natural organ pathology capable of inducing death by itself (e.g. acute myocardial infarction, cerebral haemorrhage from a ruptured aneurysm, pulmonary thromboembolism, etc.) is evidenced.

**b.** To strengthen and then confirm the hypothesis of acute lethal intoxication when there is evidence of anatomical lesions characteristic or suggestive of an acute fatal intoxication, also in light of documented clinical and laboratory findings.

The chemical-toxicological data are needed for the qualitative and quantitative demonstration of the presence of the toxicant in the biological fluids and in the tissues collected during the clinical or necroscopic ascertainment.

Retrieval of toxic substances in the living or dead body constitutes, in general, the most important criterion, often decisive to the diagnosis.

The chemical-toxicological analysis should be articulated according to two directions:

- *general unknown research*, when it arouses suspicion of intoxication, but the substance is ignored;
- *specific research*, when circumstantial and/or clinical documentary evidences consent to hypothesise an exposure to specific substances.

Autopsy sampling must include the encephalon, liver, kidneys, lungs, cardiac and peripheral blood, gastric content, bile, urine, head or body hair, and even bone. The samples collected must be stored in separated containers and filled as much as possible to minimise evaporation of volatile substances and the oxidation of drugs. The blood sample for quantitative analyses must be drawn from the femoral vein as this site is less exposed to post mortem alterations of concentrations of xenobiotics. Blood samples from different periferic sites and from the cardiac cavity, left and right, are useful for revealing the possible variation of the concentration of xenobiotics in the post-mortal period. In subjects who fall victim to fires, blood should be taken from vessels in regions spared by the fire, as the diffusion of carbon monoxide has been observed in literature. Specimens taken from different sites must be stored in different containers [5]. Urine can be taken before or during autopsy. The cerebrospinal fluid can be drawn, preferentially, by a suboccipital puncture or even aspirated from ventricles after the removal of the cranium. The gastric and intestinal content must be described in a detailed manner. Possible remains of drug tablets must be preserved in a separate container. In case subcutaneous or intravenous injection of drugs is suspected, a cutaneous sample should be taken from the site of injection and a cutaneous control sample from another region [5]. As to keratin matrices, they must preferably be natural hair cut from the posterior vertex of the head, where a lower variability of drug concentration is described [5]. The hair should be preserved at room temperature since freezing leads to a reduction of concentration. In a corpse, it is strongly advisable to take the hair sample before autopsy to avoid contamination with biological fluids, which cannot be completely removed by washings. Alternatively, sampling of pubic or axillary hairs, or nails, preferably taken from the feet, can be useful. However, nails contain lower concentrations of xenobiotics compared to hair.

In cases of corpses in an advanced state of decomposition it is necessary to collect larvae of diptera and other arthropods found on the body to perform entomotoxicological analyses, aimed at determining in the larvae the presence of xenobiotics originally present in the dead body fluids/tissues. Since living larvae rapidly metabolize the xenobiotics after removal from the corpse, they must be rapidly frozen and analysed as soon as possible. In addition, to avoid environmental contamination, the larvae must be washed before the analyses [6]. It is necessary to underline that, although larvae are useful as qualitative toxicological specimens, they seem to provide limited information of quantitive nature. Moreover the absence of xenobiotics in the larvae does not necessarily imply the absence of xenobiotics in their "food" source [6].

The toxicological analyses must encompass both qualitative and quantitative determinations, employing advanced technologies, using validated methods, foreseeing obligatory analyses of confirmation with certified reference standard of the xenobiotics identified. In general, two types of extraction procedures are foreseeable to separate and concentrate analytes from endogenous compounds: the liquid/liquid and the solid/liquid. The instrumental analyses will use advanced technologies able to separate analytes in the gaseous or liquid phase (gas

http://dx.doi.org/10.5772/60445

chromatography, GC, or liquid chromatography, LC) and to identify them through specific detectors such as UV, IR, FID, fluorescence, mass spectrometry and multiple mass spectrometry (GC-MS, HPLC-MS, MS/MS, etc). Particularly, the use of high or low resolution mass spectrometry coupled with chromotographic technique is considered the gold standard of analytical techniques. It will also be necessary to determine concentration ratios of parenchyma-haematic, urinary-haematic, parent/metabolite compound, in order to perform a correct assessment of results from the historic, biological and statistical epidemiological points of view.

The laboratory of Forensic Toxicology has the primary task of assuring the accuracy of the results through processes of controls of the analytical and organizational quality. The organizational or logistic quality assurance implies the adoption of a protocol intended to preserve the chain of custody of biological specimens from the sampling, through analyses and reporting. Particular attention must be paid to the preservation procedures of the biological samples, both "in short term" (2°-4°C in the refrigerator) and "in long term" (freezer at a maximum temperature of -18°C/-20°C).

The analytical quality assurance must be achieved through the validation of methods, applying principles of selectivity, specificity, precision, accuracy and linearity. The analytical method must also be characterized by its LOD (limit of detection) and by its LOQ (limit of quantification). It is also necessary that the "cut-off "of the method be declared, an arbitrary measure that is adopted in order to discriminate between the results to be considered negative and the results to be considered positive. The cut-off is not therefore just a technical-analytical measure, but is also determined according to the specific diagnostic objective. The "purpose" of the research and the "aim" of the analytical element greatly influence and condition the choice of "cut off" values. Finally, it is important to remember that every analytical procedure must distinguish and appropriately use screening methods and methods of confirmation. The concept of the "confirmation" in Forensic Toxicology is indispensable, and the confirmation technique must necessarily be based on different analytical principals and/or chemical-physical characteristics from the screening procedure.

However, a positive or negative chemical-toxicological report is not sufficient proof to affirm or exclude a death by intoxication. In the first case, for example, one might identify an insufficient concentration of the toxin, arising from accidental contact or environmental contamination. A second possible explanation can be found, for example, in the method of analysis used (high limit of detection and intrinsic limitations of the analytical technique can give an apparently negative result), or in the transformation of the toxicant in metabolites or in its elimination from the organism.

For a further exemplification, the qualitative detection of a poison in the gastrointestinal tract is not sufficient evidence to establish that the substance was the cause of death. It is necessary to demonstrate that it has been absorbed and carried through general circulation, unto the organs where it has exercised its possibly lethal effect.

Similarly, the results of the urine tests are often of little significance in determining the physiopathological effects of the toxic substance, since they only allow proof that the toxic was present in the victim's body some time before death. The physiopathological effects of the majority of the xenobiotics only correlates, in fact, with their blood concentration.

The laboratory plays a crucial role in the forensic toxicological diagnostic when a correct methodology is adopted in sampling procedures and the choice of specimen to be analysed, and when interpretation of the results is well integrated with the data acquired through other types of research.

Once the ascertainment is completed in all its stages, an evaluation phase is undertaken, in which the results of different types of tests must be comparatively and critically evaluated.

Identification of intoxication as a cause of medico-legal relevance can emerge in terms of certainty or probability, which is in turn distinguished in statistical and logical probability.

In toxicology there are not often general scientific laws, of universal or statistical epidemiological coverage, which make it possible to verify or rule out exposure to toxic substances as a cause of medico- legal relevance. It follows that one must usually have recourse to the process of rational credibility, according to the best science and experience, on the basis of what is known regarding the ethio-pathogenesis of disease from toxic origin. In the appendix, the characteristics of the most common drugs of abuse, responsible of acute or chronic intoxication, are shortly summarized according to The National Institute of Drugs of Abuse (NIDA).

## 3. Alcohol, drugs and driving

The studies of "Man-Machine Interaction" [7], evaluating the complex of actions and abilities required to drive motor vehicles and complex machinery (such as industrial), demonstrate that alcohol, drugs and medication influence the psychosensorial and psychomotor functions underlying such skills.

The effects of acute intake of **ethyl alcohol** vary depending on the levels of ethanolemia (in mg%mL o g/L) and the characteristics of the subject. Alcohol can induce sedation and reduction of anxiety, dyslalia, ataxia, impaired judgement and disinhibition. Alcohol has psycho-behavioural effects linearly correlated to its blood concentration. The 50 mg%mL limit, fixed by most driving codes as the limit for drunk driving, is not predictive of the disabling effects of lower concentrations, more evident in the adolescent and elderly population. In any case, the multiplication of risk by 3, 10 and 40 times applies when haematic concentrations exceed 80, 100 and 150 mg%mL, respectively. Driving with levels greater than 150 mg%mL substantiate the identification of alcohol abuse or dependency problems, in need of social-rehabilitative intervention. In Table 1 is a summary of the dysfunctions correlating to values of blood alcohol concentration (BAC) derived from clinical observation and studies on man-machine interaction.

Knowledge of the above described effects and the observation in a real or simulated driving test, allow for the following conclusions. Alcohol consumption determines a deterioration in one's driving ability through an increase in speed, loss of awareness, impaired visual function and attention, wavering about the lane markings, slowing down of reaction time for "breaking and steering", overestimation of "collision" time, inadequate risk assessment [8,9]. Scarce experience, age, alcohol tolerance are factors enhancing alcohol related driving incapacity.

| BAC mg%mL | DYSFUNCTIONS |
|---|---|
| *20* | Insecurity; initial slowing down of the reaction time to a visible stimulus |
| *30* | Initial reduction in the sense of depth of field (stereo optometric) |
| *40* | Reduction in the corneal reflex; impoverished capacity to drive at a constant speed |
| *50* | Incapacity to drive in 25-30% of drivers, reduction in lateral visual perception, mild impairment of judgment |
| *65* | Initial alteration of balance |
| *80-120* | Reduction in the adaptability to darkness; impairment of ocular-motory coordination |
| *120-200* | Reduction in reaction times; initial diplopia; evident inebriation; serious disturbance to balance; inability to judge distances |
| *200-300* | Disorientation, mental confusion, diplopia, unstable walk |
| *300-400* | Incapacity of remaining stood up straight, state of bewilderment |
| *>400* | Coma, anesthesia, areflexia |

**Table 1.** Values of BAC and correlation with driving dysfunctions

The central nervous system is affected not only by the acute effects of ethanol abuse, but also from chronic intake. A significant percentage of alcohol dependents are affected by dementia, cerebellar degeneration, peripheral miopathies and neuropathies.

Incapacity to drive caused by *Cannabis indica* (marijuana and hashish), varies according to the dose of active ingredient taken, not excluding the accidental consumer. Alterations of performance are reported for values of tetrahydrocannabinol (THC, the active principle of Cannabis) comprised between 2 and 5 ng/ml [10]. THC leads to an increase in systolic pressure and cardiac frequency, conjunctival hyperemia, difficulty with nocturnal vision and focusing on objects, above all if in motion, reduction in awareness, distortions of space and time, delayed reactions to stimuli, anxiety, paranoia, panic attacks, motor coordination deficit and impaired judgement with a greater propensity for "risk taking" [11]. These effects, especially expressive with speed and "wavering" of the car (as demonstrated by real driving tests), are accentuated by and also affect reaction times when cannabis is consumed in combination with alcohol [8], as well as together with other psychoactive substances. The effects of cannabinoids are also found in chronic consumers in the long term.

All **hallucinogens**, of natural origin (mescaline, psilocine, psilocybine, etc.) or of synthesis (LSD, derivatives and analogues) induce driving incapacity, seriously altering all the sensitive, neurocognitive, and psychomotor functions, at any dose, either in a state of tolerance or intolerance. The hallucinogenic effects, which start from 15 minutes to 1 hour after ingestion, determine the increase of arterial pressure and of body temperature, as well as spatial-temporal distortion and depersonalisation, often leading to suicide attempts.

**Cocaine** and **amphetamines** are the most prevalent disabling psycho-stimulants, which, though causing a "HIGH" stage and initial improvement of certain psycho-motory functions (reaction time, attention, awareness), cause an incapacity by altering risk perception [12,13]. The initial stimulating effects are soon substituted by tremors, hypertension, tachycardia and, in the case of amphetamines, increase in body temperature and manifestation of epileptic convulsions. In the "DOWN" phase, debilitating effects follow such as depression, irritability, fatigue and anxiety attacks. The down phase can occur a early as 45 minutes after ingestion and has a duration of 2-4 days. As for amphetamine derivatives (e.g. ecstasy) physical and behavioural effects manifest after just a few minutes of ingestion, and protract up to six hours. Such effects, due to a generalized stimulation of the central nervous system, include: euphoria, hyperexcitability, nervousness, tachycardia, insomnia, anorexia, bruxism and mydriasis. Paradoxically, such effects are accompanied by a sense of wellbeing and relaxation and some ameliorative psychological effects. Among the chronic effects are deficits in cognitive functions (memory loss, difficulty concentrating and learning) and psychotic flashbacks. For both hallucinogens and psycho-stimulants drugs, studies of man-machine interaction demonstrate: an increase in dynamic variations of the motor vehicle, both in a lateral and longitudinal (waving) direction; maintenance of high speed; notable reduction of safety distances; reduced reaction to sound and visual stimuli (mydriasis). The above-mentioned effects, indicators of a considerable risk of road crashes and accidents [14], are accentuated or favoured by the combined intake of ethylic alcohol or the increase in drug dose (lateral undulations, increase in speed and reaction times).

The role of natural **opiates**, *Methadone* and *Buprenorphine* in the determination of road accidents is still debated. The verified effects on the incapacity to drive correlate to mood changes, reduced motor coordination, drowsiness, slower psychomotor coordination and pupillary constriction. Withdrawal symptoms and frequent association with other psychoactive substances take on considerable importance, particularly with ethyl alcohol. For some authors Methadone Maintenance Treatment is thought to impede capacity to drive, until psychic stabilisation (> 1 year) and secure absence of the co-use of other psychoactive substances. Buprenorphine in healthy subjects increases reaction time in a laboratory test but not in a simulation driving test.

Studies that have evaluated all medications employed in heroine dependence therapy have shown that the parameters of competence (deviation from the lateral standard position, speed and capacity to steer round a bend, reaction to stimuli), do not present a difference in treated patients *vs* controls, except in the case of combined intake of ethylic alcohol [15].

**Gamma hydroxybutyrate** (GHB), a natural constituent of diverse systems and apparatus of the human organism, also a drug used in anaesthesiology therapy and in the treatment of

http://dx.doi.org/10.5772/60445

alcohol dependence, is the object of abuse for its euphoric, sedative and anabolic effects. Other effects deriving from GHB intake include: disorientation, slowness to react, agitation, inability to focus attention, impaired coordination and balance, tremors, drowsiness, unconsciousness. Given the capacity of GHB to induce sedation, the possibility of determining incapacity to drive motor vehicles becomes evident. It produces collateral effects characterized by nausea, vomiting, drowsiness, vertigo, bradycardia and respiratory depression, coma. Association with alcohol exponentially increases the above described effects [16].

As far as **medicinal drugs** are concerned, there is an *ample difference* between the effects of psychotropic *medicines* belonging to the *same therapeutic class.*

Among *Antidepressants, Barbiturates, Benzodiazepines, Hypnotics* and *Neuroleptics,* are disabling medicines and medicines for which the conclusions are not definitive. Also among *Anxiolotics* and *Antihistamines* coexist disabling drugs and drugs free from effects.

In particular, psychopharmacological studies of man-machine interactions (real and simulated driving test, laboratory test) have identified: drugs that induce an incapacity to drive; drugs that determine a positive effect on the capacity to drive; drugs that do not determine any effect [17].

An analytical systematic research in the field of Alcohol, Drugs and Driving poses particular problems regarding: correct blood sampling, which requires skin disinfection with an alcohol free liquid and blood drawing with a vacutainer vial containing suitable preservatives and anticoagulants; urine sampling, carried out under visual control; use of a chain of custody that documents time, place and personnel engaged in collection and transfer of samples; written consensus to sample collection and analysis given by the subject suspected of DUI, when considered by statuary laws; analytical procedures to be adopted; conservation of specimens in case of possible contestation.

Analytical procedures for the determination of BAC must be in headspace gas-chromatography with a suitable specific detector, whereas the determination of ethanol by enzymatic methods in serum or urine is not suitable for a report of medico-legal value.

The range of substances that must be determined qualitatively and quantitatively is wide, and includes both scheduled and prescription drugs (e.g. benzodiazepines, Z drugs), depending on specific Country legislation. It is thus necessary to have more validated methods available, both in GC-MS and LC-MS, and adequate reference standards. In the evaluation phase, only concentrations identified in the blood may be related to the state of impairment, although there is no univocal approach: in some Countries, threshold values are given by law (blood cut-off) to determine riving impairment, in other Countries no values are set and every concentration is considered impairing (*zero tolerance*).

For the use of oral fluid as the biological fluid for road side DUI controls, the following problems arise: absence of standardized procedure for sample taking; frequent paucity of specimen compared to conventional matrices (e.g. blood) with consequent limitations of multi-class analyses and counter analyses; greater concentration of active compounds than their metabolites, detectable at low concentrations if not sometimes absent; variability of the relationship between salivary and blood concentrations, depending on the variability of the salivary pH, in turn dependent on the speed of saliva production; the possibility of oral contamination as a result of endonasal or inhalatory intake (smoking) of a substance, with a consequent increase of the salivary concentration, independent of the blood concentration.

In light of such criticality, analyses on saliva specimen introduce prospects of controversy connected to analytical, kinetic and evaluative problems.

## 4. Workplace Drug Testing (WDT)

The problem with the consumption of psychoactive substances in the workplace has been the object of multiple studies, characterized by investigations on diverse populations of workers (deceased or hurt in a work related injury or subjects recruited with random criteria or for a toxicological control duty) and different methodologies of research (survey, chemical-toxicological analyses on biological matrices, integrated approach) [18]. Despite the limitations of comparative interpretation, the results of the highlighted studies reveal that:

- cannabis is generally the most diffuse narcotic substance in workers subject to random and mandatory checks;
- alcohol, opiates and cannabis are the most frequently detected substances in injured and deceased workers subject to sporadic toxicological checks.

Given that such evidence does not patently allow for establishing the significance of the role of psychoactive substances, in the genesis of accidents at work, the need to implement systematic, international and national studies, including comparative analysis of anamnestic/cathamnestic, clinical/autoptic and chemical-toxicological data, extended to multiple biological matrices (blood, urine and hair), exists.

There are guidelines elaborated by International Scientific Societies and statuary legislations that provide instructions for authorized laboratories to perform toxicological analyses in the work place frame. Such indications regard: the method of specimen collection and analysis; interpretation of results, also dependent on predetermined cut-off statutory values; internal and external monitoring of analytical quality; the manner of reporting.

Organization of toxicological controls on workers presumes therefore the application of uniform and standardised toxicological assessment, aimed at safeguarding the security of work places, also through acquisition of scientific epidemiological evidence.

## 5. Doping

Doping urges for an institutional and collective attention as an underground phenomenon in rapid growth in the sporting world and social reality. Changing and refinement of substances and doping methods, their growing pharmacodynamic effectiveness, lacking or problematic

http://dx.doi.org/10.5772/60445

detectability of substances with ergogenic purposes (so called food supplements), widespread and clandestine commercialization of drugs, and the volume of annual trade, all signify a state of emergency.

In this context, death caused by doping is an event routinely reported by high level sporting competitions [19]. The scarcity of data deduced from international literature and the lack of institutional systems of epidemiological monitoring does not permit reliable estimates of the size of the phenomenon, even and above all with reference to amateur sporting activity. The intrinsic dangerousness of all doping practices, as well as the remarkable heterogeneity of protocols investigating an athlete's sudden death, contribute to the problem. The risk of death related to use of doping substances and practices is mainly associated to anabolics and stimulants, followed by erythropoietic stimulating drugs, growth hormones and diuretics [20].

However, paucity of epidemiological data relative to doping consumption and correlating cases of deaths, cannot define the real size of the phenomenon, which is certainly underestimated. The use of doping seems to be accepted by the sporting community, also because of the underestimation of the related dangers.

The inability to define the real danger is reflected in the failure to alert institutions, entrusted with the implementation of preventative, informative and repressive educational interventions.

To dam difficulties associated with the growing abundance of doping substances, laboratories must exchange their experiences and rational adjustment of procedures is needed in a process of constant renewal, in technology and analytical procedures. The renewal must involve use of systems of greater sensitivity and analytical accuracy, as well as larger systematic screenings to incorporate new banned substances in real time.

## 6. Conclusion

Activity in the field of Forensic Toxicology is identified with the detection, identification and quantification of xenobiotics in *biological* and *non biological* matter. A synopsis of such analytical phases leads to the interpretation of results through a rigorous *evaluative criteriology* in relation to different regulatory areas.

The two main areas where the analysis of biological material applies are «forensic Toxicology of the dead» and «forensic Toxicology of the living person».

Forensic Toxicology of the dead is devoted to determine the presence of xenobiotics in liquids and tissues and evaluate the possible causal or concausal role in the determination and dynamics of the death.

Forensic Toxicology of the living person is committed to determine the presence of xenobiotics in the biological specimen (blood, urine, air inhaled, hair, etc.) and in evaluating the possible causal or concausal role of incapacity and/or deviations in behaviour (see suitability to drive, WDT, doping, etc.), or rather harm to the person.

Obligation in the above-mentioned areas is complex because of «pre-analytical» and «analytical» variables. Among the pre-analytical variables are: quantity of dose ingested, frequency and means of ingestion, interval between intake and sample taking, the sample collection procedure, the interval between sample taking and analysis.

Among the analytical variables are: elevated number of analytes, large variety of chemical structures, of volatility, functional groups, hydrophilic/lipophilic ratios, values of $pK_a$ or $pK_b$; wide ranges of concentration in liquids and biological tissues, dependent on dose intake; the way the specimens are stored; the possible lack of pharmacokinetic and pharmacodynamic studies; the diversity of biological matrices and potential analytical interferences produced by exogenous, endogenic and putrefactive substances.

The complexity of those variables ensures that *every analysis may be given as an individual case for which there are no rules applicable to all xenobiotics and all situations.*

With the diffusion of environmental toxins and the clandestine drug market, the forensic toxicology laboratory is also committed to the analysis of non-biological material. In this context, Forensic Toxicology can provide to institutions and society information and awareness on the appearance of new drugs; identification of the major channels of drug distribution in the local and national black market; identification of the means adopted by traffickers to bypass systems of control; information on substances used in the cutting or treatment of the drug; suggestions for timely legislative adaptations.

With the main objective of providing scientifically based *evidence*, the complexity of all the above outlined roles of forensic toxicology entails the need for the adoption of quality assurance systems, ascertainement methodologies and evaluation criteriologies.

## 7. Addendum

### 7.1. Principal drugs of abuse

#### *7.1.1. Nicotine*

Alakloid from *Nicotiana tabacum*; found in cigarettes, cigars, and smokeless tobacco (snuff, spit tobacco, chew); it can be smoked, snorted, chewed

**Acute Effects** - Increased blood pressure and heart rate

**Health Risks** - Chronic lung disease; cardiovascular disease; stroke; cancers of the mouth, pharynx, larynx, esophagus, stomach, pancreas, cervix, kidney, bladder, and acute myeloid leukemia; adverse pregnancy outcomes; addiction

#### *7.1.2. Ethanol*

Alcohol, ethyl alchol, produced by sugar fermentation; found in liquor, beer, and wine; orally ingested (swallowed)

http://dx.doi.org/10.5772/60445

**Acute Effects** - In low doses, euphoria, mild stimulation, relaxation, lowered inhibitions; in higher doses, drowsiness, slurred speech, nausea, emotional volatility, loss of coordination, visual distortions, impaired memory, sexual dysfunction, loss of consciousness

**Health Risks** - Increased risk of injuries, violence, fetal damage (in pregnant women); depression; neurologic deficits; hypertension; liver and heart disease; addiction; fatal overdose.

#### *7.1.3. Tetraydrocannabinol*

Active principle of *Cannabis*; found in marijuana or hashish or hash oil or hemp; smoked or swallowed.

Scheduled drug.

**Acute Effects** – Euphoria; relaxation; slowed reaction time; distorted sensory perception; impaired balance and coordination; increased heart rate and appetite; impaired learning, memory; anxiety; panic attacks; psychosis

**Health Risks** - Cough, frequent respiratory infections; possible mental health decline; addiction

### 7.2. Opioids

Alkaloids from Papaverum Somniferum; found in opium (Morphine, Codeine) or derived from opium by chemical synthesis (Heroin) or chemically synthesized (Naloxone, Oxycodone, Oxymorphone etc); Heroin (diacetylmorphine) can be injected, smoked, snorted; Opium can be swallowed or smoked; scheduled drugs.

**Acute Effects** - Euphoria; drowsiness; impaired coordination; dizziness; confusion; nausea; sedation; feeling of heaviness in the body; slowed or arrested breathing

**Health Risks** - Constipation; endocarditis; hepatitis; HIV; addiction; fatal overdose

#### *7.2.1. Stimulants*

Alkaloids found in *Coca* leaves (Cocaine) or chemically synthesized (amphetamines and methamphetamines, methylenedioxyamphetamines, methylenedioxyamphe-tamines, amphetamine-like compounds, phenethylamine derivatives); Cocaine can be snorted, smoked, injected; Amphetamine derivatives can be swallowed, snorted, smoked, injected; scheduled drugs.

**Acute Effects** - Increased heart rate, blood pressure, body temperature, metabolism; feelings of exhilaration; increased energy, mental alertness; tremors; reduced appetite; irritability; anxiety; panic; paranoia; violent behavior; psychosis. **for MDMA** - Mild hallucinogenic effects; increased tactile sensitivity; empathic feelings; lowered inhibition; anxiety; chills; sweating; teeth clenching; muscle cramping

**Health Risks** - Weight loss, insomnia, sleep disturbances; cardiac or cardiovascular complications; depressions; stroke; seizures; addiction. **for MDMA** - Sleep disturbances; depression; impaired memory; hyperthermia; addiction.

**Also, for cocaine** – Nasal damage from snorting

**Also, for methamphetamine** – Severe dental problems

*7.2.2. Dissociative drugs*

**Synthetic drugs:** Ketamine (injected, snorted, smoked); Phencyclidine (PC) and analogs (swallowed, smoked, injected). **Naturally occurring**: salvinorine from *Salvia divinorum* (chewed, swallowed, smoked).

**Acute Effects** - Feelings of being separate from one's body and environment; impaired motor function

**Also, for ketamine** - Analgesia; impaired memory; delirium; respiratory depression and arrest; death

**Also, for PCP and analogs** - Analgesia; psychosis; aggression; violence; slurred speech; loss of coordination; hallucinations

**Health Risks** - Anxiety; tremors; numbness; memory loss; nausea

*7.2.3. Hallucinogens*

**Synthetic drugs**: Lysergic acid diethylamide (LSD, swallowed, absorbed through mouth tissues).

**Naturally occurring**: Mescaline, from the peyote cactus (Lophophora williamsii), the San Pedro cactus (Echinopsis pachanoi) and in the Peruvian torch (Echinopsis peruviana), (swallowed, smoked); Psilocybin, from mushrooms of genus Psilocybe, such as P. azurescens, P. semilanceata, and P. cyanescens, and from about a dozen other genera (swallowed).

**Acute Effects** - Altered states of perception and feeling; hallucinations; nausea

**Also, for LSD** - Increased body temperature, heart rate, blood pressure; loss of appetite; sweating; sleeplessness; numbness, dizziness, weakness, tremors; impulsive behavior; rapid shifts in emotion

**Also, for Mescaline** - Increased body temperature, heart rate, blood pressure; loss of appetite; sweating; sleeplessness; numbness, dizziness, weakness, tremors; impulsive behavior; rapid shifts in emotion

**Also, for Psilocybin** - Nervousness; paranoia; panic

**Health Risks, for LSD** - Flashbacks, Hallucinogen Persisting, Perception Disorder

*7.2.4. Anabolic steroids*

**inhalants**

**Acute Effects, for Anabolic steroids** - No intoxication effects.

**for Inhalants (varies by chemical)** - Stimulation; loss of inhibition; headache; nausea or vomiting; slurred speech; loss of motor coordination; wheezing

**Health Risks, for Anabolic steroids** - Hypertension; blood clotting and cholesterol changes; liver cysts; hostility and aggression; acne; in adolescents—premature stoppage of growth; in males—prostate cancer, reduced sperm production, shrunken testicles, breast enlargement; in females—menstrual irregularities, development of beard and other masculine characteristics

**for Inhalants** - Cramps; muscle weakness; depression; memory impairment; damage to cardiovascular and nervous systems; unconsciousness; sudden death.

## Author details

Donata Favretto*, Massimo Montisci and Rossella Snenghi

*Address all correspondence to: donata.favretto@unipd.it

Legal Medicine and Toxicology, University Hospital of Padova, Padova, Italy

## References

[1] Janssen W, Trubner K, Puschel K. Death caused by drug addiction: a review of the experiences in Hamburg and the situation in the Federal Republic of Germany in comparison with the literature. Forensic Sci Int. 1989,43: 223-37.

[2] Recommendation no. R (99) 3 of the Committee of Ministers to member states on the harmonization of medico-legal autopsy rules. Forensic Sci Int. 2000, 111(1-3):5-58.

[3] Basso C, Burke M, Fornes P, Gallagher PJ, de Gouveia RH, Sheppard M, Thiene G, van der Wal A; Association for European Cardiovascular Pathology. Guidelines for autopsy investigation of sudden cardiac death. Virchows Arch. 2008, 452(1):11-8.

[4] Porzionato A, Macchi V, Guidolin D, Parenti A, Ferrara SD, De Caro R. Histopathology of carotid body in heroin addiction. Possible chemosensitive impairment. Histopathology. 2005, 46(3):296-306.

[5] Skopp G. Preanalytic aspects in postmortem toxicology. Forensic Sci Int. 2004, 142(2-3):75-100.

[6] Introna F, Campobasso CP, Goff ML. Entomotoxicology.Forensic Sci Int. 2001, 120(1-2):42-7

[7] Ferrara SD, Giorgetti R, Methodology in man-machine interaction and epidemiology on drugs and traffic safety. Experiences and Guidelines from an International Workshop. Padova: ARFI Research. Monograph 6, 1992.

[8] Ogden EJ, Moskowitz H. Effects of alcohol and other drugs on driver performance. Traffic Inj Prev. 2004, 5(3): 185-98.

[9] Laapotti S, Keskinen E. Fatal drink-driving accidents of young adult and middle-aged males--a risky driving style or risky lifestyle? Traffic Inj Prev. 2008, 9(3):195-200.

[10] MacDonald S, Mann R, Chipman M, Pakula B, Erickson P, Hathaway A, MacIntyre P. Driving behavior under the influence of cannabis or cocaine. Traffic Inj Prev. 2008, 9(3):190-4.

[11] Lane SD, Cherek DR, Tcheremissine OV, Lieving LM, Pietras CJ. Acute marijuana effects on human risk taking. Neuropsychopharmacology. 2005, 30(4): 800-9.

[12] Fillmore MT, Rush CR, Hays L. Acute effects of oral cocaine on inhibitory control of behavior in humans. Drug Alcohol Depend. 2002, 67(2): 157-67.

[13] Kuypers KP, Samyn N, Ramaekers JG. MDMA and alcohol effects, combined and alone, on objective and subjective measures of actual driving performance and psychomotor function. Psychopharmacology. 2006, 187(4):467-75.

[14] Smink BE, Ruiter B, Lusthof KJ, De Gier JJ, Uges DR, Egberts AC. Drug use and the severity of a traffic accident. Accid Anal Prev. 2005, 37(3): 427-33.

[15] Schindler SD, Ortner R. Maintenance therapy with synthetic opioids and driving aptitude. Eur Addict Res. 2004, 10(2): 80-7.

[16] Couper FJ, Logan BK. GHB and driving impairment. J Forensic Sci. 2001, 46(4): 919-23.

[17] Walsh J, De Gier JJ, Christopherson AS, Verstraete AG. Drugs and driving. Traffic Inj Prev. 2004, 5(3): 241-53.

[18] Bunn TL, Slavova S, Bernard AC. Work-related injuries in a state trauma registry: relationship between industry and drug screening. J Trauma Acute Care Surg. 2014, 77(2):280-5.

[19] Marijon E, Tafflet M, Antero-Jacquemin J, El Helou N, Berthelot G, Celermajer DS, Bougouin W, Combes N, Hermine O, Empana JP, Rey G, Toussaint JF, Jouven X. Mortality of French participants in the Tour de France (1947-2012). Eur Heart J. 2013, 34(40): 3145-50.

[20] Montisci M, El Mazloum R, Cecchetto G, Terranova C, Ferrara SD, Thiene G, Basso C. Anabolic androgenic steroids abuse and cardiac death in athletes: morphological and toxicological findings in four fatal cases. Forensic Sci Int. 2012; 217(1-3):e13-8.

Chapter 5

# Tramadol Poisoning

Omid Mehrpour, Mohammaddavood Sharifi and
Nasim Zamani

Additional information is available at the end of the chapter

http://dx.doi.org/10.5772/60439

## 1. Introduction

Poisoning is one of the leading causes of mortality and morbidity in many countries. In 1955, poisoning was the most common cause of death in patients aged between 35 and 44 years [1]. Tramadol was first manufactured in Germany in 1970 to relieve post-surgical and chronic pains [2]. It is currently the most commonly prescribed opioid in the world [3]. According to the Australian studies, tramadol use has increased almost 10 times between 1998 and 2004 [4].

Although tramadol is very commonly prescribed, it should be administered with the consideration of the risk to benefit ratio [5]. Tramadol is one of the most common causes of poisoning in adult male patients with the previous history of drug addiction and psychological problems and suicide is the most common motivation for its use in this group of the patients [1,3,6-8]. The aim of this review is to evaluate all possible clinical manifestations and life-threatening signs/symptoms of tramadol poisoning.

## 2. Pharmacology

Tramadol is a synthetic analogue of codeine with central effects [2,6,9-13]. It is not an opioid derivative or non steroidal anti-inflammatory (NSAID) medication. Actually, tramadol has low affinity for opioid receptors [14,15] and has a hydrochloride structure (Figure 1) [1,16].

Tramadol is used as a racemic mixture in the treatments [15]. This mixture is a 1:1 ratio of two enantiomers with synergistic analgesic effects [17]. The (+) and (-) enantiomers weakly connect to mu opioid receptors [18]. Enantiomer (+) is the opioid part but increases serotonin release and inhibits its re-uptake, as well. Enantiomer (-) is a noradrenaline re-uptake inhibitor [17-19].

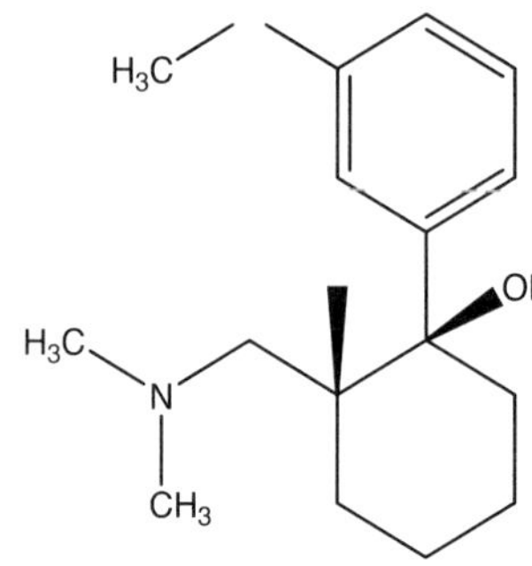


**Figure 1.** Tramadol structure

Most of the analgesic effects of tramadol are likely secondary to its monoaminergic central pathways [3,10,20]. Tramadol acts through some different pathways including:

**a.** Affecting mu receptors causing the opioid-like effects;

**b.** Affecting noradrenergic pathways causing inhibition of norepinephrine reuptake in central nervous system (CNS);

**c.** Affecting serotonergic pathways causing inhibition of serotonin reuptake in the CNS;

**d.** Affecting GABAergic pathways causing increased GABA neurotransmitter in the brain [2,8,13,17,21,22].

Tramadol is currently available as tablets, oral drops, solution for injection, and suppository [8] with the oral rout being the most common rout of its administration. Tramadol has a high volume of distribution (3 L/kg) [3,7]. Bioavailability of an oral dose of tramadol is 75% which can reach almost 100% with a programmed schedule [7]. The common therapeutic dose of tramadol is 50 to 100 mg (50 mg oral, 50-100 mg intramuscular [IM], and/or100 mg rectal; 1.5 mg/kg/day in a 60-kg patient) three to four times a day. Doses higher than 400 mg/day are generally not necessary [8,17,23]. However, evaluation of five rheumatologic disorder patients over 65 years of age revealed that a daily tramadol dose of 300 to 1200 mg was needed for them to relieve their pain [24].

Analgesic effects of tramadol are dose-related. The relation between serum level and analgesic effect is not the same among different people. It is estimated that the normal therapeutic serum level of tramadol and its metabolite are 0.1 to 0.3 mg/L and 0.03 to 0.04 mg/L, respectively [3,25-27]. According to the information from International Association of Forensic Toxicologists, therapeutic, toxic, and fatal levels of tramadol in adults are 0.1-0.8 mg/L, 1-2 mg/L, and over 2 mg/L, respectively [26]. Tramadol is completely and rapidly absorbed after oral use. Sustained-release tablets affect within 12 hours and their serum level peaks at 4-9 hours postingestion [6]. In the mice, tramadol is more available and effective at the final phase of the darkness and most of the mortalities happen at the mid phase of the darkness; such an effect has not been detected in human volunteers [28,29].

In postmortem evaluations using gas chromatography, tramadol level is at the most in heart, liver, peripheral blood, urine, kidney, lung, spleen, bile, and brain without any distribution into the muscles [6,25,30].

Tramadol is generally metabolized through N-demethylation, O-demethylation, glucuronidation, and/or sulfation. Metabolization of tramadol is performed by cytochrome P450 enzymes. CYP2D6 is responsible for O-demethylation while N-demethylation is done by CY2B6 and CY3A4 [6,31,32]. Tramadol can be used in renal failure although decreased doses are recommended in renal problems and liver cirrhosis [33].

In a study on six alpacas (some kind of camel), the half-life of all three metabolites of tramadol (O-, N-, and Di-desmethyltramadol) was reported to be more than the parent drug [34]. The main metabolite (O-desmethyltramadol) has a 200-time affinity for mu receptors and its analgesic effect is twice the parent medication, as well [2,15,26].

## 3. Tramadol toxicity

Tramadol is considered to be a safe drug. However, mortality has been reported with its use [35,36]. Toxicity can happen accidentally. Patients with the previous history of addiction are at extreme danger for such toxicity and according to FDA warnings, tramadol administration should be performed cautiously in these patients [6,37].

Toxicity of tramadol can be predicted by P450 polymorphism [38,39]. Few studies have shown the difference in the postsurgical analgesic serum levels of tramadol among people which is probably due to the genetic polymorphism in the activity of CYP2D6 [40,41]. Diversity in the response depends on the CYP2D6 genotype. Ultra-rapid metabolizers have a higher risk of tramadol toxicity with higher plasma levels of O-desmethyltramadol. They experience higher analgesic effects and nausea in comparison to the group who are extensive metabolizers [38].

## 4. Epidemiology of tramadol toxicity

Most of the tramadol-intoxicated patients are male (63% to 89.3%) [3,21,37,42-48] and single [1,8,21]. However, in few studies, female patients were more (55% to 59%) [49,50]. Most of the patients were in their 3$^{rd}$ decade of life. This is while the age range of the patients was reported to be between 5-week-old and 87-year-old in different studies [1,3,8,37,44,45,47-51]. Patients generally ingested tramadol [6,8,45,52]. Almost 51.9% to 98.7% of the patients had intentionally overdosed on tramadol; 27.8% to 29.6%, 0.87% to 3.7%, and 0.2% to 7.4% had recreationally, accidentally, or medically overdosed on tramadol, respectively [1,3,6,8,23,45].

In a recent study, university students with the previous history of cigarette smoking and consumption of addicting opioids were more prone to abuse tramadol [24]. In another study, 22.2% of the hospitalized patients had a history of admission due to tramadol overdose [3]. It has been said that in almost 90%, 7.9%, and 2.1% of the tramadol toxicities, poisoning is due to acute, chronic, and acute on chronic overdoses [3]. Most of the patients refer within the first 6 hours postingestion [21,45,49] with a hospitalization period of 15 minutes to 21 days [8,21]. Signs/symptoms of toxicity recover within 24 hours and almost 42% of the patients will need ICU admission [49,50,53].

## 5. Biologic characteristics

Tramadol is used as the first-line treatment in musculoskeletal pains [15,54-57] and as an alternative treatment in osteoarthritis (OA) patients in whom NSAIDs are contraindicated or those with resistant pain to oral analgesics [58].

Tramadol analgesic effects are due to the inhibition of norepinephrine and serotonin reuptake as well as agonism of mu receptors which cause blockage of the pain impulses in the spinal cord [7,56,59]. Direct administration of tramadol on the sciatic nerve can reduce the amplitude and speed of spinal somatosensory evoked potential in the rats emphasizing the analgesic effects of tramadol on the peripheral nerves [60].

In tramadol-induced anesthesia, the patient become conscious rapidly, has amnesia during the surgery, and experiences few side effects [61]. Controlled release of tramadol through polyhydroxybutyrate (PHB) microspheres is also available which induces longer anesthesia after epidural use in comparison with tramadol alone [62].

According to a study performed on the rats, tramadol reinforces the immune system by increasing phagocytosis. Use of tramadol is therefore favored as an analgesic in immune-compromised patients [63].

## 6. Side effects and clinical/paraclinical findings

Tramadol is an analgesic with less side effects in comparison with other opioids [64]. It has the least gastrointestinal and renal toxicities [65]. Drug screening for opioids is generally negative in the patients with tramadol overdose [66].

In overdose, lethargy, nausea, tachycardia, agitation, seizure, coma, hypotension, hypertension, respiratory depression, dysuria, constipation, dizziness, facial paresthesia, ataxia, headache, edema, movement disorders, perspiration, blurred vision, hallucination, itching, vertigo, palpitation, hypo- and hyper-reflexia, diplopia, multi-organ failure, acute liver failure due to fulminant liver necrosis, renal failure, and urine retention have been reported [8,17,23, 48-51,64,67,68]. Dizziness, nausea, constipation, vertigo, and headache are the most common symptoms [57,69,70]. Miosis is not as common as that in toxicities with other opioids and is detected in up to one-thirds of the patients probably due to serotonin and norepinephrine reuptake inhibition [71].

## 7. CNS manifestations of tramadol toxicity

The CNS manifestations are of the most common signs/symptoms of tramadol overdose ranging from CNS depression to lethargy and deep coma [6]. O-desmethyltramadol impairs consciousness and causes electrocardiographic (ECG) changes and seizure [44]. n a study by Spiller et al, significant neurologic toxicity was seen in tramadol overdose [49] which was mainly due to the monoamines reuptake inhibition [3,72].

In sub-acute and chronic toxicities, clinical manifestations are mostly behavioral disorders and seizure and may occur with doses of 25mg/kg or higher [17]. Seizure is an important problem in tramadol toxicity with its frequency being reported between 8% and 14% in different social studies and 15% to 55.3% in hospital studies. Most of the patients experience only one episode of seizure [44,47, 49,50]. Seizure is more common in young males (mean age of 22 – 39.5 y) [8,23,43,44,52]; however, some studies reported no significant difference in the frequency of seizure between different genders [3,47,72,73].

Seizure happens in less than 1% of the patients with therapeutic levels [23,74]. It seems that tramadol causes seizure in a dose-dependent manner [3,21,23] while some other studies have not confirmed this [43,44,75]. The least tramadol amount that has resulted in seizure is 100 mg. Tramadol neurotoxicity generally occurs within the first 24 hours postingestion (mainly in the first 6 hours) and seizures are usually tonic-clinic [3,6-8,11,21,23,50,75-78]. Status epilepticus has also been reported [6,11,59,76]. This shows that tramadol can cause seizure at both therapeutic and toxic levels [43,52,77,79].

Brain computed tomography (CT) of the tramadol-intoxicated patients has often been reported to be normal [43,77]. Künig and assistants reported two cases of fluctuating dizziness and cognitive problems due to long-term treatment with tramadol who recovered with cessation of the drug [80]. In a study performed to evaluate the risk of idiopathic seizure in tramadol users, only 17 cases of idiopathic seizure were found among 10917 patients, all of whom, used tramadol in combination with some other medication; it, therefore, is difficult to relate their seizure to tramadol use [71]. Seizure is less frequent in the patients who use tramadol with benzodiazepines. Psychological and somatic complications (hepatitis C and liver injury) were detected in those who had seized. Ethanol can reduce the seizure threshold in tramadol use. Seizure is also more common in younger patients who have abused tramadol for a long period of time [23].

Background seizing disorders, medications causing seizure, ethanol withdrawal, CNS depressants, or head injury can affect seizure occurrence in tramadol overdose, as well [45]. Mydriasis and tachycardia can accompany with a higher risk of seizure [44].

In a cohort study comparing 9218 tramadol users and 37232 non-users, less than 1% of the users experienced seizure after the first use. Risk of seizure was 2-to 6-fold in the patients who had background diseases or consumed other medications. The risk was also higher in those between 25 and 54 years of age, those who use tramadol for more than 4 times, or those with the history of alcohol abuse, infarction, or head injury [74].

In another study on 97 patients with seizure, electroencephalographic (EEG) evaluations were normal in seven and isolated sharp slow-wave feature of EEG was seen in one patients. Brain CT was normal in all and magnetic resonance imaging (MRI) was normal in five patients [77]. Tramadol-induced seizure can cause trauma, intra-articular dislocation, and tongue laceration [67,81,82].

In a study on 70 rats, it was revealed that tramadol could inhibit electron transfer cycle (ETC), cause ATP depletion, and disrupt the mitochondrial integrity. Apoptosis may also happen due to tramadol use [83]. In the neonates, tramadol can trigger pentylenetetrazole-induced seizure in an age-dependant manner causing fewer seizures in the neonatal period and more seizures after the lactating period [84].

Administration of tramadol hydrochloride to a zebrafish caused abnormal behaviors, reduced activity, and reduced brain and body weight. In the zebrafish brain, functional cytoskeletal proteins engaged in the energy metabolism had changed due to tramadol. Lower levels of ATP synthetase, creatine kinase, pyruvate dehydrogenase, kinase, and aldolase C could be due to the impaired production of energy because of tramadol. Weak regulation of the proteins engaged in the oxidative stress, mitochondrial functional abnormalities, and impaired production and destruction of the proteins represented the neurotoxicity of tramadol (Table 1) [85].

| Authors | Publication year | Number of patients | Cause of ingestion | Sex | Co-administration or comorbidity | Dosage |
|---|---|---|---|---|---|---|
| Raigeret al. [139] | 2012 | 1 | Prescribed by physician | Female | History of seizure | 100 mg IV |
| Petramfar et al.[140] | 2010 | 106 | Prescribed by physician in 18.9% Abuse in 81.1% | 96% M | History of epilepsy in 13.2%, abuse of antidepressant in 5.8%, alcohol in 5.8%, opiate in 23.3% | 50-1500 mg IV or oral |
| Mehrpour M [141] | 2005 | 2 | Prescribed by physician | F/M | _ | 100 mg IV |

**Table 1.** Studies on tramadol-induced seizures

## 8. Cardiopulmonary effects of tramadol

Acute pulmonary hypertension and right heart failure are the uncommon presentations reported in a young tramadol-overdosed patient [86]. Cardiopulmonary arrest was reported in some cases that had ingested more than 5 g of tramadol [8]. Higher doses of tramadol can block sodium channels and cause Brugada pattern in the ECG [11,47] which can be accompanied by ventricular dysrhythmias including ventricular fibrillation [11]. In a study on 479 tramadol-poisoned patients, up to 73% of the patients had ECG changes due to blockage of the sodium channels. Almost one-thirds of the patients had terminal 40 msec frontal plane axis deviation and one-fourth had QT prolongation (more than 0.44 sec) [47]. Some cases of right heart failure, resistant shock, asystole, hypotension (especially systolic), and sinus tachycardia have also been recorded [6,35,44,49]. Hypertension has also been reported. The least tramadol dose that has resulted in hypertension and agitation is 500 mg [49].

Eleven suspected cases of tramadol-related angioedema have been reported from Sweden. Involvement of the mouth/pharynx and upper respiratory system can progress to acute respiratory distress and airway obstruction [87]. Tramadol causes respiratory depression with less frequency in comparison with other opioids [28,57,88]. Renal failure is a probable risk factor for respiratory depression [28,89]. Tramadol overdose can cause respiratory depression; but in therapeutic oral doses, it does not cause respiratory complications. In a study on IV administration of 50 to 75 mg of tramadol, no significant changes were detected in the respiratory rate, respiratory volume per minute, and arterial PaO2 [90].

## 9. Hepatic system

Sixteen cases of non-fatal hepatobiliary dysfunction due to tramadol ingestion have been reported [74]. Tramadol has caused centrilobular congestion and focal necrosis of the liver cells and minimal vacuolization in the kidney tubular cells of the rats. No changes were detected in the lactate dehydrogenase, blood urea nitrogen (BUN), aspartate aminotransferase (AST), and malondialdehyde (MDA); however, alanine aminotransferase (ALT) increased significantly showing the possible hepatotoxicity of tramadol [91]. It was shown that acute or chronic toxicity did not affect liver weight or cause histopathological changes in its tissue [17,92].

In the rats, mu receptor activation increases glucose use or decreases the liver gluconeogenesis which results in the low levels of plasma glucose in diabetic rats [88,93]. It has been shown that tramadol improves the peripheral metabolism of glucose by central activation of the mu receptors. Therefore, central and peripheral metabolisms of glucose unite and cause hypoglycemia. It has also been suggested that tramadol changes the liver glucose output regulated by other organs (likely CNS) [93].

## 10. Gastrointestinal system

Although tramadol is fairly tolerated after ingestion, nausea and vomiting may happen in 14% to 75 % of the cases after its oral use [8,49]. Some patients discontinue tramadol consumption because of nausea and vomiting. It has been shown that slow titration decreases the frequency of tramadol discontinuation due to these complications [94].

## 11. Carcinogenic effects

In long-term studies on rats and mice, no tramadol-attributed carcinogenic changes were detected. Histopathologic evaluations showed increased risk of hepatic adenoma in the males and non dose-related pulmonary adenoma in females. No specific mutations or chromosomal impairments were detected in rats, mice, or hamsters due to tramadol use. In skin and eye tests, tramadol had weak corrosive effects on the white rabbits' eyes but no irritating changes on their skin [2]. Oral administration of tramadol was reported to have no carcinogenic effects on the mice and rats. No mutations or increased risk of gene toxicity were detected in human-beings, either [17].

Tramadol can cause urinary retention because of opioid agonistic effects that can increase the tonicity of the bladder sphincter [68]. Also, it was shown to have hazardous effects on the growth, survival, and reproduction system of Daphnia Magna with the most effects on the latter. Long-term exposures decreased expression of the *vtg* gene which is an important biomarker in the reproduction of the oviparous animals [64,95].

In a study by Matthiesen et al, low dose of tramadol had no effect on the fertility, giving birth, and lactation of the rats and had no teratogenic effects on the fetus [17]. These results are however in contrast to the results withdrawn by Bornas who mentioned that laboratory studies had confirmed the teratogenic effects of tramadol on the animals. Tramadol and M1 metabolite can cross the placenta easily because of their low molecular weights [55].

## 12. Biochemical findings of tramadol

Bleeding time (BT), clotting time (CT), prothrombin time, partial thromboplastin time, and body temperature were not affected by tramadol [17]. But, leukocytosis has been reported [44]. Tramadol overdose may result in increased creatine phosphokinase (CPK) which may be seen with or without seizure and can be accompanied by acute renal failure (Table 2) [13].

| Authors | Publication year | Number of patients | Sex | Co-administration or comorbidity | Mortality | Findings | Dosage or concentration |
|---|---|---|---|---|---|---|---|
| Afshari and Ghooshkhanehee [14] | 2009 | Case report | male | _ | _ | Seizure, confusion, miosis, dramatic rise of CPK, LDH, Cr | 4000 mg |
| Eizadi -Mood et al. [21] | 2011 | 186 | Male=76.6% | Addiction history in 41%, psychotic disorder in 30.4%, cardiac disease in | 1.1% | CNS depression in 57%, bradypnea in 18%, tachycardia in | Mean dosage of 2006±7466 mg |

| Authors | Publication year | Number of patients | Sex | Co-administration or comorbidity | Mortality | Findings | Dosage or concentration |
|---|---|---|---|---|---|---|---|
| | | | | 15%, renal disease and epilepsy in few patients | | 25%, hypertension in 6% | |
| Talaie et al. [43] | 2009 | 132 | Male=73.5% | _ | _ | Seizure in 46.2% | 100-4000 mg |
| Hassanian-Moghaddam et al. [45] | 2012 | 525 | Male=70.1% | History of addiction In 16.4% | 2.68% | Seizure in 46.1% Apnea in 3.6% | Mean dose of 1358.4±1071.8 mg |
| Nasif et al. [142] | 2010 | Case report | female | _ | _ | Headache, dizziness, nausea, drowsiness, visual hallucinations | 500 mg |
| Khan et al. [143] | 2010 | Case report | male | _ | _ | Rhabdomyolysis, ARF | 1000 mg |
| El-Hussuna et al. [144] | 2010 | Case report | female | _ | _ | Loss of consciousness, hypothermia, tachycardia, atrial fibrillation in ECG, hyperamylasemia | 3750 mg |
| Ahmadi et al. [145] | 2012 | 1023 | Male=78.5% | 26.6% with history of addiction 21.6% with coingested drugs (specially benzodiazepines) | 0.97% | Seizure in 41.8% of patients | Most of patients less than 5000 mg |
| Pothiawala et al. [146] | 2011 | Case report | female | _ | _ | Sinus tachycardia | Cr=4 mg/L Dose=700 mg |
| Taromsari et al. [147] | 2012 | 306 | Male=83% | Not mentioned | 0.003% | Seizure in 20.3%, agitation in 25.2% prolonged PT in 18.3%, increased ALT in 5.6%, hypotension in 10.5%, Mydriasis in 8.2%, apnea in 2.3% | Mean dose 746±453mg |

| Authors | Publication year | Number of patients | Sex | Co-administration or comorbidity | Mortality | Findings | Dosage or concentration |
|---|---|---|---|---|---|---|---|
| Elkalioubie et al. [148] | 2011 | Case report | female | _ | _ | Hypoglycemia hypothermia, renal and liver failure, cardiac arrest, coagulopathy | 4500 mg |

**Table 2.** Studies on patients with tramadol poisoning

## 13. Serotonin syndrome

Serotonin syndrome (SS) is a potentially fatal syndrome due to increased synthesis, decreased metabolism, increased release, and reuptake inhibition of serotonin or direct agonism at the serotonin receptors [5,53]. This syndrome is often due to complex interactions between the consumed medications. Three key clinical features of this syndrome include:

1. Neuromuscular hyperactivity (tremor, clonus, myoclonus, hyper-reflexia, stiffness, impaired coordination).
2. Autonomic hyperactivity (profuse sweating, fever, tachycardia, tachypnea, chills, nausea, diarrhea, vomiting).
3. Mental status changes (agitation, confusion, restlessness, hypomania and/or visual or auditory hallucinations).

The exact rate of SS is unclear but is generally not expected to occur in more than 5% of the hospitalized patients [5,44,53,96-98]. The (+) enantiomer of tramadol inhibits re-absorption of serotonin [99]. Usually, SS happens after tramadol overdose or its concurrent use with other medications especially antidepressants; however, it may happen even after a single therapeutic dose of tramadol [5,98,100].

Patients who consume mono amine oxidase (MAO) inhibitors are at the risk of development of SS [66,101]. SS has been reported after concurrent use of tramadol with serotonin reuptake inhibitors (SSRIs), venlafaxine, atypical antipsychotics, fluoxetine, sertraline, paroxetine, citalopram, fluvoxamine, moclobemide, clomipramine, mirtazapine, and tricyclic antidepressants [5,7,53,97,102].

In patients who develop lethargy, hypotension, hypoxia, agitation, tachycardia, hypertension, confusion, hyperthermia, or hyper-reflexia, diagnosis of SS should be borne in mind [7,101,103]. Treatment is conservative and includes cessation of the culpable medication as well as administration of the antiserotonergics (ciproheptadine, metisergide, propranolol, and chlorpromazine). Clinical manifestations recover within 24 hours except in those who have consumed medications with longer half-lives [5,53,97]. Up to 42% of the patients may need

ICU admission [48,53]. Pretreatment with chlordiazepoxide may prevent tramadol-induced SS [48].

## 14. Drug interactions

Opioids metabolized by CYP450 (including tramadol) may induce many drug-drug interactions [104]. In an Australian study, unwanted drug interactions were evaluated in 46859 patients who consumed antidepressants. In 8.1% of the patients who had experienced such complications, the most common consumed medication was tramadol (3.6%). As previously clarified, tramadol is similar to venlafaxine in structure and is believed to have antidepressant effects. Venlafaxine can even cause false positive results for tramadol in urine tests [5]. Co-administration of tramadol and antidepressants especially TCAs, SSRIs, venlafaxine, bupropion, and phenothiazines should be performed cautiously because of the increased risk of seizure [6,25,72]. Hallucinations and SS have been reported after co-administration of tramadol and SSRIs [87]. Concurrent administration of tramadol and NSAIDs can result in gastrointestinal hemorrhages due to severe platelet inhibition [105]. Fatal toxicities have been reported after tramadol-TCA overdoses [106]. It has been shown that tramadol-related mortality is more common after co-ingestion of benzodiazepines [8,26]. Co-administration of tramadol and CNS depressants, TCAs, and MAO inhibitors are therefore contraindicated [23]. Tramadol can also interact with antitumor medications. For instance, tramadol decreases the efficacy of cisplatin by affecting gap junctions [107]. In a case report, combination of paroxetine, dosulepin, and tramadol caused hallucination which improved after cessation of the medications [108].

## 15. Tramadol-related mortalities

Fatalities have been reported after tramadol overdose or its co-ingestion with other medications. In most cases, death occurred after ingestion of high doses within 24 hours post-ingestion with really high blood levels [70]. However, death due to tramadol overdose is rare and consists up to 1% of the hospitalized cases [1,10,44,88]. Blood levels of tramadol have been between 0.03 to 134 mg/L in different fatal cases [26,32,109,110].

The most common mechanisms of death after tramadol overdose are cardio-respiratory depression, resistant shock, asystole, and liver failure [111]. Apnea may increase the risk of tramadol intoxication-related deaths [45]. Fatal toxicity of tramadol has been reported after co-administration of other medications including propranolol, trazodone, ethanol, and especially CNS depressants including benzodiazepines, barbiturates, and serotonergic drugs [88]. M1/M2 (ODT/NDT) metabolite ratio of higher than one in biologic liquids and organs represents more sudden deaths while M1/M2 < 1 shows that death will occur at later stages after the tramadol use [32,112]. In fatal cases of tramadol, femoral blood samples are the best since they have the least redistribution changes after death [113]. Tramadol may remain undetected in muscle samples after death due to its overdose [114].

## 16. Miscellaneous side effects

Mannocchi and assistants reported a case of death due to tramadol and propofol due to advanced severe dyspnea [115]. A report showed nine deaths due to consumption of krypton (a plant material containing ODT and mitragynine) in whom the concentration of ODT was between 0.4 to 4.3 µg/g [116]. Another study reported death due o tramadol because of respiratory depression accompanying GABA A and GABA B1 alpha1 over-expression in the ambiguus nucleus and medulla oblongata solitary. (Table 3) [117].

| Author | Publication year | Number of patients | Cause of ingestion | Cause of death | Co-administration or comorbidity | Dosage or concentration(C) |
|---|---|---|---|---|---|---|
| Barbera et al. [32] | 2013 | Case report | Suicide | Respiratory depression and cardiac arrest | Carbamazepine | C= 61.83 mg/l |
| De Decker et al. [88] | 2007 | Case report | Intentional overdose | Asystole and multiple organ failure | Munchausen's syndrome, benzodiazepine | C=8 mg/L |
| Solarino et al. [149] | 2009 | Case report | Suicide | Cardiorespiratory failure | Nicotine, diphenhydramine | C= 6.6 mg/L |
| Ripple et al. [150] | 2000 | Case report | Prescribing multiple drugs | Seizure activity | Alcohol, venlafaxine, trazodone, quetiapine, lithium, acetaminophen | C= 0.7 mg/L |
| Gheshlaghi et al. [151] | 2009 | Case report | Suicide | Cardiopulmonary arrest | _ | Dose=1000 mg |
| Häkkinen et al. [152] | 2012 | 117 | Accidental in 54.8% Suicide in 31.3% Unclear 13.9% | Not mentioned | Other opioids detected in 18.8% Benzodiazepines in 85.5% and alcohol in 14.5% | Median concentration of 5.3 mg/L |
| Randall and Crane et al. [153] | 2014 | 127 | Suicide in 38% Accidental in 27% Unknown in 35% | Mostly multi organ or liver failure and aspiration pneumonia | Other drug/ medicine in 49%, alcohol in 36% | C= 1.85-88.8 mg/L |

**Table 3.** Studies on deaths related to tramadol poisoning

## 17. Toxicity in children

Accidental ingestion of tramadol is well tolerated by children [50,71,111]. Side effects of tramadol seem to be more common but milder in children. Vomiting is especially common in them [118]. Riedel and Stockhausen reported that tramadol could cross the blood brain barrier (BBB) in children and suppress the brain [119]. Rectal administration of tramadol resulted in severe CNS depression in a 5-week-old infant which was explained to be due to the decreased kinetic elimination and increased permeability of the BBB [51]. Mazor et al. reported two cases of tramadol toxicity with abnormal neurological findings (both seizures and seizure-like activities) in children [9]. Seizure has been reported after accidental ingestion of 4 mg/kg of tramadol in children [23].

Short-term use of tramadol in lactating mother is not dangerous [120] and the risk of neonatal dependency is low.

Tramadol can cause SS without the effect of any other medication while in the adults the risk is increased if a SSRI is also taken [40]. In an 8-month-old infant with SS, the cause of hospital presentation was epistaxis. Sinus tachycardia, hyperthermia, hypertension, agitation, drowsiness, and hyper-reflexia of the lower extremities occurred within the first 24 hours after ingestion of 200 mg of tramadol. Neurologic and cardiovascular effects recovered in two days. The infant was discharged after five days in good condition [121].

## 18. Treatment

Treatment should focus on conservative approaches including maintenance of airway, breathing, and circulation, oxygen therapy, fluid resuscitation, and diazepam administration to control agitation and seizure [6,14,36]. Patients should be monitored for increased CPK and possible acute renal failure that may happen within the next two days [6,14]. Hemodialysis should be considered in cases with acute renal failure and severe creatinine increase [14]. They may need intubation and ICU admission. Gastrointestinal decontamination should be performed in the patients who have referred within the first two hours post-ingestion and have no contraindications [8,49,50].

In severe toxicities due to ingestion of large amounts of sustained-release drug, multiple dose activated charcoal should be considered if no contraindication exists [6,122]. In cases with resistant shock or asystole, extracorporeal methods may be needed [6,35]. Treatment of liver failure is conservative, as well, and urgent liver transplantation is not feasible in many cases [18]. Intubation/ventilation and administration of naloxone are the treatments for tramadol-induced apnea [45]. In severe cases who have not even seized, experimental therapy with diazepam can be performed which can be of help in mild undiagnosed SS [6,44]. Treatment of SS in also conservative and includes withdrawal of the culpable drug and external cooling. Up to 42% of the patients may need ICU and most of them recover within 12-24 hours [70].

In a clinical study on 122 patients, naloxone administration could induce seizure in tramadol-intoxicated patients [75]. Therefore, naloxone should not routinely be administered to treat decreased level of consciousness in tramadol toxicity unless respiratory depression has developed [21,45]. Seizures due to tramadol do not respond to naloxone but improve with administration of benzodiazepines. Naloxone can be considered for treatment of post-seizure complaints [123].

Shadnia et al suggested that because of the low risk of multiple seizures in tramadol toxicity, anticonvulsant treatment should not be routinely given even in those with initial seizures [52]. Stoops et al evaluated naltrexone and showed that it could reverse the opioid-induced effects such as miosis; but, increased the serotonergic and adrenergic effects such as mydriasis [56].

Intravenous lipid emulsion (ILE) can reduce mortality due to acute toxicity of tramadol in rabbits, but increasing the ILE dose may cause reverse effects. In a study on 30 rabbis, ILE reduced tramadol-induced tachycardia when administered within 30 minutes of poisoning and showed positive effects on normalizing mean arterial pressure and diastolic blood pressure but it did not have major effect on systolic blood pressure. Intralipid also prevented tramadol-related seizures in low doses and reduced the frequency of increased CPK with higher doses [124].

## 19. Dependency and withdrawal

Although tramadol has less side effects, addicting capacity, and respiratory depression power in comparison with other opioids, many cases of dependency, abuse, intentional overdose, or poisoning have been reported following its use [20,27,48,56,70,113,125,126]. Tramadol withdrawal lasts longer compared with other opioids [111]. Where ultrarapid metabolizers are high in number, people are expected to have a higher risk of dependency to tramadol [127].

Tramadol is as potent as heroin to cause euphoria [2,55,112]. Withdrawal occurs after rapid abrupt discontinuation of tramadol with clinical manifestations including abdominal cramps, anxiety, skeletal pain, depression, diarrhea, goose flesh, insomnia, lacrimation, nausea, restlessness, rhinorrhea, and sweating. The manifestations may sometimes be atypical and include hallucination, paranoia, panic attack, confusion, and atypical sensational experiences such as paresthesia, itching, tingling, delusion, depersonalization, derealization, and tinnitus [22,55].

Tramadol dependency happens faster in those who abuse it with other analgesics or ethanol [55]. Clinical therapeutic doses of tramadol may affect psychomotor and physiologic capacities of the patients who recreationally abuse it [128].

Tramadol abuse in pregnancy may cause preterm labor and withdrawal manifestations in the newborn baby depending on the age of pregnancy, time elapsed since the beginning of tramadol use, dose of tramadol, CYP450 D2 polymorphism, development of the liver conjugation, and renal function of both mother and baby. Attempts have been performed to treat this syndrome in neonates using clonidine alone or in combination with the thin opioid tinctures, chloral hydrate, benzodiazepines, and methadone [55]. In a study on patients with chronic non-cancer pain, it was shown that the frequency of abuse and dependency on tramadol and NSAIDs were the same and significantly less than hydrocodone [129].

## 20. Conclusion

Weak opioids such as tramadol can be used in the treatment of reumatologic pains after development of complications following use of NSAIDs or if they are unable to alleviate the patients' pain [130]. It is less dangerous to the organs in comparison with selective and nonselective NSAIDs and very powerful in the treatment of chronic pains [131]. Tramadol can also be used in moderate to severe toothaches alone or in combination with acetaminophen or codeine [132,133]. In opioid-addicted patients, tramadol can be used for the treatment of withdrawal pain [68]. Tramadol in combination with paracetamol has a fair efficacy, immunity, and acceptance rate by the patients without development of dependency syndrome [131,134,135].

Complications can be decreased by adding tramadol to the controlled medications [136]. Monitoring of the liver function especially when the maximum daily doses are given is mandatory. Also, because of drug-drug interactions and differences in the individual metabolism and the chance of dependency, tramadol administration should be controlled by the treating physician. If the patient is an opioid-addict, tramadol should not be administered unless absolutely indicated [137,138].

## Acknowledgements

This Chapter is supported by Medical Toxicology and Drug Abuse Research Center in Birjand University of Medical Sciences, Birjand, Iran.

## Author details

Omid Mehrpour[1*], Mohammaddavood Sharifi[2] and Nasim Zamani[3]

*Address all correspondence to: omid.mehrpour@yahoo.com

1 Medical Toxicology and Drug Abuse Research Center, Birjand University of Medical Sciences, Birjand, Iran

2 Department of Emergency medicine, Mashhad University of Medical Sciences, Iran

3 Department of Clinical Toxicology, Loghman Hakim Hospital, Shahid Behehshti University of Medical Sciences, Tehran, Iran

The authors declare that they have no competing interests.

## References

[1] Ahmadi H, Hosseini J, Rezaei M. Epidemiology of tramadol overdose in Imam Khomeini hospital, Kermanshah, Iran (2008). Journal of Kermansha University of Medical Sciences. 2011;15(1):72-7.

[2] Shamsi Meymandi M, Nakhaee N, Shojaee Baghini M, Mazhari S, Sharifi S, Sharifi F. Evaluation of general practitioners' knowledge about Tramadol, Kerman, 1383. Journal of Kerman University of Medical Sciences. 2005;12(3):202-8 (Persian).

[3] Taghaddosinejad F, Mehrpour O, Afshari R, Seghatoleslami A, Abdollahi M, Dart RC. Factors related to seizure in tramadol poisoning and its blood concentration. Journal of medical toxicology. 2011;7(3):183-8.

[4] Pearson S, Ringland C, Kelman C, Mant A, Lowinger J, Stark H, et al. Patterns of analgesic and anti inflammatory medicine use by Australian veterans. Internal medicine journal. 2007;37(12):798-805.

[5] Sansone RA, Sansone LA. Tramadol: seizures, serotonin syndrome, and coadministered antidepressants. Psychiatry (Edgmont). 2009;6(4):17.

[6] Afshari R, Afshar R, Mégarbane B. Tramadol overdose: review of the literature. Réanimation. 2011;20(5):436-41.

[7] Goodarzi F, Mehrpour O, Eizadi-Mood N. A study to evaluate factors associated with seizure in Tramadol poisoning in Iran. Indian Journal of Forensic Medicine & Toxicology. 2011;5(2).

[8] Shadnia S, Soltaninejad K, Heydari K, Sasanian G, Abdollahi M. Tramadol intoxication: a review of 114 cases. Human & experimental toxicology. 2008;27(3):201-5.

[9] Mazor SS, Feldman KW, Sugar NF, Sotero M. Pediatric tramadol ingestion resulting in seizurelike activity: a case series. Pediatric emergency care. 2008;24(6):380-1.

[10] Moore KA, Cina SJ, Jones R, Selby DM, Levine B, Smith ML. Tissue distribution of tramadol and metabolites in an overdose fatality. The American journal of forensic medicine and pathology. 1999;20(1):98-100.

[11] Cole JB, Sattiraju S, Bilden EF, Asinger RW, Bertog SC. Isolated tramadol overdose associated with Brugada ECG pattern. Pacing and Clinical Electrophysiology. 2012;35(8):e219-e21.

[12] Shipton E. Tramadol--present and future. Anaesthesia and intensive care. 2000;28(4):363-74.

[13] Raffa R. Pharmacological aspects of successful long-term analgesia. Clinical rheumatology. 2006;25(1):9-15.

[14] Afshari R, Ghooshkhanehee H. Tramadol overdose induced seizure, dramatic rise of CPK and acute renal failure. JPMA The Journal of the Pakistan Medical Association. 2009;59(3):178-.

[15] Goeringer K, Logan B, Christian G. Identification of tramadol and its metabolites in blood from drug-related deaths and drug-impaired drivers. J Anal Toxicol. 1997;21(7):529-37.

[16] Levine B, Ramcharitar V, Smialek JE. Tramadol distribution in four postmortem cases. Forensic science international. 1997;86(1):43-8.

[17] Matthiesen T, Wöhrmann T, Coogan T, Uragg H. The experimental toxicology of tramadol: an overview. Toxicology letters. 1998;95(1):63-71.

[18] Grond S, Meuser T, Uragg H, Stahlberg HJ, Lehmann KA. Serum concentrations of tramadol enantiomers during patient-controlled analgesia. British journal of clinical pharmacology. 1999;48(2):254-7.

[19] Wang H, Wang L, Guan D, Wang M. [Tramadol intoxication and its toxicological effect]. Fa yi xue za zhi. 2008;24(4):293-6.

[20] Babalonis S, Lofwall MR, Nuzzo PA, Siegel AJ, Walsh SL. Abuse liability and reinforcing efficacy of oral tramadol in humans. Drug and alcohol dependence. 2013;129(1):116-24.

[21] Eizadi-Mood. N, Sabzghabaee. AM, Safdari. A, Yaraghi. A.. Clinical Signs, Hospitalization Duration and Outcome of Tramadol Intoxication. Jornal Of Isfahan Medical School. 2011;28(117):1187-93.

[22] Senay EC, Adams EH, Geller A, Inciardi JA, Muñoz A, Schnoll SH, et al. Physical dependence on Ultram (tramadol hydrochloride): both opioid-like and atypical withdrawal symptoms occur. Drug and alcohol dependence. 2003;69(3):233-41.

[23] Jovanovic-Cupic V, Martinovic Z, Nešic N. Seizures associated with intoxication and abuse of tramadol. Clinical Toxicology. 2006;44(2):143-6.

[24] Paiva A, Lobo M, Chainho J. P. 5.036 Dependence on tramadol—a case series. European Neuropsychopharmacology. 2003;13:S421-S2.

[25] Liang M, Cai X, Jin M. [Distribution of tramadol in acute poisoned rats]. Fa yi xue za zhi. 2010;26(6):436-9.

[26] Clarot F, Goulle J, Vaz E, Proust B. Fatal overdoses of tramadol: is benzodiazepine a risk factor of lethality? Forensic science international. 2003;134(1):57-61.

[27] Radbruch L, Glaeske G, Grond S, Munchberg F, Scherbaum N, Storz E, et al. Topical review on the abuse and misuse potential of tramadol and tilidine in Germany. Subst Abus. 2013;34(3):313-20.

[28] Warnke A, Schug B, Vanderbist F, Blume H. [Importance of the formulation for a chronopharmacologically optimised way of pain therapy. Results of a comparative bioavailability study of tramadol extended-release capsules after single-dose evening versus morning administration]. MMW Fortschritte der Medizin. 2008;150:36-42.

[29] Liu X, Song J. [Chronopharmacology of tramadol in mice]. Yao xue xue bao= Acta pharmaceutica Sinica. 2001;36(8):561-4.

[30] Musshoff F, Madea B. Fatality due to ingestion of tramadol alone. Forensic science international. 2001;116(2):197-9.

[31] Levo A, Koski A, Ojanperä I, Vuori E, Sajantila A. Post-mortem SNP analysis of CYP2D6 gene reveals correlation between genotype and opioid drug (tramadol) metabolite ratios in blood. Forensic science international. 2003;135(1):9-15.

[32] Barbera N, Fisichella M, Bosco A, Indorato F, Spadaro G, Romano G. A suicidal poisoning due to tramadol. A metabolic approach to death investigation. Journal of forensic and legal medicine. 2013;20(5):555-8.

[33] Murphy E. Acute pain management pharmacology for the patient with concurrent renal or hepatic disease. Anaesthesia and intensive care. 2005;33(3):311-22.

[34] Edmondson M, Duran S, Boothe D, Stewart A, Ravis W. Pharmacokinetics of tramadol and its major metabolites in alpacas following intravenous and oral administration. Journal of veterinary pharmacology and therapeutics. 2012;35(4):389-96.

[35] Daubin C, Quentin C, Goullé J-P, Guillotin D, Lehoux P, Lepage O, et al. Refractory shock and asystole related to tramadol overdose. Clinical toxicology. 2007;45(8): 961-4.

[36] Tobias JD. Seizure after overdose of tramadol. Southern medical journal. 1997;90(8): 826-7.

[37] Tjäderborn M, Jönsson AK, Hägg S, Ahlner J. Fatal unintentional intoxications with tramadol during 1995–2005. Forensic science international. 2007;173(2):107-11.

[38] 38.Johansson I, Ingelman-Sundberg M. Genetic polymorphism and toxicology—with emphasis on cytochrome p450. Toxicological Sciences. 2011;120(1):1-13.

[39] Samer CF, Daali Y, Wagner M, Hopfgartner G, Eap CB, Rebsamen M, et al. Genetic polymorphisms and drug interactions modulating CYP2D6 and CYP3A activities have a major effect on oxycodone analgesic efficacy and safety. British journal of pharmacology. 2010;160(4):919-30.

[40] Rollason V, Samer C, Piguet V, Dayer P, Desmeules J. Pharmacogenetics of analgesics: toward the individualization of prescription. 2008.

[41] Musshoff F, Madea B, Stuber F, Stamer UM. Enantiomeric determination of tramadol and O-desmethyltramadol by liquid chromatography-mass spectrometry and application to postoperative patients receiving tramadol. Journal of analytical toxicology. 2006;30(7):463-7.

[42] Bergheim M, Gieré R, Kümmerer K. Biodegradability and ecotoxicitiy of tramadol, ranitidine, and their photoderivatives in the aquatic environment. Environmental Science and Pollution Research. 2012;19(1):72-85.

[43] Talaie H, Panahandeh R, Fayaznouri MR, Asadi Z, Abdollahi M. Dose-independent occurrence of seizure with tramadol. Journal of medical toxicology. 2009;5(2):63-7.

[44] Tashakori A, Afshari R. Tramadol overdose as a cause of serotonin syndrome: a case series. Clinical Toxicology. 2010;48(4):337-41.

[45] Hassanian-Moghaddam H, Farajidana H, Sarjami S, Owliaey H. Tramadol-induced apnea. The American journal of emergency medicine. 2013;31(1):26-31.

[46] Fathi Y, Bashrian S, Barati M, Hazavei S. Tramadol Abuse Status and Related Factors among Three College Students in Hamadan. Sci J Hamadan Univ Med Sci. 2012;19(3):23-9.

[47] Emamhadi M, Sanaei-Zadeh H, Nikniya M, Zamani N, Dart RC. Electrocardiographic manifestations of tramadol toxicity with special reference to their ability for prediction of seizures. The American journal of emergency medicine. 2012;30(8):1481-5.

[48] Mansouripour SM, Afshari R. Chlordiazepoxide preventive effect on tramadol overdose induced serotonin syndrome evaluated by Hunter and Radomski criteria: A clinical trial. Toxicology international. 2013;20(2):126.

[49] Spiller HA, Gorman SE, Villalobos D, Benson BE, Ruskosky DR, Stancavage MM, et al. Prospective multicenter evaluation of tramadol exposure. Clinical Toxicology. 1997;35(4):361-4.

[50] Marquardt KA, Alsop JA, Albertson TE. Tramadol exposures reported to statewide poison control system. Annals of Pharmacotherapy. 2005;39(6):1039-44.

[51] Bianchetti M, Beutler A, Ferrier P. [Acute poisoning with a narcotic (Tramadol) in an infant of five weeks]. Helvetica paediatrica acta. 1988;43(3):241-4.

[52] Shadnia S, Brent J, Mousavi-Fatemi K, Hafezi P, Soltaninejad K. Recurrent seizures in tramadol intoxication: implications for therapy based on 100 patients. Basic & clinical pharmacology & toxicology. 2012;111(2):133-6.

[53] Kitson R, Carr B. Tramadol and severe serotonin syndrome. Anaesthesia. 2005;60(9): 934-5.

[54] Wang S-Q, Li C-S, Song Y-G. Multiply organ dysfunction syndrome due to tramadol intoxication alone. The American journal of emergency medicine. 2009;27(7):903. e5-. e7.

[55] Borna H, Borna S. Tramadole withdrawal in a neonate: a case report. Tehran University Medical Journal. 2012;70(6).

[56] Stoops WW, Lofwall MR, Nuzzo PA, Craig LB, Siegel AJ, Walsh SL. Pharmacodynamic profile of tramadol in humans: influence of naltrexone pretreatment. Psychopharmacology (Berl). 2012;223(4):427-38.

[57] Schug SA. The role of tramadol in current treatment strategies for musculoskeletal pain. Therapeutics and clinical risk management. 2007;3(5):717.

[58] Schnitzer TJ. Update of ACR guidelines for osteoarthritis: role of the coxibs. Journal of pain and symptom management. 2002;23(4):S24-S30.

[59] Raffa RB, Buschmann H, Christoph T, Eichenbaum G, Englberger W, Flores CM, et al. Mechanistic and functional differentiation of tapentadol and tramadol. Expert Opin Pharmacother. 2012;13(10):1437-49.

[60] Tsai Y-C, Chang P-J, Jou I-M. Direct tramadol application on sciatic nerve inhibits spinal somatosensory evoked potentials in rats. Anesthesia & Analgesia. 2001;92(6): 1547-51.

[61] Rothhammer A, Weis K, Skrobek W. [The clinical usefulness of Tramadol-infusion anaesthesia (author's transl)]. Der Anaesthesist. 1981;30(12):619-22.

[62] Salman M, Sahin A, Onur M, Öge K, Kassab A, Aypar Ü. Tramadol encapsulated into polyhydroxybutyrate microspheres: in vitro release and epidural analgesic effect in rats. Acta anaesthesiologica scandinavica. 2003;47(8):1006-12.

[63] Shirzad H, Dehghanian SL, Yousefi M, Nikookar M, Rafieian M. Effects of tramadol on activity of peritoneal phagocytes in Balb/C mice. ISMJ. 2011;14(4):214-9.

[64] Agrawal A, Diwan S, Mahajan R. Severe delirium following single dose of tramadol. Indian journal of medical sciences. 2009;63(2):80-1.

[65] Garcia J, Altman RD, editors. Chronic pain states: pathophysiology and medical therapy. Seminars in arthritis and rheumatism; 1997: Elsevier.

[66] In: Goldfrank LR, Flomenbaum N, Lewis NA, Howland MA, Hoffman RS, Nelson LS, editors. Goldfrank's Toxicologic Emergencies. 7 ed. New York: McGraw-Hill Medical; 2000:916

[67] Sanaei-Zadeh H. Tramadol intoxication and shoulder pain. European review for medical and pharmacological sciences. 2014;18(2):285.

[68] Lofwall MR, Babalonis S, Nuzzo PA, Siegel A, Campbell C, Walsh SL. Efficacy of extended-release tramadol for treatment of prescription opioid withdrawal: a two-phase randomized controlled trial. Drug Alcohol Depend. 2013;133(1):188-97.

[69] El-Naggar M, El-Sehly WM, Morad GM, Eeed M, Hassan M. P19: The toxic effect of prolonged Ultram administration on cerebral cortex of albino rats: Toxicological and histological study. Experimental and Toxicologic Pathology. 2009;61(3):290.

[70] Loughrey M, Loughrey C, Johnston S, O'Rourke D. Fatal hepatic failure following accidental tramadol overdose. Forensic science international. 2003;134(2):232-3.

[71] Jick H, Derby LE, Vasilakis C, Fife D. The risk of seizures associated with tramadol. Pharmacotherapy: The Journal of Human Pharmacology and Drug Therapy. 1998;18(3):607-11.

[72] Gasse M, Derby L, Vasilakis Scaramozza C, Jick H. Incidence of FirstTime Idiopathic Seizures in Users of Tramadol. Pharmacotherapy: The Journal of Human Pharmacology and Drug Therapy. 2000;20(6):629-34.

[73] Farajidana H, Hassanian-Moghaddam H, Zamani N, Sanaei-Zadeh H. Tramadol-induced seizures and trauma. Eur Rev Med Pharmacol Sci. 2012;16(Suppl 1):34-7.

[74] Gardner JS, Blough D, Drinkard CR, Shatin D, Anderson G, Graham D, et al. Tramadol and seizures: a surveillance study in a managed care population. Pharmacotherapy: The Journal of Human Pharmacology and Drug Therapy. 2000;20(12):1423-31.

[75] Esmail Farzaneh, Mehdi Samadzadeh, Bita Shahbazzadegan, Iraj Sayadrezai, Babak Mostafazadeh, Azam Sarbandi Farahani, et al. Comparing the Frequency of Seizure in Patients Intoxicated with Tramadol Treated with or without Naloxone. Journal of Isfahan Medical School. 2012;30(197).

[76] Thundiyil JG, Kearney TE, Olson KR. Evolving epidemiology of drug-induced seizures reported to a Poison Control Center System. Journal of medical toxicology. 2007;3(1):15-9.

[77] Labate A, Newton MR, Vernon GM, Berkovic SF. Tramadol and new-onset seizures. The Medical Journal of Australia. 2005;182(1):42-3.

[78] Lota A, Dubrey S, Wills P. Profound hyponatraemia following a tramadol overdose. QJM. 2012;105(4):397-8.

[79] Bekjarovski N, Chaparoska D, Radulovikj-Bekjarovska S. Seizures after use and abuse of tramadol. Prilozi/Makedonska akademija na naukite i umetnostite, Oddelenie za bioloski i medicinski nauki= Contributions/Macedonian Academy of Sciences and Arts, Section of Biological and Medical Sciences. 2012;33(1):313-8.

[80] Künig G, Dätwyler S, Eschen A, Gasser US. Unrecognised Long-Lasting Tramadol-Induced Delirium in Two Elderly Patients. Pharmacopsychiatry. 2006;39(05):194-9.

[81] Sanaei-Zadeh H. Is prophylactic administration of the anticonvulsants necessary in tramadol-intoxicated patients after an initial seizure? DARU Journal of Pharmaceutical Sciences. 2013;21(1):60.

[82] Rehni AK, Singh I, Kumar M. Tramadol-Induced Seizurogenic Effect: A Possible Role of Opioid-Dependent $\gamma$-Aminobutyric Acid Inhibitory Pathway. Basic & clinical pharmacology & toxicology. 2008;103(3):262-6.

[83] Mohamed TM, Ghaffar HMA, El Husseiny RM. Effects of tramadol, clonazepam, and their combination on brain mitochondrial complexes. Toxicology and industrial health. 2013:0748233713491814.

[84] Gholami M, Hajizadeh-Moghaddam A, Saboory E. Comparison of the effects of chronic administration of morphine and tramadol in infancy on acute Pentylenetetrazol–induced seizure in prepubertal rats. Tehran University Medical Journal. 2013;70(10).

[85] Zhuo HQ, Huang L, Huang HQ, Cai Z. Effects of chronic tramadol exposure on the zebrafish brain: a proteomic study. J Proteomics. 2012;75(11):3351-64.

[86] Garrett P. Tramadol overdose and serotonin syndrome manifesting as acute right heart dysfunction. Anaesthesia and intensive care. 2004;32(4):575-7.

[87] Hallberg P, Brenning G. Angioedema induced by tramadol—a potentially life-threatening condition. European journal of clinical pharmacology. 2005;60(12):901-3.

[88] De Decker K, Cordonnier J, Jacobs W, Coucke V, Schepens P, Jorens PG. Fatal intoxication due to tramadol alone: case report and review of the literature. Forensic science international. 2008;175(1):79-82.

[89] Stamer UM, Stüber F, Muders T, Musshoff F. Respiratory depression with tramadol in a patient with renal impairment and CYP2D6 gene duplication. Anesthesia & Analgesia. 2008;107(3):926-9.

[90] Aronson MD. Nonsteroidal anti-inflammatory drugs, traditional opioids, and tramadol: constrating therapies for the treatment of chronic pain. Clinical therapeutics. 1997;19(3):420-32.

[91] Atici S, Cinel I, Cinel L, Doruk N, Eskandari G, Oral U. Liver and kidney toxicity in chronic use of opioids: an experimental long term treatment model. Journal of biosciences. 2005;30(2):245-52.

[92] Tolman KG. Hepatotoxicity of non-narcotic analgesics. Am J Med. 1998;105(1b):13s-9s.

[93] Mugunthan N, Davoren P. Danger of Hypoglycemia Due to Acute Tramadol Poisoning. Endocrine Practice. 2012;18(6):e151-e2.

[94] Petrone D, Kamin M, Olson W. Slowing the titration rate of tramadol HCl reduces the incidence of discontinuation due to nausea and/or vomiting: a double-blind randomized trial. J Clin Pharm Ther. 1999;24(2):115-23.

[95] Le TH, Lim ES, Lee SK, Park JS, Kim YH, Min J. Toxicity evaluation of verapamil and tramadol based on toxicity assay and expression patterns of Dhb, Vtg, Arnt, CYP4, and CYP314 in Daphnia magna. Environmental toxicology. 2011;26(5):515-23.

[96] El-Okdi NS, Lumbrezer D, Karanovic D, Ghose A, Assaly R. Serotonin Syndrome After the Use of Tramadol and Ziprasidone in a Patient With a Deep Brain Stimulator for Parkinson Disease. Am J Ther. 2013.

[97] Lange-Asschenfeldt C, Weigmann H, Hiemke C, Mann K. Serotonin syndrome as a result of fluoxetine in a patient with tramadol abuse: plasma level-correlated symptomatology. J Clin Psychopharmacol. 2002;22(4):440-1.

[98] Hernandez AF, Montero MN, Pla A, Villanueva E. Fatal moclobemide overdose or death caused by serotonin syndrome? Journal of forensic sciences. 1995.

[99] Mason BJ, Blackburn KH. Possible serotonin syndrome associated with tramadol and sertraline coadministration. Ann Pharmacother. 1997;31(2):175-7.

[100] Pilgrim J, Gerostamoulos D, Drummer OH. Deaths involving serotonergic drugs. Forensic science international. 2010;198(1):110-7.

[101] Gillman P. Monoamine oxidase inhibitors, opioid analgesics and serotonin toxicity. British Journal of Anaesthesia. 2005;95(4):434-41.

[102] Ghiculescu R, Choong K. Iatrogenic neuropsychiatric syndromes. Australian family physician. 2008;37(8):627.

[103] Gnanadesigan N, Espinoza RT, Smith R, Israel M, Reuben DB. Interaction of serotonergic antidepressants and opioid analgesics: is serotonin syndrome going undetected? Journal of the American Medical Directors Association. 2005;6(4):265-9.

[104] Overholser BR, Foster DR. Opioid pharmacokinetic drug-drug interactions. The American journal of managed care. 2011;17:S276-87.

[105] Hersh EV, Pinto A, Moore PA. Adverse drug interactions involving common prescription and over-the-counter analgesic agents. Clinical therapeutics. 2007;29(11): 2477-97.

[106] Bynum ND, Poklis JL, Gaffney-Kraft M, Garside D, Ropero-Miller JD. Postmortem distribution of tramadol, amitriptyline, and their metabolites in a suicidal overdose. Journal of analytical toxicology. 2005;29(5):401-6.

[107] He B, Tong X, Wang L, Wang Q, Ye H, Liu B, et al. Tramadol and flurbiprofen depress the cytotoxicity of cisplatin via their effects on gap junctions. Clinical Cancer Research. 2009;15(18):5803-10.

[108] Devulder J, De Laat M, Dumoulin K, Renson A, Rolly G. Nightmares and hallucinations after long-term intake of tramadol combined with antidepressants. Acta Clinica Belgica. 1995;51(3):184-6.

[109] Clarkson JE, Lacy JM, Fligner CL, Thiersch N, Howard J, Harruff RC, et al. Tramadol (Ultram®) Concentrations in Death Investigation and Impaired Driving Cases and Their Significance. Journal of forensic sciences. 2004;49(5):1101-5.

[110] Michaud K, Augsburger M, Romain N, Giroud C, Mangin P. Fatal overdose of tramadol and alprazolam. Forensic science international. 1999;105(3):185-9.

[111] Sharawy NE. Toxicity of Tramadol.Protocol submitted for fulfillment of master degree in forensic medicine and clinical toxicology.Faculty of medicine Benha university 2012.

[112] Zhang H, Liu Z. The Investigation of Tramadol Dependence with No History of Substance Abuse: A Cross-Sectional Survey of Spontaneously Reported Cases in Guangzhou City, China. BioMed research international. 2013;2013.

[113] Costa I, Oliveira A, de Pinho PG, Teixeira HM, Moreira R, Carvalho F, et al. Postmortem Redistribution of Tramadol and O-Desmethyltramadol. Journal of analytical toxicology. 2013;37(9):670-5.

[114] Klingmann A, Skopp G, Pedal I, Poetsch L, Aderjan R. [Distribution of morphine and morphine glucuronides in body tissue and fluids--postmortem findings in brief survival]. Archiv fur Kriminologie. 1999;206(1-2):38-49.

[115] Mannocchi G, Napoleoni F, Napoletano S, Pantano F, Santoni M, Tittarelli R, et al. Fatal self administration of tramadol and propofol: A case report. Journal of forensic and legal medicine. 2013;20(6):715-9.

[116] Kronstrand R, Roman M, Thelander G, Eriksson A. Unintentional fatal intoxications with mitragynine and O-desmethyltramadol from the herbal blend Krypton. Journal of analytical toxicology. 2011;35(4):242-7.

[117] Zhang S, Guan DW, Wang L, Wang HX, Zhang GH, Zhao R, et al. [The expression of GABA(A) receptor alpha1 and GABA(B) receptor 1 in medulla oblongata solitary nucleus and ambiguous nucleus in the cases of tramadol intoxication]. Fa Yi Xue Za Zhi. 2011;27(6):401-4.

[118] Tramadol oral solution: new drug. Poorly evaluated and potentially dangerous in children. Prescrire Int. 2005;14(77):83-5.

[119] Riedel F, Stockhausen H-Bv. Severe cerebral depression after intoxication with tramadol in a 6-month-old infant. European journal of clinical pharmacology. 1984;26(5):631-2.

[120] Hendrickson RG, McKeown NJ. Is maternal opioid use hazardous to breast-fed infants? Clinical Toxicology. 2012;50(1):1-14.

[121] Maréchal C, Honorat R, Claudet I. Serotonin syndrome induced by tramadol intoxication in an 8-month-old infant. Pediatric neurology. 2011;44(1):72-4.

[122] Raffa RB, Wu C, Stone Jr DJ, Borenstein MR, Codd EE, Coogan TP. Determination of the adsorption of tramadol hydrochloride by activated charcoal in vitro and in vivo. Journal of pharmacological and toxicological methods. 2000;43(3):205-10.

[123] Saidi H, Ghadiri M, Abbasi S, Ahmadi S-F. Efficacy and safety of naloxone in the management of postseizure complaints of tramadol intoxicated patients: a self-controlled study. Emergency Medicine Journal. 2010;27(12):928-30.

[124] Vahabzadeh M, Moshiri M, Mohammadpour AH, Hosseinzadeh H. Promising effects of intravenous lipid emulsion as an antidote in acute tramadol poisoning. Regional anesthesia and pain medicine. 2013;38(5):425-30.

[125] Zhang M, Jing L, Liu Q, Wen RT, Li JX, Li YL, et al. Tramadol induces conditioned place preference in rats: interactions with morphine and buprenorphine. Neurosci Lett. 2012;520(1):87-91.

[126] McDiarmid T, Mackler L. What is the addiction risk associated with tramadol? Clinical Inquiries, 2005 (MU). 2005.

[127] Mehrpour O. Addiction and seizure ability of tramadol in high-risk patients. Indian J Anaesth. 2013;57(1):86-7.

[128] Zacny JP. Profiling the subjective, psychomotor, and physiological effects of tramadol in recreational drug users. Drug and alcohol dependence. 2005;80(2):273-8.

[129] Adams EH, Breiner S, Cicero TJ, Geller A, Inciardi JA, Schnoll SH, et al. A comparison of the abuse liability of tramadol, NSAIDs, and hydrocodone in patients with chronic pain. J Pain Symptom Manage. 2006;31(5):465-76.

[130] Bertin P. Current use of analgesics for rheumatological pain. European journal of pain (London, England). 1999;4:9-13.

[131] Schug SA. Combination analgesia in 2005—a rational approach: focus on paracetamol–tramadol. Clinical rheumatology. 2006;25(1):16-21.

[132] Desmeules J, Rollason V, Piguet V, Dayer P. Clinical pharmacology and rationale of analgesic combinations. Eur J Anaesthesiol Suppl. 2003;28:7-11.

[133] Mehlisch DR. The efficacy of combination analgesic therapy in relieving dental pain. J Am Dent Assoc. 2002;133(7):861-71.

[134] McQuay H, Edwards J. Meta-analysis of single dose oral tramadol plus acetaminophen in acute postoperative pain. European journal of anaesthesiology Supplement. 2002;28:19-22.

[135] Edwards JE, McQuay HJ, Moore RA. Combination analgesic efficacy: individual patient data meta-analysis of single-dose oral tramadol plus acetaminophen in acute postoperative pain. Journal of pain and symptom management. 2002;23(2):121-30.

[136] Spiller HA, Scaglione JM, Aleguas A, Foster H, Durback-Morris L, Scharman EJ, et al. Effect of scheduling tramadol as a controlled substance on poison center exposures to tramadol. Ann Pharmacother. 2010;44(6):1016-21.

[137] Bertsche T, Mikus G. [Adverse drug reactions and drug interactions in analgesic therapy]. Therapeutische Umschau Revue therapeutique. 2011;68(1):19-26.

[138] Patt S, McDiarmid T. Tramadol addiction. J Fam Pract. 2005;54(4):356.

[139] Raiger LK, Naithani U, Bhatia S, Chauhan SS. Seizures after intravenous tramadol given as premedication. Indian journal of anaesthesia. 2012;56(1):55.

[140] Petramfar P, Haghighi AB. Tramadol induced seizure: report of 106 patients. Iranian Red Crescent Medical Journal. 2010;12(1):49-51.

[141] Mehrpour M. Intravenous tramadol-induced seizure: two case reports. Iranian Journal of Pharmacology & Therapeutics (IJPT). 2005;4(2):146-7.

[142] Nasıf İ, ÇELİK Y, BALCI K, İNAL MT, MEMİŞ D. Visual Hallucinations InducedBy Tramadol Overdose: Case Report. Turkiye Klinikleri Journal of Medical Sciences. 2010;30(3):1105-7.

[143] Khan FY, Yousef H, Errayes M. Tramadol toxicity-induced rhabdomyolysis. Journal of Emergencies, Trauma and Shock. 2010;3(4):421.

[144] El-Hussuna A, Arnesen RB, Rosenberg J. Unusual association of diseases/symptoms: Tramadol poisoning with hyperamylasemia. BMJ case reports. 2010;2010.

[145] Ahmadi H,Rezaie M,Hoseini J. Epidemiology Analysis of Poisonings with Tramadol. Journal of Forensic Research 2012; 3:151.

[146] Pothiawala S, Ponampalam R. Tramadol Overdose: A Case Report. Proceedings of Singapore Healthcare 2011;20(3):219-223.

[147] Taromsari MR, Badsar AR, Bahrami F, Jahanseir K, Fallah Karkan M. Clinical and Laboratory Findings in Patients with Tramadol Intoxication Referred to Razi Hospital During 2005-06. Iranian Journal of Toxicology. 2012;6(16):605-9.

[148] Elkalioubie A, Allorge D, Robriquet L, Wiart J-F, Garat A, Broly F, et al. Near-fatal tramadol cardiotoxicity in a CYP2D6 ultrarapid metabolizer. European journal of clinical pharmacology. 2011;67(8):855-8.

[149] Solarino B, Rießelmann B, Buschmann CT, Tsokos M. Multidrug poisoning involving nicotine and tramadol. Forensic science international. 2010;194(1):e17-e9.

[150] Ripple MG, Pestaner JP, Levine BS, Smialek JE. Lethal combination of tramadol and multiple drugs affecting serotonin. The American journal of forensic medicine and pathology. 2000;21(4):370-4.

[151] Gheshlaghi F, Eizadi-Mood M, Fazel K, Behjati M. An unexpected sudden death by oral tramadol intoxication: a case not reported earlier. Iranian Journal of Toxicology. 2009;2(4):292-4.

[152] Häkkinen M, Launiainen T, Vuori E, Ojanperä I. Comparison of fatal poisonings by prescription opioids. Forensic science international. 2012;222(1):327-31.

[153] Randall DC, Crane PJ. Tramadol deaths in Northern Ireland: A review of cases from 1996 to 2012. J Forensic Leg Med. 2014;23:32-6

Section 3

# Environmental Toxicology

Chapter 6

# How to Answer the Question — Are Drugs Real Threats to Biological Systems or Overrated Innocuous Chemicals?

Bruno Nunes

Additional information is available at the end of the chapter

http://dx.doi.org/10.5772/59886

## 1. Introduction

Recent years have brought a new awareness about the potential deleterious environmental impacts of a multiplicity of anthropogenic substances. We have now reached a scientific/technological standpoint that allows the prediction of most likely effects posed by large groups of substances, including pharmaceutical drugs, and their effects on exposed biota. However, as is the case of pharmaceutical drugs, scarce are the studies and unequivocal data that establish a direct linkage between their environmental presence and dispersal, and toxicity in exposed organisms. Several drawbacks are systematically invoked by detractors of the issue of pharmaceutical contamination when considering this issue, from the unmistakable low levels in which drug residues are found, to the absence of effects caused by metabolites being excreted from biologic systems. However, one cannot discard the evidences: drug residues are present in most environmental matrices, including the particular case of the aquatic compartment; the number of drugs, their metabolites and degradation products detected in these environmental matrices is alarmingly high, and never stopped increasing since their first detections; some of these drugs are not characterized in terms of toxicity towards the majority of exposed organisms, and their toxic outcomes are unpredictable; the use, release and presence of these substances will not end, or be decreased in a near future, a factor that should, at least, work as an additional stimulus for the development of research into this field.

Therapeutic agents, both human and veterinary, are modern commodities that make part of the developed society. These chemicals are usually developed to fulfil a series of criteria, mainly effectiveness, safety, comfort of use, therapeutic success, and low incidence of side effects. However, the issue of environmental fate of these molecules has only recently been raised, and the main approach established in international guidelines (e.g. European Medicines Agency, EMA) takes only in consideration the expected levels in which these compounds may occur in the aquatic compartment. Thus, a consensual precautionary principle was adopted, considering only the levels of dispersion, based on estimates of consumption, that drugs may undergone. No specific guidelines or testing protocols were ever developed to analyse the biological effects of pharmaceuticals in the environment, and efforts devoted so far to this problematic have always relied on the quest, validation and proposal of more accurate and reliable analytical methodologies. However, rather than quantifying the presence or levels of drugs in the environment, an integrative approach that characterizes their toxic effects on multiple components of the ecosystem is now much required. Only with results from a comprehensive, well-suited battery of multi-species biotests, complemented by a systematic survey of published data, it will be possible to answer to the big question: are drugs in the environment real threats to biological systems, or overrated innocuous chemicals?

The main drawback of studying the potential deleterious effects of drugs in the environment is the type of compound that one might expect to find. Considering that a rough estimate of the number of distinct substances presently in use in Europe is around 3000, it is possible to sustain the complexity of this task. Taking into consideration that a considerable number of these substances share a similar pharmacology/toxicology, we can reduce this number surely to a certain hundreds; however, being metabolised and excreted, the formation of metabolites and degradation products will increase again the number of substances that one can find in the wild. An additional factor to consider is the absence of toxicity data for the majority of metabolites and degradation products. For all the given reasons, the ecotoxicological profile of most therapeutic drugs is largely unknown, and a large effort must be devoted to the proposal, validation and use of a comprehensive set of biomarker tools. This effort will be mandatory to diagnose exposure to pharmaceuticals for a vast number of species, and to predict the magnitude of the threat posed by pharmaceutical compounds to non-target organisms.

Even if this approach is satisfactorily followed, the discrepancy of experimental data can be another factor to consider. For some drugs, a considerable amount of scientific data is now available, which should facilitate the interpretation of their ecotoxicological profiles and risks. However, this is not always a simple and immediate task to perform. In fact, for some drugs, the already compiled information is sparse, contradictory and based on erroneous assumptions, making extremely difficult the interpretation of data. This is the case of paracetamol, as shown by Nunes et al. [1]. According to this study, the toxicity of paracetamol is highly variable, even among species of the same phylogeny; however, this situation is even more complicated if one considers the variations of magnitude in responses obtained with standardized bioassays.

More than being an exhaustive attempt to establish a comprehensive review of what has been done in recent years regarding the diagnostic of effects of drugs in the wild, the present chapter intends to summarize the new evidences showing that therapeutic drugs and their residues/metabolites can indeed work as environmental pollutants, and may constitute additional sources of chemical stress to already polluted areas. It is also our intention to show the linkage between exposures to low, almost vestigial, levels of pollutants, and the most significant biological deleterious effects, in several biological models, mainly from the aquatic environ-

http://dx.doi.org/10.5772/59886

ment. Both field and laboratory studies will serve as case studies of particular importance to demonstrate that pharmaceuticals, despite their almost negligible concentrations, can be of environmental concern for sensitive key elements of the ecosystem. On the other hand, one of the main purposes of this review is the establishment of key guidelines, for the development, implementation and validation of toxicological biomarker tools to assess the subtle effects elicited by pharmaceuticals.

The issue of pharmaceuticals as contaminants has been a hot topic in environmental sciences for more than two decades [2]. However, this is not a novel issue, and early studies conducted during the mid 70s already showed the presence of significant amounts of clofibric acid (the pharmacologically active metabolite of several fibrates that explains their activity as lipid lowering agents), in water from the sewage systems of a North American town, Kansas City [3]. This same compound was again found in water quality monitoring studies, initially aimed to quantify pesticide residues, in Germany [4], almost twenty years after their initial detection. This apparent coincidence meant that compounds such as clofibric acid might have a general and ubiquitous presence, being highly dispersed among water compartments [5]. This was then confirmed by subsequent studies, showing that the dispersion of these pharmaceutical substances was not limited in any way to sewage or even freshwater, since it could also be detected in the North Sea. Clofibric acid has an undisputable historical importance, that was not followed by the confirmation of its (eco)toxicogical significance [7, 8]; nevertheless, and from a merely retrospective analysis, its detection in several water samples was a major event that served as basis for a new area of environmental toxicology, devoted to the study of the presence and effects of therapeutic drugs in the environment.

Given the enormous body of evidence that was compiled since the mid 90s to the present day, from studies involving all possible aquatic matrices (freshwater, sea water, sewage effluents, drinking water, groundwater) it is almost impossible not to consider the issue of drugs and their ecotoxicological effects one of the most challenging scenarios for years to come. Consequently, the presence of pharmaceutical residues in the wild is nowadays a matter of interest, among the scientific community and the general public [1, 9, 10, 11]. This interest derives from the intrinsic features that these compound possess. Pharmaceuticals are biologically active, capable of exerting effects in a large number of organisms, even when in extremely low concentrations. Drugs are widely used and dispersed, being ubiquitously found in the aquatic environment, as a result of the overall low degradation efficiency of sewage treatment plants; drugs are present in surface water, groundwater, and even oceans; furthermore, these substances are refractory to biological degradation or can assume other forms after metabolism [2, 9, 12], largely toxicologically uncharacterised especially for wild organisms. An adequate lipophylicity allows drugs to be slightly water soluble, but readily absorbed by living organisms [8, 13]. Aquatic organisms are by far more exposed to pharmaceutical residues. The deleterious impact of specific therapeutic compounds on aquatic organisms has already been shown to occur, even under real scenarios of contamination [13, 14, 15].

Drugs reach the aquatic compartment mainly via sewage systems. The use of pharmaceutical drugs requires its ultimate elimination from the patients' organisms, which results in its presence in the sewage treatment system, when it is present [2]. In modern western societies, sewage treatment plants (STPs) are common and generally efficient. However, the purpose of conventional STPs is reducing the amount of organic pollution, and not the elimination of often-recalcitrant compounds such as drugs. This results frequently in extremely low removal rates in STPs when it concerns to pharmaceuticals [16], requiring the implementation of novel and usually expensive technologies. This results in the continuous release of drugs an their metabolites into the receiving waters. Given that the amount introduced into the wild generally equals the sum of drug that is naturally degraded by natural pathways, it is possible to sustain that pharmaceuticals are environmentally pseudopersistent [17, 18]. Other alternative routes can also explain the presence of pharmaceuticals in the aquatic compartment, but in a lesser extent, such as release from manufacturing industries, and leachates from landfills [19]. Despite the existence of distinct routes by which pharmaceutical substances reach water bodies, it is important to stress that the majority of the residues result from human use and release, and from the inefficacy of treatments systems. Consequently, the issue of aquatic contamination by drugs is intrinsically connected to the personal use made by human consumers, which cannot be stopped or prevented, even if more advanced solutions to mitigate the presence of drugs are developed and implemented.

As a consequence of human use, several classes of drugs are routinely detected and quantified in the most varied water matrices. The most prominent classes of drugs found in the wild include non steroidal anti-inflammatories, antibiotics, anticonvulsants, antidepressants and oral contraceptives, which are systematically reported in monitoring surveys [20, 21] of the aquatic environment. However, this corresponds to a generic assumption and the reality shows that almost all substances (or their metabolites/degradation products) used in human therapeutics can be virtually detected, mainly in sewage or even in receiving waters. It is also noteworthy to observe that representatives of all these pharmacotherapeutic classes co-occur, simultaneously, in the same sample or matrix. Despite co-occurring in extremely low amounts, usually ranging from the ng to the µl per litre, it is not possible to discard the possibility of exertion of effects, mediated or not by the same receptors activated during human therapy. This poses important challenges, not only in analytical terms (which are out of the scope of this chapter), but especially in terms of the toxicological deleterious outcomes resulting from exposure to such complex mixtures, in individual terms (altered physiology of exposed organisms) and to the ecosystem [22]. Given these main topics, the major scientific question addressed here can be described as an interconnected two-tier approach: do pharmaceutical drugs, or metabolites/residues, exert deleterious effects in wildlife? If so, what is the type of effects to be expected, and what the extent to be considered? To answer these two issues, it will be necessary to adopt new strategies to surpass the usual difficulties in obtaining responses or measurable biological effects. Until the present day, few studies clearly showed the relationship between realistic conditions of exposure and deleterious effects caused by pharmaceuticals in non-target organisms. Considering the most frequently adopted toxicological endpoints (e.g. death, growth impairment) and the levels, concentrations or dosages required to elicit such effects, it is possible to state that traditional approaches are not suited, for most cases, to address the effects of drugs in aquatic organisms. Thus, it is mandatory to select an additional set of tools that may address the issues initially raised, and constitute future testing guidelines for pharmaceuticals in the wild. The combination of standardized methods, well-established analytical techniques, and new biochemical strategies (including gene

http://dx.doi.org/10.5772/59886

expression/epigenetics) might result in the establishment of a link between the low levels of exposure and biological responses in non target, environmentally exposed biota.

## 2. Effects to be expected from drug exposure

It is impossible to predict the effects of drugs in the wild, given their sheer number and the possible interactions among them in the wild. The mere quantity of different drugs in use in modern human therapeutics is overwhelming, and prevents the establishment of any plausible prediction in terms of toxicity of complex mixtures, such as urban effluents. The human use of pharmaceutical drugs in the European Union is vast, and approximately 3000 distinct substances are used, including substances from different pharmaco-therapeutic classes such as anti-inflammatories, β-blockers, oral contraceptives, blood lipid regulators, antibiotics and others [23]. This is a brief, albeit comprehensive summary of the therapeutic classes one can find in the aquatic compartment, from an empirical perspective of only considering classes of drugs that are used in extremely high amounts. However, this is a criterion that is not exempt of drawbacks or criticisms, since the mentioned classes, those that are used and dispersed in the highest amounts, are not necessarily representative of drugs with the highest biological or toxicological activity. For instance, cytostatic or anticancer drugs are extremely active and biologically aggressive, despite not being extensively used [24]; however, these substances are among the most active environmental drugs [25]. It is thus extremely difficult to prioritise substances only based on simple criteria of use and consumption; more difficult is the task to develop and validate markers of toxicological interest to be used in routine analysis.

Furthermore, the presence of an even larger number of metabolites [26], and products of degradation by natural or anthropogenic means (photodegradation, hydrolysis, microbial degradation, chemical treatment processes at STPs, chemical reaction among drug residues and with other substances) implies the need to include the possibility of toxicological interactions among all compounds that may be present in a given environmental (especially water) sample; these interactions, that may result in increased toxicological activity, has been already shown to be a possibility in the wild [27, 28]. It is not just a matter of selecting a biological response, but to choose the one most likely to respond to this vast group of compounds, in a specific organism that may be successfully analysed, both in field surveys and in laboratory-based bioassays. It is not just feasible to study all pharmaceutical compounds, on all putative model organisms.

## 3. Typology of toxic effects elicited by drugs and its relation with pharmacology

The toxicity of pharmaceutical drugs in exposed aquatic biota is frequently determined by their intrinsic pharmacology and toxicology, and outcomes that are already described for other species are also possible to occur in aquatic organisms [29]. Additionally, other toxic effects may not derive at all from the known pharmacology of these substances, and can indeed result from specific biochemical and physiological pathways that are over-stimulated in highly responsive species. Thus, it is possible to expect a wide range of toxic effects, which difficult the process of selection of adequate and responsive toxicological endpoints to be observed and studied, both in monitoring and in laboratory based assays.

Despite the multiplicity of effects drugs can cause on non-target aquatic organisms, the selection of a marker of toxicity is sometimes extremely difficult. It is impossible to select a single biomarker that will be equally responsive to all drugs, considering the diversity of pharmacological mechanisms involved in the activities of such a large number of substances. Consequently, it must be emphasized that a thorough process of selection of adequate markers of toxicity is mandatory. However, the quest for a putative toxic effect of a drug can be directly connected to its mode of action, in pure pharmacological terms. This was the case of anticholinesterasic compounds of therapeutic use, such as pyridostigmine and neostigmine, as shown by Rocha et al. [30]. This study showed that the most likely effects of environmental contamination by these two substances could be related to cholinesterasic impairment, a key factor encompassing other effects at the individual and population level, such as reduced feeding behaviour and decrease offspring production. However, this study was not followed by other successful attempts to establish relationships between drug exposure and potential ecotoxicological effects, and very scarce is the number of published papers that point this possibility. The study conducted by Rodrigues et al. [15] evidenced that the same drug, pyridostigmine, could elicit similar results in the fish species *Lepomis gibbosus*, in terms of cholinesterasic inhibition; however, this pattern of response was not reflected by behavioural modifications, despite the occurrence of neurotoxicity. Drugs can act by pathways that are also shared by other classes of compounds, which share with drugs the same aquatic matrix. Cholinesterasic inhibition was again the target of the study by Nunes et al. [31], when studying the combination effects of a pharmaceutical drug, pyridostigmine, and two common environmental contaminants (the metal copper, and the organophosphate pesticide chlorfenvinphos), well known for their ability to impair cholinesterasic activity of exposed aquatic organisms. This study showed that the combination of the three compounds, even for realistic levels, could result in a toxicological outcome that constitutes the exacerbation of the pharmacological pathway activated by the drug pyridostigmine.

The environmental effects of other substances of therapeutic use are also related with their intrinsic effects. One of the most thoroughly characterized examples is the one of antibiotics. By being discharged into the aquatic environment, often maintaining intact their pharmacological properties, antibiotics still exert their effects on wild bacterial species [32]. This favours the selection of resistant strains, by means of dispersing resistance genes among susceptible bacteria. This phenomenon has been extensively characterized, and derives from the anthropogenic pressure exerted by human residues containing drugs that are released into the environment, favouring the dispersion of ancient natural genes that encode resistance mechanisms [33, 34]. To address the issue of antibiotic presence and effects in the environment, namely those that can increase gene transfer among bacterial strains, a common strategy is to analyse where these genes can be found, especially in the water compartment, which is the most vulnerable to this issue. The review by Zhang et al. [35] summarizes the efforts recently devoted to the development of new methodologies to characterize the dissemination of resistance genes in the wild following antibiotic release from human activities. It is thus possible to conclude that the mere analysis of genes encoding resistance factors can be considered an effective tool to analyse the effects of antibiotics in the wild.

Effects of other drugs can involve alterations in the regulation of the endocrine system. The use of synthetic oral contraceptives, glucorticoids and others is one of the main causes for the ubiquitous presence of these classes in most aquatic matrices, where they maintain their biological effects [36]. Some of these compounds have already been demonstrated to exert potential endocrine effects in exposed wildlife, even in the ranges of concentrations in which they were found [37]. Despite their present levels of contamination, which are indisputably low, the large use and liberation of these compounds into the aquatic compartment will not exempt this endocrine disrupting substances from exerting deleterious effects on exposed biota, as reviewed by Runnalls et al. [38]. In fact, the effects caused by this class of compounds have already been documented, especially in terms of development, metamorphosis, and sexual dimorphism, in amphibians [39], fish [40, 41], molluscs [42], and also crustaceans [43]. It is not surprising that these compounds, even after excretion, maintain their initial pharmacological properties. However, effects elicited are well distinct from those caused in humans, and can include feminization and significant alterations in individual features and population structures, which constitutes a major effect in ecological terms. So, it is possible to conclude that the assessment of endocrine disrupting effects is another valid example on how to use the pharmacological properties of a given class of chemical drugs to search for their effects in the environment. The study conducted by Velasco-Santamaría et al. [44] evidenced that the presence of such compounds in the wild can also be potentiated by the concomitant presence of other substances with similar pharmacological properties and therapeutic use. The synthetic oestrogen ethinylestradiol can exert increased toxic endocrine effects in the presence of another endocrine active pharmaceutical, such as trenbolone, in the marine fish species *Zoarces viviparous*.

# 4. Mortality, growth impairment an other classic tools

Despite their traditional use for the toxicity assessment of a large number of substances, mortality and growth impairment endpoints have been extensively used to describe the toxicity of pharmaceutical substances towards wild biota. In fact, more than reflecting real scenarios of contamination, the validity of calculating and interpreting mortality data relies on the establishment of sublethal toxicity criteria and to analyse in comparative terms, the ecotoxicity of substances that act by unknown (or largely uncharacterised) mechanisms of toxic action. In fact, $LC_{50}$ values of pharmaceutical drugs are well suited to establish rankings of ecotoxicity among very distinct compounds, and these criteria are straightforward to implement and interpret. However, these endpoints are not a first choice if one requires the establishment of complex mechanisms, or even effects at extremely low levels, which are likely to cause alterations other than death, immobilization, or impairment of the population growth. These responses are not fine tuned alterations, and may be seen as blunt tools for toxicity characterization, with poor of even null ecological relevance.

The number of ecotoxicity studies analysing lethality or growth impairment is thus considerable. The study published by Carlsson et al. [45], showed that antiparasitic drugs could exert extreme toxicity, when compared to antibiotics, thus threatening the survival of zebrafish embryos. The crustacean species *Daphnia magna* was very sensitive to the antidepressant sertraline, as shown by Minagh et al. [46]; this compound was capable of inducing strong alterations in the population of this crustacean species, after 21 days of exposure. Population changes were also observed after chronically exposing *D. magna* to the compounds testosterone and 4-hydroxyandrostenedione, even for ecologically relevant levels [47], reinforcing the possibility of exertion of deleterious effects in the wild. Another crustacean, namely *Neocaridina denticulate*, demonstrated to be extremely sensitive in terms of lethality to a combination of pharmaceutical drugs (paracetamol and ibuprofen) commonly found in the aquatic environment [48]. The ecotoxicological effects of mefenamic acid on *D. magna* and *Moina macrocopa* were evaluated by Collard et al. [49]. This study showed that lethal effects were not likely to occur for already reported levels of this compound; however, the chronic exposure to this compound showed that changes in reproduction are possible, especially in the case of *M. macrocopa*.

On the other hand, the absence of potential risk posed by the presence of clofibric acid was evidenced by the study by Nunes et al. [50] and by Emblidge and DeLorenzo [51], in multi-species assessments that focused on mortality and growth impairment as toxicity endpoints. Similarly, the work by Ferreira et al. [52] evidenced the absence of potential lethal effects posed by antibiotics (oxytetracycline and florfenicol) on the crustacean species *Artemia parthenogenetica*. Despite not exerting lethal effects, several combinations of pharmaceutical drugs (including an ecologically relevant mixture) were capable of causing significant alterations in zebrafish embryos, as shown by Madureira et al. [53]. The antibiotic oxytetracycline was shown to be reasonably safe towards the fish species *Labeo rohita*, since the lethal levels were well above concentrations that are not likely to be found in the wild, as shown by Ambili et al. [54].

Growth of autothrophic organisms is another endpoint likely to respond to exposure to human use drugs; the study conducted by Berninger et al. [55] showed the refractivity of the aquatic plant species *Lemna minor* to the drug diphenhydramine. Somewhat similarly, the work conducted by Nunes et al. [56] evidenced the occurrence of an oxidative-based response of two species of the genus *Lemna* (*L. minor* and *L. gibba*) elicited by the drug paracetamol, which resulted in significant growth alterations. On the other hand, the study conducted by Ferreira et al. [52] presented evidences concerning the toxicity of the antibiotics oxytetracycline and florfenicol on the microalgae species *Tetraselmis chuii*.

## 5. The quest for new biomarker tools: Oxidative stress

As seen before, the transformation of a pharmacological effect into a biomarker, can thus work as a reliable indicator of exposure of wild organisms to several classes of pharmaceutical drugs. Despite the presented evidences, describing successful cases in which the pharmacology of a drug (or a group of drugs) may also be used to study its toxicity, the majority of therapeutic drugs do not exert effects that can be interpreted as reliable environmental biomarkers. There are two major drawbacks of this approach: the first reason is related with the levels in which these substances are found, and the second most important, is the absence of a counterpart response in wild organisms of the response elicited in human patients.

http://dx.doi.org/10.5772/59886

Toxicity is a matter of dose, and can be generally described by a dose-response relationship. Assuming that these compounds are found in extremely low levels, the exertion of a clear toxic response (e.g. death, immobilization, impairment of reproduction) is not always possible. It is thus important to know in detail the mechanisms by which the drugs not only exert their pharmacological activities, but also those involved in adverse effects, metabolism and detoxification processes, and other accessory or side-effects that the drugs may cause. Only by means of knowing these fundaments of pharmacology and toxicology it is possible to select biomarkers that will respond satisfactorily at extremely low levels of exposure. Given the extremely low levels in which drugs are found in the aquatic compartment, effects are sometimes minor and negligible, or may even be considered null or absent if an adequately responsive biomarker is not employed. This can be a real challenge for ecotoxicologists, since specific biomarkers, others than the main pharmacological effect, that signal a biological alteration following an exposure to drugs in concentrations between the ng/l to μg/l are not abundant.

On the other hand, drugs are designed to be safe for human patients, and it is possible to suggest that this somewhat harmless nature can also prevent drugs from causing extreme toxicity in other organisms. However, drugs can indeed cause multiple effects, which do not occur by activation of specific single receptors, but reflect major changes in the homeostasis of exposed organisms. The presence of pharmaceutical compounds can cause changes at many different levels, including in the redox cycle of exposed organisms; these may cause the formation of reactive chemical species, capable of inducing damages to biological structures. Therefore, the quantification of oxidative stress biomarkers is important to evaluate the redox status of the exposed organisms. Several studies have already shown that, even for realistic levels of contamination, some compounds can exert pro-oxidative effects, measurable mostly in terms of modification of the antioxidant defence mechanism of exposed aquatic organisms; in many cases, membrane lipid peroxidation is a likely outcome of oxidative damage, and this event can be also quantified [8, 13, 56, 57, 58, 59]. The exertion of oxidative stress is a factor to consider when evaluating long term, thus realistic, exposures. Considering that exposure to anthropogenic therapeutic drugs can occur during a significant portion of the entire life cycle of a given organism, it is not possible to exclude the occurrence of cumulative processes ending up in irreversible conditions. In fact, oxidative stress, if sustained for long period, can also be the cause of genotoxicity. Data from the literature sustain the exertion of deleterious effects of specific pharmaceutical compounds, including genotoxicity on fish [60], and in crustaceans (e.g. *D. magna*) [61, 62]. Consequently, it is possible to use oxidative stress not only as an indicator of exposure to a broad series of compounds, but also as a predictor of other subsequent effects, that may derive from oxidative alterations and damages.

The extended knowledge concerning the metabolic pathways required for the bioactivation or detoxification of therapeutic compounds can also function as a valid source of analytic tools for the assessment of effects. The activation by over-expression of metabolic enzymes, involved in the detoxification of pharmaceuticals, is a probable event whenever a biological system is challenged by exposure to drugs in the wild. Among metabolic enzymes prone to over-expression, one can identify mainly those involved in the direct metabolism of drugs. The activities of phase I metabolic enzymes, for example (such as cytochrome P450), and phase II metabolic reactions (namely isoenzymes glutathione-S-transferases, GSTs), can also be increased in aquatic organisms by exposure to pharmaceutical drugs [7, 8, 13]. Being routinely quantified in modern ecotoxicological laboratories, the activities of such enzymes are intrinsically interesting to quantify not only the level of exposure to drugs, but also the likely consequences of drug exposure. This may be justified since these enzymatic forms are not only involved in the bioactivation/detoxification of drugs, but do also participate in numerous endogenous processes, which can be altered following an environmentally drug-induced chemical insult. The broad spectrum of these analytical tools is also a factor to consider, being highly unspecific, effects both phase I and II metabolic enzymes can indeed respond to a multiplicity of therapeutic classes.

## 6. Alternative tools to assess the environmental effects of drugs: Toxicity, pharmacology and other effects

Several toxicity assessment projects have relied in the development and validation of new tools to quantify the extent of the toxic response. As previously stated, known pharmacological properties can serve as a comprehensive source of biomarkers to be used in ecotoxicity assessments. However, some of the responses of wild organisms to drugs may be based on physiological mechanisms that are not directly related (activated or impaired) following patterns included in the pharmacology of pharmaceutical substances. Some of these responses are purely paradoxical, while others are only the reflex of the activation of mechanisms and receptors in wild organisms that were never studied and/or identified in common experimental models.

This is the case of behavioural alterations in several wild organisms. The work by Berninger et al. [55] showed that the fish species *Pimephales promelas* was highly sensitive to the antihistaminic drug diphenhydramine in terms of feeding behaviour. The feeding behaviour was also modulated after exposure of the fish *Perca fluviatilis* to the antidepressant sertraline, as evidenced by Hedgespeth et al. [63]. Behaviour is also a trait that can be significantly changed after exposure to pharmaceuticals, both in fish [64], and in crustacean species [65]. Strong behavioural alterations were also reported by Nunes et al. [13] after the exposure of the fish *Gambusia holbrooki* to the neuroactive compound diazepam, with impairment of the swimming capability. An opposite pattern has been presented by crustacean species, which seem not to be equally responsive to pharmaceutical drugs. As evidenced by Nieto et al [66], the food ingestion behaviour of the freshwater crustacean *Atyaephyra desmarestii* was not affected by ecologically relevant levels of several therapeutic drugs, such as diclofenac, ibuprofen, and carbamazepine. Food ingestion was also affected following exposure of *Xenopus laevis* to fluoxetine, as demonstrated by Conners et al. [67], thus conditioning the development of this organism during its early life stages. Antidepressants that exert their therapeutic activity through the selective inhibition of serotonin reuptake are likely to be adequate candidates to alter the behaviour of a large number of aquatic organisms, considering that the most prominent pathway involved in their activity is highly conserved. According to the editorial by Ford [68], specific compounds including sertraline and fluoxetine, can dramatically alter the feeding behaviour profile of a large number of aquatic organisms, from fish to crustaceans.

http://dx.doi.org/10.5772/59886

The endocrine disrupting effects of several human use drugs has been the subject of research for several years, and quite a few studies report the occurrence of significant effects caused by drugs (e.g. anti-inflammatories) on fish [69]. Endocrine disruptive effects caused by pharmaceuticals are not exclusive to fish, since invertebrates, such as crustaceans, are also prone to be affected in their endocrine functions by exposure to pharmaceutical drugs, as reviewed by Hutchinson [70]. Neuroendocrine effects are another aspect of this issue. Considering that a large number of pharmaceutical drugs act by altering the expression and effects of biological compounds of high physiological importance (e.g. neuropeptides, neurotransmitters, or neurohormones), it is with no surprise that similar mechanisms can be impaired in non-target species environmentaly exposed to these same drugs. The consequences are not only so far uncharacterised, but also, unpredictable. Consequences to be expected will naturally include alterations in the physiology of exposed wildlife, affecting behavioural traits, or the hormonal homeostasis, which are of fundamental importance to the organisms and to the ecosystem. It is thus expectable to observe impairments at several levels, such as reproduction, development, growth, response to chemical aggression or other sources of stress [71, 72]. The neuroendocrine effects of specific compounds, such as sertraline, were shown by Conners et al. [67] in tadpoles of the species *Xenopus laevis*. This antidepressant substance caused significant developmental impairments during the early life stages of this organism, which occurred for ecologically relevant levels. Another antidepressant drug, such as fluoxetine, was also capable of inducing strong alterations in the reproductive physiology of the fish species, *Carassius auratus*. Another antidepressant, mianserin, was also related to estrogenic activity in fish (*Danio rerio*) by inducing molecular biomarkers of estrogenicity (such as vitellogenin1 and zona pellucida proteins), as evidenced by van der Ven et al. [73]. The study conducted by Mennigen et al. [74]concluded that exposure to relevant levels of this substance could alter the expression and release of several physiological hormones, thus compromising the sexual behaviour of this fish species. Therapeutic drugs such as paracetamol and lincomycin are also involved in endocrine disruption effects. The study conducted by Kim et al. [75] showed that these two pharmaceuticals could affect the steroidogenic pathway and increase estrogenicity, in crustaceans (*D. magna* and *Moina macrocopa*), but also in fish (*Oryzias latipes*). These effects were translated into a significant reduction in juvenile survival of fish, and on a significant increase in the vitellogenin levels in male fish. Other substances, such as furosemide and several fibrates (e.g. bezafibrate, fenofibrate and gemfibrozil) can also exert this type of endocrine effects. According to the data obtained by Isidori et al. [76], these substances were shown to activate the human estrogenic receptor $\alpha$, thus favouring estrogenic responses in wild organisms. Mefenamic acid is another example of an endocrine compound whose pharmacology in most experimental organisms does not include this aspect. However, the data compiled by Collard et al. [49] showed its involvement in endocrine effects in fish (*D. rerio*), evidenced by alterations in vitellogenin and its mRNA expression, overexpression of genes of the hypothalamus–pituitary–gonad axis, and histological changes in ovaries of exposed females.

Epigenetic effects can also derive from the environmentally-driven impact of specific compounds; exposure to persistent organic pollutants (including pharmaceuticals) or endocrine disrupting chemicals are examples of classes of chemicals that have been related to alterations in epigenetic marks, including in fish and cladocerans (Vandegehuchte and Janssen, 2011) [77].

Several published papers refer that deleterious effects of transient chemical exposure (namely, via environment) of *D. magna* can result in the transference to nonexposed generations through epigenetic inheritance [78, 79, 80], which is a decisive factor to link ecotoxicological effects observed at the levels of communities to alterations at the ecosystem levels [81]. The effects of chemical pollutants on the epigenetics of fish is also significant, as shown by the screening of pollution resistance of north American fish species [82]. Alteration of gene expression is also another factor to consider after environmental exposure to chemical stressors; several papers show the responsiveness of aquatic organisms to environmental pharmaceuticals, demonstrating the validity of this approach [83, 84].

Specific drugs, not anticholinesterasic by nature, can also impair neurotransmission, by cholinesterasic inhibition [85]. One of the most significant examples is the one represented by zinc pyrithione. According to the work developed by Sánchez-Bayoa and Goka [86], this antidandruff compound is extremely toxic to several aquatic organisms, including the crustacean *D. magna*. Despite being photodegradable, recent studies show that zinc pyrithione may exert important toxic effects on aquatic organisms (e.g. *Paracentrotus lividus* and *Mytilus edulis*), even at extremely low levels [87]. Effects of zinc pyrithione are not restricted to invertebrates, since fish species are also extremely sensitive to the presence of this compound [88]. The products of degradation of zinc pyrithione can be of great environmental concern per se, since the effects of such compounds on several marine organisms are well known. The toxicity of zinc pyrithione has been documented for organisms such as the algae species *Skeletonema costatum*, the crustacean *Tigriopus japonicus*, and the fish *Pagrus major* [89]. The mechanism of toxic action of zinc pyrithione metabolites includes AChE inhibition, as shown by Mochida et al. [90].

The energy metabolism of wild organisms is a putative target for pharmaceutical toxicity. As shown by Mennigen et al. [91], exposure to the drug fluoxetine could result in significant alterations in the fish species *Carassius auratus*, namely in terms of energy metabolism. Low levels of exposure were causative of anorectic effects, while higher levels could directly compromise the hepatic glucose metabolism, by means of depressing the activity of the gluconeogenic enzyme fructose-1,6-bisphosphatase. Chronic exposure of marine mussels (*Mytilus* sp.) to two therapeutic drugs, genfibrozil and diclofenac, showed the interference of these substances on several parameters, including energy metabolism features [92]. The respiratory activity of exposed organisms is another function that can be altered after exposure to anthropogenic compounds, which interfere with metabolic pathways used by organisms to obtain energy (anaerobiosis vs. aerobiosis) [7]. This study evidenced the roles of both clofibrate and clofibric acid, hypolipidemic fibrates used in human therapeutics, in the increase in muscle lactate dehydrogenase activity, thus favouring the less energetically efficient anaerobiotic pathway.

## 7. Future directions: A combination of tools

From the previous sections, it was made clear that it is extremely difficult to search and define without any shadow of doubt the biological effects to be expected from a large number of

http://dx.doi.org/10.5772/59886

extremely different chemical substances, exerted on a vast multiplicity of organisms. Not only are the substances very different per se, thus exerting distinct effects, but also the organisms can have alternative pathways and receptors that make them more or less prone to the exertion of those same effects. It is not possible always to rely on the well-described human pharmacology, despite the large number of studies that sustain the most common effects, since humans are not environmentally exposed to the majority of these substances or to their residues. However, some of the effects are shared both by humans and by other organisms in the wild, a decisive factor when one tries to select an adequate tool to quantify an effect elicited by a pharmaceutical drug in the environment.

The present scenario shows us that we are halfway between the total lack of data concerning pharmaceutical effects in the wild, and a full and comprehensive knowledge about their faith and ultimate consequences. A large effort has been undertaken and toxicity of several pharmaceutical classes is nowadays already characterized in a vast number of organisms. Despite the validity of this effort, other pharmaceutical classes are not fully understood in their interaction with biota, thus requiring the development of additional attempts until a definite light is shed on this issue. Presently, environmental scientists dealing with this issue still have to face a significant array of drawbacks, from the simple lack of data for some drugs/organisms, unpredictability of data and, of the biological responses in somewhat exotic species, confounding factors that already occur for other studies, but whose influence is exponentially increased in this specific area, lack of analytical tools, such as biomarkers with enough sensitivity to face the extremely low levels found in the wild and that are able to understand highly subtle biological responses, lack of test protocols or species well adapted to be used in ecotoxicological testing under conditions of brackish water, tropical or artic climates, or extreme environments, in which drugs are also likely to occur.

Despite not being the core of this chapter, the quantification of the levels of pharmaceutical drugs in the wild, especially in the aquatic environment, is crucial. It is important to know in detail the compounds that may exist (or co-exist) in the same matrix, since these compounds are important to select an analytical tool/biomarker that will allow the prediction of biological effects. It is also of fundamental importance to know which are the most representative compounds (or pharmacotherapeutic classes) in a given sample also to establish causal relationships between their levels and the extent of the observed biological response. Only with a complimentary approach comprising hydrology, water analytical chemistry and biological assessment of effects it will be possible to fully characterize the impact of drugs on the wildlife.

The typology of exposure is also a matter of concern. From the previously mentioned studies, two main types of exposure were adopted in the majority of studies: acute (short-term) and chronic (long term). The use of short-term exposure periods is somewhat neglected, but this is not a totally invalid strategy. Despite not having the relevance of a long period of exposure, which reflects the most likely conditions of exposure in the wild, short exposure periods are also of extreme importance, and must be included in bioassays for the assessment of the effects of pharmaceutical drug. Acute assays are important since they allow researchers to test the responsiveness of a specific test species towards a given drugs, Acute exposure can also be of importance to define rankings of comparative toxicity for several substances, independently from their mode of action and toxicity. Data from acute tests can also be useful to determine ranges of concentrations representing sublethal levels to which organisms may be exposed. Finally, the entire set of information potentially gathered from this type of test may serve to prioritise compounds to be studied under chronic conditions of exposure. However, and if one considers the need to increase the ecological relevance of data obtained from ecotoxicity tests, chronic assays are likely to represent a more credible simulation of what happens in the wild. Organisms are frequently subjected to contamination during considerable periods of their entire life cycle, or may even contact with chemical pollution of anthropogenic origin for different generations. It is thus important to prioritise a testing strategy that simulates these conditions, and the most adopted type of bioassay, despite its inherent difficulties, is the chronic exposure. Chronic exposures can more easily mimic real events, occurring under realistic low levels of contaminants, and can consequently increase the ecological relevance of the obtained data. Furthermore, the selection of chronic exposures can permit the proposal of multispecies assessments (e.g. mesocosms), which are obviously advantageous if one intends to simulate real environmental conditions. On the other hand, multispecies assessments are a valid approach, since the sensitivity of distinct organisms towards pharmaceuticals is frequently very diverse.

From the majority of the cited studies, it is possible to conclude that a biomarker-based approach is valid to obtain information regarding specific pathways involved in the toxic response. This does not necessarily imply that more traditional approaches (including mortality, or growth/population effects) are fully inadequate to assess the ecotoxicological effects of drugs. Nevertheless, the low levels of exposure make difficult the exertion of such effects, and the resultant toxicity often occurs by impairment of specific, subtler, biochemical pathways. It is thus important to analyse the sub-individual level, and more biomarkers must be proposed and fully validated. Effects at the molecular level, including enzymes, must be interpreted as signalling tools for effect or damage in biological systems. Given their overall importance, specific pathways must be primary sources of analytical tools. It is possible to suggest that novel biomarkers can derive from analysis of the enzymatic machinery involved in the energetic metabolism, gene expression and epigenetics, and damage (e.g. of oxidative nature) repair. These will be the most likely biomarkers of contamination of the future.

The next step will be transposing laboratory biomarker-based assays, with a combination of chronic-acute exposure of multiple species to other alternative models, namely under field conditions. It is now mandatory to propose new test species, well adapted to conditions that do not represent standard settings: species from tropical/polar (or otherwise extreme) regions must be analysed following the above-described strategy, and their use for ecotoxicological purposes validated. This will be of crucial importance to transfer bioassays from the laboratory to the field, increasing the validity of data and of the conclusions drawn.

Finally, a last step will combine the simultaneous analysis of complex mixtures of drugs. Frequently, environmental matrices are contaminated by a large number of distinct pharmaceuticals; any analytical procedure based on the quantification of effects caused by a single chemical will always be unsatisfactory, and will underestimate the actual toxicity of complex

http://dx.doi.org/10.5772/59886

but realistic mixtures. To avoid this underestimation, it will be of the uttermost importance to know the general interaction profiles that may occur for a large number of test species, caused not by isolated single compounds, but by the main representatives of known therapeutic classes: not being possible to test the potential interactions occurring by the simultaneous presence of hundreds or even thousands of compounds in the same matrix, a more systematic approach may involve the definition and characterization of putative biological relations of pharmacotherapeutic classes among each other.

## 8. The effects of drugs in the wild

Despite the considerable number of cited research articles so far, the present chapter would not be satisfactorily summarized without a critical evaluation of the potential ecological damages posed by pharmaceutical residues. The major drawbacks for the analysis of effects caused by pharmaceuticals are also the most important defence against their risks: their extremely low levels. Being present in residual amounts, sometimes below the ng/l range, the majority of drugs do not attain levels capable of exerting effects. However, the simultaneous presence of compounds that act via a similar pathway may favour the exertion of effects. Still, few are the examples of substances for which this behaviour has been described. Despite the lack of reported effects, and the impossibility so far of establishing a direct, unequivocal relationship between pharmaceutical exposure and deleterious effects in wildlife, an increasing number of studies has brought the issue of ecological relevance of data to the discussion. By testing already reported levels of contaminants, some researchers have already claimed having demonstrated the putative effects of drugs in exposed organisms that are also likely to occur in the wild. This has been the case of several fibrates [7], synthetic hormones [93], ivermectin [94], paracetamol [1, 57, 59], ibuprofen [95], neostigmine and pyridostigmine [15, 30, 31], fluoxetine and other antidepressants [93, 96]. However, the majority of studies published so far do not demonstrate this intrinsic association between pharmaceuticals contamination and deleterious effects. Nevertheless, research studies on this matter have clearly demonstrated the responsiveness of a large number of species towards drugs, evidencing the potential for toxic effects if a threshold level is attained and surpassed. This is of the uttermost importance, since it clearly shows that some of the highly conserved pathways used and activated by pharmaceutical drugs in humans, are also present in a significant number of wild organisms; this increases the possibility of biological-chemical interaction, with sometimes totally unpredicted overall effects. The protection created against the effects of human drugs by their low levels can thus be simply temporary, considering the ever-increasing amount of drugs and their residues in the wild.

## 9. Conclusions

The need to understand the potential effects of a large number of biologically active substances in the wild, has driven researchers to the development of new assessment methodologies.

Unlike other substances with human origin, pharmaceutical drugs are active, and may pose significant risks even after their elimination and for long periods. Being excreted in extremely high amounts and on a daily basis, such substances are pseudopersistent and recalcitrant. Not even the implementation of dedicated sewage treatment systems endured to reduce the global amounts of drugs entering especially the aquatic environment. Consequently, the presence of such substances is now a global reality, needing to be dully characterized. Non-target species are the most likely and vulnerable targets for the exertion of deleterious effects. The study of putative toxic effects requires the development, implementation and validation of novel analytic tools, specifically devoted to the particularities of drug contamination. From the revised literature, it is possible to anticipate that ecotoxicological analysis, in the future, will require the combination of distinct tools, on a complementary basis. The tools to be used in the future will not only respond to extremely low levels of contamination, but will include signalling responses well suited to diagnose exposure to specific classes of drugs. Despite not being entirely adapted to the issue of contamination by low levels of pharmaceutical drugs, standardized bioassays can be a valuable tool, if complemented with adequate molecular and subindividual endpoints. Being impossible to characterize the entire set of toxic responses elicited by single, individual compounds, it will be important to know the most important toxic responses of common pharmacotherapeutic classes, to allow the prediction of potential interactions. The use of multispecies assessments will also be important, since the sensitivity towards specific compounds is not necessarily comparable among distinct test organisms. Long-term studies, favouring phenomena of bioaccumulation during important periods of the organisms' life cycles will allow knowing in detail the potential endocrine effects elicited by specific compounds. Behaviour is another feature likely to be altered after pharmaceuticals exposure, thus requiring the development of new testing methodologies to address this issue.

## Acknowledgements

This work was supported by funding FEDER through COMPETE- Programa Operacional Factores de Competitividade, and by National funding through FCT-Fundação para a Ciência e Tecnologia.

## Author details

Bruno Nunes*

Address all correspondence to: nunes.b@ua.pt

Departamento de Biologia, Centro de Estudos Ambientais e do Mar (CESAM), Universidade de Aveiro, Campus Universitário de Santiago, Aveiro, Portugal

## References


[1] Nunes B, Antunes SC, Santos J, Martins L, Castro BB (in press). Toxic Potential of Paracetamol to Freshwater Organisms: a Headache to Environmental Regulators? Ecotoxicology and Environmental Safety.

[2] Halling-Sørensen B, Nors Nielsen S, Lanzky PF, Ingerslev F, Holten Lützhøft HC, Jørgensen SE (1998). Occurrence, fate and effects of pharmaceutical substances in the environment--a review. Chemosphere 36(2):357-93.

[3] Hignite C, Azarnoff DL (1977). Drugs and drug metabolites as environmental contaminants: chlorophenoxyisobutyrate and salicyclic acid in sewage water effluent. Life Sciences 20(2): 337-341.

[4] Stan HJ, Heberer T (1997). Pharmaceuticals in the Aquatic Environment. Analusis Magazine 25(7): 20-23.

[5] Heberer T, Stan H-J (1997). Determination of Clofibric Acid and N-(phenylsulfonyl)-Sarcosine in Sewage, River, and Drinking Water. International Journal of Environmental Analytical Chemistry 67: 113-124.

[6] Buser H-R, Muller MD (1998). Occurrence of the Pharmaceutical Drug Clofibric Acid and the Herbicide Mecoprop in Various Swiss Lakes and in the North Sea. Environmental Science and Technology 32(1): 188-192.

[7] Nunes B, Carvalho F, Guilhermino L (2004). Acute and chronic effects of clofibrate and clofibric acid over *Gambusia holbrooki*. Chemosphere 57: 1581 –1589.

[8] Nunes B, Carvalho F, Guilhermino L (2006). Effects of widely used pharmaceuticals and a detergent on oxidative stress biomarkers of the crustacean Artemia parthenogenetica. Chemosphere 62: 581 – 594.

[9] Daughton CG, Ternes TA (1999). Pharmaceuticals and personal care products in the environment: agents of subtle change? Environ Health Perspect. 107(6): 907-38.

[10] Jones OAH, Voulvoulis N, Lester JN (2002). Aquatic environmental assessment of the top 25 English prescription pharmaceuticals. Water Res 36:5013–5022.

[11] Miao XS, Koenig BG, Metcalfe CD (2002). Analysis of acidic drugs in the effluents of sewage treatment plants using liquid chromatography-electrospray ionisation tandem mass spectrometry. J Chromatogr A 952:139–147.

[12] Daughton CG, Jones-Lepp TL (2001). Pharmaceuticals and Personal Care Products in the Environment: Scientific and Regulatory Issues. Daughton, C.G. and Jones-Lepp, T. (eds.), ACS/Oxford University Press, Washington, D.C.

[13] Nunes B, Carvalho F, Guilhermino L. (2008) Behaviour and biomarkers of oxidative stress in Gambusia holbrooki after acute exposure to widely used pharmaceuticals

and a detergent. Ecotoxicology and Environmental Safety Ecotoxicology and Environmental Safety 71(2): 341-354.

[14] Nunes B, Carvalho F, Guilhermino L (2005). Characterization and use of the total head soluble cholinesterases from mosquitofish (Gambusia holbrooki) for screening of anticholinesterasic activity. J Enzym Inhib Med Ch 20(4): 369-376.

[15] Rodrigues S, Antunes SC, Brandão FP, Castro BB, Gonçalves F, Nunes B (2012). Effects of anticholinesterase drugs on biomarkers and behavior of pumpkinseed, *Lepomis gibbosus* (Linnaeus, 1758). J Environ Monit. 14(6):1638-44.

[16] Ibáñez M, Gracia-Lora E, Bijlsma L, Morales E, Pastor L, Hernández F (2013). Removal of emerging contaminants in sewage water subjected to advanced oxidation with ozone. Journal of Hazardous Materials 260: 389–398.

[17] Daughton CG (2002). Environmental stewardship and drugs as pollutants. Lancet 360: 1035–1036.

[18] Daughton CG (2003). Cradle-to-cradle stewardship of drugs for minimizing their environmental disposition while promoting human health. I. Rationale for and avenues toward a green pharmacy. Environ Health Perspect 111: 757–774.

[19] Lubick N (2010). Drugs in the Environment: Do Pharmaceutical Take-Back Programs Make a Difference? Environmental Health Perspectives 118(5): A211-A214.

[20] Okuda T, Yamashita N, Tanaka H, Matsukawa H, Tanabe K (2009). Development of extraction method of pharmaceuticals and their occurrences found in Japanese wastewater treatment plants. Environ Int. 35(5):815-20.

[21] Sui Q, Huang J, Deng SB, Yu G, Fan Q (2010). Occurrence and removal of pharmaceuticals, caffeine and DEET in wastewater treatment plants of Beijing, China. Water Res 44:417–26.

[22] Rosi-Marshall EJ, Royer TV (2012). Pharmaceutical Compounds and Ecosystem Function: An Emerging Research Challenge for Aquatic Ecologists. Ecosystems 15: 867–880.

[23] Huschek G, Hansen PD, Maurer HH, Krengel D, Kayser A (2004). Environmental risk assessment of medicinal products for human use according to European Commission recommendations. Environ Toxicol 19(3): 226-240.

[24] Gómez-Canela C, Ventura F, Caixach J, Lacorte S (2014). Occurrence of cytostatic compounds in hospital effluents and wastewaters, determined by liquid chromatography coupled to high-resolution mass spectrometry. Analytical and Bioanalytical Chemistry 406(16): 3801-3814.

[25] Parrella A, Lavorgna M, Criscuolo E, Russo C, Fiumano V, Isidori M (2014). Acute and chronic toxicity of six anticancer drugs on rotifers and crustaceans. Chemosphere 115: 59–66.

[26] Heberer T, Dunnbier U, Reilich C, Stan HJ (1997). Detection of drugs and drug metabolites in ground water samples of a drinking water treatment plant. Fresenius Environ. Bull. 6: 438–443.

[27] Cleuvers M (2004). Mixture toxicity of the anti-inflammatory drugs diclofenac, ibuprofen, naproxen, and acetylsalicylic acid. Ecotoxicol Environ Saf. 59(3): 309-15.

[28] De Liguoro M, Fioretto B, Poltronieri C, Gallina G (2009). The toxicity of sulfamethazine to *Daphnia magna* and its additivity to other veterinary sulfonamides and trimethoprim. Chemosphere 75(11): 1519–1524.

[29] Fent K, Weston AA, Caminada D (2006). Ecotoxicology of human pharmaceuticals Aquatic Toxicology 76(2): 122–159.

[30] Rocha R, Gonçalves F, Marques C, Nunes B (2014). Environmental effects of anticholinesterasic therapeutic drug on a crustacean species, Daphnia magna. Environ Sci Pollut Res 21: 4418–4429.

[31] Nunes B, Barbosa AR, Antunes SC, Gonçalves F (2014). Combination effects of anticholinesterasics in acetylcholinesterase of a fish species: effects of a metallic compound, an organophosphate pesticide and a pharmaceutical drug. Environmental Science and Pollution Research 21(9): 6258-62.

[32] Kümmerer K (2009). Antibiotics in the aquatic environment – A review – Part II Chemosphere 75(4): 435–441.

[33] Wright GD (2010). Antibiotic resistance in the environment: a link to the clinic? Current Opinion in Microbiology 13(5): 589–594.

[34] Finley R, Collignon P, Larsson JDG, McEwen S, Li X-Z, Gaze WH, Reid-Smith R, Timinouni M, Graham D, Topp E (2013). The Scourge of Antibiotic Resistance: The Important Role of the Environment. Clinical Infectious Diseases 57(5): 704-710.

[35] Zhang X-X, Zhang T, Fang HHP (2009). Antibiotic resistance genes in water environment. Appl Microbiol Biotechnol 82:397–414.

[36] Liu Z-H, Ogejo JA, Pruden M, Knowlton KF (2011). Occurrence, fate and removal of synthetic oral contraceptives (SOCs) in the natural environment: A review. Science of The Total Environment 409(24): 5149–5161.

[37] Arcand-Hoy LD, Nimrod AC, Benson WH (1998). Endocrine-modulating substances in the environment: estrogenic effects of pharmaceutical products. International Journal of Toxicology 17 (2): 139-158.

[38] Runnalls TJ, Margiotta-Casaluci L, Kugathas S, Sumpter JP (2010). Pharmaceuticals in the Aquatic Environment: Steroids and Anti-Steroids as High Priorities for Research. Human and Ecological Risk Assessment 16: 1318–1338.

[39] Hogan NS, Lean DRS, Trudeau VL (2006). Exposures to estradiol, ethinylestradiol, and octylphenol affect survival and growth of *Rana pipiens* and *Rana sylvatica* tadpoles. Journal of Toxicology and Environmental Health, Part A 69 (16): 1555-1569.

[40] Larsson DGJ, Adolfsson-Erici M, Parkkonen J, Pettersson M, Berg AH, Olsson P-E, Forlin L (1999). Ethinylestradiol - an undesired fish contraceptive? Aquatic Toxicology (1999), 45 (2-3), 91-97.

[41] Jobling S, Williams R, Johnson A, Taylor A, Gross-Sorokin M, Nolan M, Tyler CR van Aerle R, Santos E, Brighty G (2006). Predicted exposures to steroid estrogens in U.K. rivers correlate with widespread sexual disruption in wild fish populations. Environmental health perspectives 114 (1): 32-9.

[42] Ciocan CM, Cubero-Leon E, Puinean AM, Hill EM, Minier C, Osada M, Fenlon K, Rotchell JM (2010). Effects of estrogen exposure in mussels, *Mytilus edulis*, at different stages of gametogenesis. Environmental Pollution 158(9): 2977–2984.

[43] Souza MS, Hallgren P, Balseiro E, Lars-Anders Hansson L-A (2013). Low concentrations, potential ecological consequences: Synthetic estrogens alter life-history and demographic structures of aquatic invertebrates. Environmental Pollution 178: 237–243.

[44] Velasco-Santamaría YM, Bjerregaard P, Kor B (2013). Evidence of small modulation of ethinylestradiol induced effects by concurrent exposure to trenbolone in male eelpout *Zoarces viviparous*. Environmental Pollution 178: 189–196.

[45] Carlsson G, Patring J, Kreuger J, Norrgren L, Oskarsson A (2013). Toxicity of 15 veterinary pharmaceuticals in zebrafish (*Danio rerio*) embryos. Aquatic Toxicology 126: 30– 41.

[46] Minagh E, Hernan R, O'Rourke K, Lyng FM, Davoren M (2009). Aquatic ecotoxicity of the selective serotonin reuptake inhibitor sertraline hydrochloride in a battery of freshwater test species. Ecotoxicology and Environmental Safety 72(2): 434–440.

[47] Barbosa IR, Nogueira AJA, Soares AMVM (2008). Acute and chronic effects of testosterone and 4-hydroxyandrostenedione to the crustacean *Daphnia magna*. Ecotoxicology and Environmental Safety 71(3): 757–764.

[48] Sung H-H, Chiu Y-W, Wang S-Y, Chen C-M, Huang D-J (2014). Acute toxicity of mixture of acetaminophen and ibuprofen to Green Neon Shrimp, *Neocaridina denticulate*. Environmental Toxicology and Pharmacology 38(1): 8–13.

[49] Collard HJ, Ji K, Lee S, Liu X, Kang S, Kho Y, Ahn B, Ryu J, Lee J, Choi K (2013) Toxicity and endocrine disruption in zebrafish (*Danio rerio*) and two freshwater invertebrates (*Daphnia magna* and *Moina macrocopa*) after chronic exposure to mefenamic acid. Ecotoxicology and Environmental Safety 94: 80–86.

[50] Nunes B, Carvalho F, Guilhermino L (2005). Acute toxicity of widely used pharmaceuticals in aquatic species: *Gambusia holbrooki, Artemia parthenogenetica* and *Tetraselmis chuii*. Ecotoxicology and Environmental Safety 61 (3): 413 – 419.

[51] Emblidge JP, DeLorenzo ME (2006). Preliminary risk assessment of the lipid-regulating pharmaceutical clofibric acid, for three estuarine species. Environmental Research 100(2): 216–226.

[52] Ferreira CSG, Nunes B, Henriques-Almeida JMM, Guilhermino L (2007). Acute toxicity of oxytetracycline and florfenicol to the microalgae *Tetraselmis chuii* and to the crustacean *Artemia parthenogenetica*. Ecotoxicology and Environmental Safety 67 (2007) 452–458.

[53] Madureira TV, Cruzeiro C, Rocha MJ, Rocha E (2011). The toxicity potential of pharmaceuticals found in the Douro River estuary (Portugal)—Experimental assessment using a zebrafish embryo test. Environmental Toxicology and Pharmacology 32(2): 212–217.

[54] Ambili TR, Saravanan M, Ramesh M, Abhijith DB, Poopal RK (2013). Toxicological Effects of the Antibiotic Oxytetracycline to an Indian Major Carp *Labeo rohita*. Archives of Environmental Contamination and Toxicology 64(3): 494-503.

[55] Berninger JP, Du B, Connors KA, Eytcheson SA, Kolkmeier MA, Prosser KN, Valenti Jr TW, Chambliss CK, Brooks BW (2011). Effects of the antihistamine diphenhydramine on selected aquatic organisms. Environmental Toxicology and Chemistry 30(9): 2065–2072.

[56] Nunes B, Pinto G, Martins L, Gonçalves F, Antunes SC (2014). Biochemical and Standard Toxic Effects of Acetaminophen on the Macrophyte Species *Lemna minor* and *Lemna gibba*. Environmental Science and Pollution Research 21(18): 10815-10822.

[57] Brandão FP, Pereira JL, Gonçalves F, Nunes B (2011). The impact of paracetamol on selected biomarkers of the mollusc species *Corbicula fluminea*. Environmental Toxicology: 1-10.

[58] Antunes SC, Freitas R, Figueira E, Gonçalves F, Nunes B (2013). Biochemical Effects of Acetaminophen in Aquatic Species: Edible Clams *Venerupis decussata* and *Venerupis philippinarum*. Environmental Science and Pollution Research Environmental Science and Pollution Research 20 (9): 6658-6666

[59] Ramos AS, Correia AT, Antunes S, Gonçalves F, Nunes B (2014). Effect of Acetaminophen Exposure in *Oncorhynchus mykiss* Gills and Liver: Detoxification Mechanisms, Oxidative Defence System and Peroxidative Damage. Environmental Toxicology and Pharmacology 37(3): 1221–1228.

[60] Ragugnetti M, Adams ML, Guimarães ATB, Sponchiado G, Vasconcelos EC, Oliveira CMR (2011). Ibuprofen Genotoxicity in Aquatic Environment: An Experimental Model Using Oreochromis niloticus. Water Air Soil Poll 218(1-4): 361-364

[61] Zounkova R, Kovalova L, Blaha L, Dott W (2010). Ecotoxicity and genotoxicity assessment of cytotoxic antineoplastic drugs and their metabolites. Chemosphere 81(2): 253-60.

[62] Temussi F, DellaGreca M, Pistillo P, Previtera L, Zarrelli A, Criscuolo E, Lavorgna M, Russo C, Isidori M (2013). Sildenafil and tadalafil in simulated chlorination conditions: Ecotoxicity of drugs and their derivatives. Sci Total Environ 463–464: 366–373.

[63] Hedgespeth ML, Nilsson PA, Berglund O (2014). Ecological implications of altered fish foraging after exposure to an antidepressant pharmaceutical. Aquatic Toxicology 151: 84–87.

[64] Brandão FP, Rodrigues S, Castro BB, Gonçalves F, Antunes SC, Nunes B (2013). Short-term effects of neuroactive pharmaceutical drugs on a fish species: biochemical and behavioural effects. Aquatic Toxicology 144-145: 218-229.

[65] Bossus MC, Guler YZ, Short SJ, Morrison ER, Ford AT (2014). Behavioural and transcriptional changes in the amphipod *Echinogammarus marinus* exposed to two antidepressants, fluoxetine and sertraline. Aquatic Toxicology 151: 46–56.

[66] Nieto E, Blasco J, González-Ortegón E, Drake P, Hampel M (2013). Is *Atyaephyra desmarestii* a useful candidate for lethal and sub-lethal toxicity tests on pharmaceutical compounds? Journal of Hazardous Materials 263 Part 1: 256–265.

[67] Conners DE, Rogers ED, Armbrust KL, Kwon J-W, Black MC (2009). Growth and development of tadpoles (*Xenopus laevis*) exposed to selective serotonin reuptake inhibitors, fluoxetine and sertraline, throughout metamorphosis. Environmental Toxicology and Chemistry 28(12): 2671–2676.

[68] Ford AT (2014). From gender benders to brain benders (and beyond!). Aquatic Toxicology 151: 1–3.

[69] Ji K, Liu X, Lee S, Kang S, Kho Y, Giesy JP, Choi K (2013). Effects of non-steroidal anti-inflammatory drugs on hormones and genes of the hypothalamic-pituitary-gonad axis, and reproduction of zebrafish. Journal of Hazardous Materials 254–255: 242–251.

[70] Hutchinson TH (2002). Reproductive and developmental effects of endocrine disrupters in invertebrates: in vitro and in vivo approaches. Toxicology Letters 131(1–2): 75–81.

[71] Mennigen JA, Stroud P, Zamora JM, Moon TW, Trudeau VL (2011). Pharmaceuticals as Neuroendocrine Disruptors: Lessons Learned from Fish on Prozac. Journal of Toxicology and Environmental Health, Part B, 14:387–412.

[72] Waye A, Trudeau VL (2011). Neuroendocrine Disruption: More than Hormones Are Upset. Journal of Toxicology and Environmental Health, Part B, 14: 270–291.

[73] van der Ven K, Keil D, Moens LN, Van Hummelen P, van Remortel P, Maras M, De Coen W (2006). Effects of the antidepressant mianserin in zebrafish: Molecular markers of endocrine disruption. Chemosphere 65: 1836–1845.

[74] Mennigen JA, Lado WE, Zamora JM, Duarte-Guterman P, Langlois VS, Metcalfe CD, Chang JP, Moon TW, Vance L. Trudeau VL (2010). Waterborne fluoxetine disrupts the reproductive axis in sexually mature male goldfish, Carassius *auratus*. Aquatic Toxicology 100(4): 354–364.

[75] Kim PG, Park Y, Ji K, Seo J, Lee S, Choi K, Kho Y, Park J, Choi K (2012). Effect of chronic exposure to acetaminophen and lincomycin on Japanese medaka (Oryzias latipes) and freshwater cladocerans *Daphnia magna* and *Moina macrocopa*, and potential mechanisms of endocrine disruption. Chemosphere 89(1): 10–18.

[76] Isidori M, Bellotta M, Cangiano M, Alfredo Parrella A (2009). Estrogenic activity of pharmaceuticals in the aquatic environment. Environment International 35: 826–829.

[77] Vandegehuchte MB, Janssen CR (2011). Epigenetics and its implications for ecotoxicology. Ecotoxicology 20: 607–624

[78] Vandegehuchte MB, Lemière F, Janssen CR (2009). Quantitative DNA-methylation in *Daphnia magna* and effects of multigeneration Zn exposure. Comp Biochem Phys C 150: 343–348.

[79] Vandegehuchte MB, De Coninck D, Vandenbrouck T, De Coen WM, Janssen CR (2010a) Gene transcription profiles, global DNA methylation and potential transgenerational epigenetic effects related to Zn exposure history in *Daphnia magna*. Environ Poll 158: 3323-3329.

[80] Vandegehuchte MB, Lemière F, Vanhaecke L, Vanden Berghe W, Janssen CR (2010b). Direct and transgenerational impact on *Daphnia magna* of chemicals with a known effect on DNA methylation. Comp Biochem Phys C 151: 278–285

[81] Miner BE, De Meester L, Pfrender ME, Lampert W, Hairston Jr NG (2012). Linking genes to communities and ecosystems: Daphnia as an ecogenomic model. Proc. R. Soc. B 279: 1873–1882.

[82] Wirgin I, Waldman JR (2004). Resistance to contaminants in North American fish populations. Mut Res 552: 73–100.

[83] Hinfray N, Baudiffier D, Leal MC, Porcher JM, Aït-Aïssa S, Le Gac F, Schulz RW, Brion F (2011). Characterization of testicular expression of P450 17$\alpha$-hydroxylase, 17,20-lyase in zebrafish and its perturbation by the pharmaceutical fungicide clotrimazole. Gen Comp Endocrinol. 174(3):309-17.

[84] Thomas MA, Klaper RD (2012). Psychoactive Pharmaceuticals Induce Fish Gene Expression Profiles Associated with Human Idiopathic Autism. PLoS ONE 7(6): e32917. doi:10.1371/journal.pone.0032917

[85] Nunes B (2011). The Use of Cholinesterases in Ecotoxicology. Rev Environ Contam T 212: 29-59.

[86] Sánchez-Bayo F, Goka K (2005). Unexpected effects of zinc pyrithione and imidacloprid on Japanese medaka fish (*Oryzias latipes*). Aquat Toxicol. 74(4): 285-93.

[87] Bellas J, Granmo A, Beiras R (2005). Embryotoxicity of the antifouling biocide zinc pyrithione to sea urchin (*Paracentrotus lividus*) and mussel (*Mytilus edulis*). Mar Pollut Bull 50(11): 1382–1385.

[88] Mochida K, Ito K, Harino H, Kakuno A, Fuji K (2006). Acute toxicity of pyrithione antifouling biocides and joint toxicity with copper to red sea bream (Pagrus major) and toy shrimp (Heptacarpus futilirostris). Environ Toxicol Chem 25(11): 3058–3064.

[89] Onduka T, Mochida K, Harino H, Ito K, Kakuno A, Fujii K (2010). Toxicity of metal pyrithione photodegradation products to marine organisms with indirect evidence for their presence in seawater. Arch Environ Contam Toxicol 58(4): 991–997.

[90] Mochida K, Ito K, Harino H, Tanaka H, Onduka T, Kakuno A, Fujii K (2009). Inhibition of acetylcholinesterase by metabolites of copper pyrithione (CuPT) and its possible involvement in vertebral deformity of a CuPT-exposed marine teleostean fish. Comp Biochem Phys C 149(4): 624–630.

[91] Mennigen JA, Sassine J, Trudeau VL, Moon TW (2010b). Waterborne fluoxetine disrupts feeding and energy metabolism in the goldfish *Carassius auratus*. Aquatic Toxicology 100(1): 128–137.

[92] Schmidt W, Rainville L-C, McEneff G, Sheehan D, Quinn B (2014). A proteomic evaluation of the effects of the pharmaceuticals diclofenac and gemfibrozil on marine mussels (*Mytilus* spp.): evidence for chronic sublethal effects on stress-response proteins. Drug Testing and Analysis 6: 210–219.

[93] Luna TO, Plautz SC, Salice CJ (2013). Effects of 17$\alpha$-ethynylestradiol, fluoxetine, and the mixture on life history traits and population growth rates in a freshwater gastropod. Environmental Toxicology and Chemistry 32(12): 2771–2778.

[94] Brinke M, Heininger P, Traunspurger W (2013). Effects of a bioassay-derived ivermectin lowest observed effect concentration on life-cycle traits of the nematode *Caenorhabditis elegans*. Ecotoxicology 22:148–155.

[95] Han S, Choi K, Kim J, Ji K, Kim S, Ahn B, Yun J, Choi K, Khim JS, Zhang X, Giesy JP (2010). Endocrine disruption and consequences of chronic exposure to ibuprofen in Japanese medaka (*Oryzias latipes*) and freshwater cladocerans *Daphnia magna* and *Moina macrocopa*. Aquatic Toxicology 98(3): 256–264.

[96] Hazelton PD, Du B, Haddad SP, Fritts AK, Chambliss CK, Brooks BW, Bringolf RB (2014). Chronic fluoxetine exposure alters movement and burrowing in adult freshwater mussels. Aquatic Toxicology 151: 27–35.

Chapter 7

# Estrogenic Compounds in Estuarine and Coastal Water Environments of the Iberian Western Atlantic Coast and Selected Locations Worldwide — Relevancy, Trends and Challenges in View of the EU Water Framework Directive

Maria João Rocha and Eduardo Rocha

Additional information is available at the end of the chapter

http://dx.doi.org/10.5772/59885

## 1. Introduction

Water is vital to life and thus its availability and quality has increasingly been the object of intense concern and disputes by multiple agents that include from people directly relying on ecological services, or simply living in impacted zones, to influential non-governmental environmental organizations and regulatory governmental authorities. The scientific community has increasingly intervened, particularly through the production of sound diagnostic and mechanistic data and also prognostic models, which fundamentally rely on both chemical and biological environmental monitoring. Despite the global increasing of pollution and its impacts, it appears that there is an uncontrollable expansion of anthropogenic activities, mainly in countries where there are no strict environmental policies. Therefore, pollution continues to negatively affect the quality of water and, in consequence, the vast ecosystems associated with it. Presently, it is estimated that hundreds of new chemicals with harmful potential are recorded daily in the CAS® (Chemical Abstracts Service, http://www.cas.org/cashome). Thus, the subject "Water Quality" has been the target of many reflections, particularly in Europe, where in general, all state members of the European Union (EU) have shown their concern about the near future possibility of water shortages, for all, both in quantity and quality [1]. Related to this aspect, it is also recognized as of major importance the need to protect biodiversity and natural ecosystems; an example of such recognition is depicted in the 2012 European Parliament resolution on the "EU Biodiversity Strategy 2020" [2].

In line with the referred intentions, at the beginning of the millennium the EU adopted legislation — the EU "Water Framework Directive" (WFD) [3] — that was considered very innovative at the time. The WFD called for a comprehensive and integrated approach of water protection and management, having as its ultimate goal that all European waters (continental surface waters, transitional waters, coastal waters and groundwaters) reached good chemical and ecological status within a 15 years period, since the date of publication of that directive. To achieve these requirements, temporal incremental goals were established amongst all EU states to ensure the success of this program. Thus, it was decided *inter alia* to: (*i*) apply all necessary measures to avoid the damage of superficial water bodies; (*ii*) impose fines on violators responsible for deteriorating the status of surface water bodies; (*iii*) achieve good ecological and chemical status for all artificial or heavily modified water bodies; (*iv*) progressively reduce the pollution of priority compounds, some of these focused in this Chapter, by limiting their emissions, their discharge and/or runoff into the environment.

However, as the water situation in each EU state was different and unique, since 2000 and up to the present, it has been necessary to make adjustments to overcome this aspect. Indeed, just one year after the WFD 2000/60/EC publication, this directive was updated [4]. In the renovated document (2455/2001/EC), among other measures, it was published a list containing thirty-three harmful compounds which presence in surface waters should be limited or at least/ reduced under limit values [4]. Among these compounds stands out the persistent organic pollutants (POPs), such as, pesticides, polycyclic aromatic hydrocarbons and alkylphenols. Later, the number of harmful compounds were expanded up to forty five and additional environmental quality standards were included in (2008/105/EC) [5]. Nonetheless, because further toxicity details each pollutant are becoming known, the number of compounds in the WFD list tends to increase. In this vein, the current directive 2013/39/EU integrates new substances in its watch lists [6]. Among those are EDCs such as the extremely potent 17β-oestradiol ($E_2$) and 17α-ethinylestradiol ($EE_2$), as discussed in this Chapter.

## 2. Estrogenic endocrine disrupting compounds in surface waters

Accordingly to the National Institute of Environmental Health Sciences (USA), endocrine disrupting compounds are natural or man-made compounds that may mimic or interfere with the function of hormones in the body, producing a variety of adverse effects over the reproductive, the neurological and the immune systems of humans and both domestic and wild animals [7]. In the case of EDCs with oestrogenic activity, these substances can act: (*i*) on the hypothalamus, inhibiting the release of gonadotropin releasing hormones [8]; (*ii*) on the pituitary, inhibiting the release of gonadotropins [8]; (*iii*) on the gonads, interfering with the production of steroid hormones, namely $E_2$ [9]; (*iv*) on the circulation of endogenous hormones, as these compounds have the ability to bind to the same plasmatic carriers [8]; (*v*) on the same cellular receptors used by the endogenous hormones causing important structural changes [10]. In males of various fish species, situations of *ovotestis*, *i.e.*, presence of oocytes in testes, were reported in polluted systems that include some in Portugal [11].

http://dx.doi.org/10.5772/59885

Here, it is exposed the environmental concentrations of sixteen oestrogenic EDCs, which were chosen taking in account the following features: (*i*) *in vivo* and *in vitro* potency, such as the natural oestrogens and $EE_2$ [12]; (*ii*) abundance in terms of incidence and concentration), such as bisphenol A and the alkylphenols (and their ethoxylates) [13, 14], and (*iii*) the ubiquitous, but paradoxically less studied, phytoestrogens [14, 15].

## 2.1. Oestrogens

### 2.1.1. *Main characteristics and environmental origins*

Both natural and synthetic oestrogens, including oestrone ($E_1$), $E_2$ and $EE_2$ (Figure 1) may induce, even in low (ng/L) concentrations, from mild to extremely harmful effects over the endocrine system [16]. In particular, these compounds have been associated with the occurrence of endocrine disorders such as those over the reproductive system of a wide range of species, including molluscs, crustaceans, fish, birds and mammals [17-22]. Another disruption effect observed in animals, collected from waters containing high levels of oestrogenic contamination, is the decrease of their immune system responses disorders [23]; this phenomenon also seems to occur when humans are exposed to the same type of EDCs [24, 25]. These observations, together with the abovementioned facts, justified the recent incorporation of these compounds in the WFD watching lists [6]. In this sense, and in order to be aware about the concentrations of $E_1$, $E_2$ and $EE_2$ in surface waters, studies were initiated to monitor their presence and appraise their temporal evolution. It is known that the primary sources of these three EDCs are their excretion by urine and faeces [26]. So, these compounds reach the rivers, estuaries and coastlines either through the discharge of effluents coming from sewage treatment plants (STPs) — or directly from sewages (hence untreated) that deliver their content into waterways.

| Class | Example | Chemical structure | Origin |
|---|---|---|---|
| Natural oestrogens | Oestrone ($E_1$) | 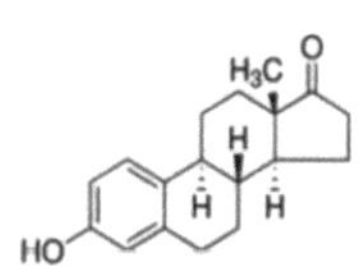 | Urine and faeces excretion [26]. |
| | 17β-Oestradiol ($E_2$) | 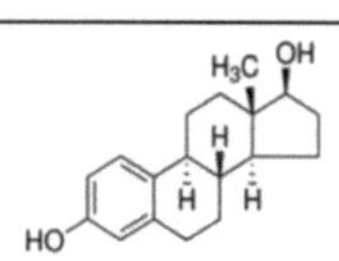 | |
| Synthetic oestrogens | 17α-Ethinylestradiol ($EE_2$) | 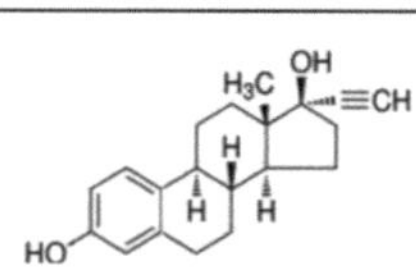 | Urine and faeces of women consuming birth control pills [26]. |

**Figure 1.** Natural and synthetic oestrogens included ($E_2$ and $EE_2$) or to be included ($E_1$) in the watch list of compounds under surveillance by the WFD [6].

Although the concentrations of the referred EDCs are typically in the order of few ng/L (Table 1), it has been experimentally proven that such amounts are potentially harmful [12]. For example, just 4 ng/L of $E_2$ resulted in the formation of *ovotestis* in male Japanese medaka (*Oryzias latipes*) [27]. Also the male mummichog (*Fundulus heteroclitus*) exposed to 100 ng/L of $EE_2$ showed a large increase in the gonadosomatic index, decrease in testosterone production and liver synthesis of vitellogenin [28].

### *2.1.2. Oestrogens in surface waters*

The highest concentrations of $E_1$ in surface waters were reported in Japan (Tama River) [29], Taiwan (Shui-Dan River) [30] and, China (Pearl Rivers) [31, 32] where its levels ranged from78.7 ng/L to 85.6 ng/L. The highest amounts of $E_2$ were measured in Italy (Venice Lagoon), Japan (Tama River) and Taiwan (Shui-Dan River) where its levels ranged from12 ng/L to175 ng/L. Finally the highest levels of $EE_2$ were found in Spain (Ebre River) [33], China (Pearl Rivers) [31, 32] and Italy (Venice Lagoon) [34] where its levels ranged from 34 to 130 ng/L. From the *in vivo* and *in vitro* experiments referred in section 3.1.1., among many other, it is concluded that those levels are environmental conditions for the occurrence of endocrine disrupting events. In north/central Europe, the surface water concentrations of these compounds are typically lower than those described in Asia and Brazil (Table 1). Even so, significant biological impacts associated with pollution were detected in Europe. For example, roach (*Rutilus rutilus*) and gudgeon (*Gobio gobio*) males caught in rivers and estuaries of the United Kingdom showed high occurrence of *ovotestis* [35-38]. In Portugal, in the early 2000s, *ovotestis* was observed in flounder (*Platichthys flesus*) and mullets (*Mugil cephalus*) caught from Douro estuary [11]. However, as it can be seen from Table 1, at that time no information existed about the degree of oestrogenic contamination in Iberian western Atlantic coast surface waters - this led to our integrated studies shown in this Chapter, which first data were published in 2009 (Table 2).

| EDC | Sampling area | Concentration (ng/L) | References |
|---|---|---|---|
| | Estuarine and coastal waters, The Netherlands | 0.1 - 3.4 | [26] |
| | Scheldt Estuary, Belgium – The Netherlands | ND - 10.0 | [39] |
| | The Netherlands (surface water) | <0.30 - 7.2 | [40] |
| | Rivers in Germany | 0.10 - 4.1 | [41] |
| | Coastal area of Baltic Sea, Germany | 0.08 - 0.54 | [42] |
| | Seine River, France | 1.0 - 3.2 | [43] |
| $E_1$ | Tiber River, Italy | 5.0 - 12 | [44] |
| | Venice Lagoon, Italy | <1.20 - 10 | [34] |
| | Ebro River, Spain | ND - 4.9 | [56] |
| | Llobregat River, Spain | <LOD - 22 | [45] |
| | Llobregat River, Spain | 0.82 - 5.81 | [46] |
| | Thermaikos Gulf, Nothern Aegean Sea, Greece | <LOD | [47] |
| | Buyukcekme watershed, Istambul, Turkey | 1.40 - 5.74 | [48] |

http://dx.doi.org/10.5772/59885

| EDC | Sampling area | Concentration (ng/L) | References |
|---|---|---|---|
| | Acushnet Estuary, USA | 0.73 - 1.20 | [49] |
| | South Florida, USA | 0.88 - 5.20 | [50] |
| | Brazilian surface water | ND - 39 | [51] |
| | Tama River, Japan | 6.4 - 85.6 | [29] |
| | Dan-Shui River, Taiwan | 22.4 - 66.2 | [30] |
| | Yellow River, China | ND - 15.6 | [52] |
| | Pearl rivers, South China | ND - 78.7 | [31, 32] |
| | Yangtze River estuary, China | ND - 1.43 | [53] |
| | Songhua River, Northern China | ND - 3.05 | [54] |
| | Tamagawa River, Japan | 3.4 - 6.6 | [55] |
| $E_2$ | Estuarine and coastal waters, The Netherlands | 0.3 - 5.5 | [26] |
| | Scheldt Estuary, Belgium - The Netherlands | ND | [39] |
| | The Netherlands (surface water) | <0.8 - 1.0 | [40] |
| | Rivers in Germany | 0.15 - 2.0 | [41] |
| | Coastal area of Baltic Sea, Germany | ND | [42] |
| | Seine River, France | 1.0 - 3.2 | [43] |
| | Tiber River, Italy | 2.0 - 6.0 | [44] |
| | Ebro River, Spain | ND - 1.9 | [56] |
| | Llobregat River, Spain | ND | [46] |
| | Thermaikos Gulf, Nothern Aegean Sea, Greece | ND | [47] |
| | Buyukcekme watershed, Istambul, Turkey | 1.10 - 5.39 | [48] |
| | Acushnet Estuary, USA | 0.56 - 0.83 | [49] |
| | South Florida, USA | ND - 1.80 | [50] |
| | Brazilian surface water | ND - 7.3 | [51] |
| | Tama River, Japan | 0.5 - 12 | [29] |
| | Dan-Shui River, Taiwan | 1.4 - 33.9 | [30] |
| | Yellow River, China | ND - 2.3 | [52] |
| | Pearl rivers, South China | ND - 7.72 | [32] |
| | Yangtze River estuary, China | ND - 1.4 | [53] |
| | Songhua River, Northern China | ND - 1.16 | [54] |
| | Tamagawa River, Japan | 0.6 - 1.0 | [55] |
| $EE_2$ | Estuarine and coastal waters, The Netherlands | 0.1 - 4.3 | [26] |
| | Scheldt Estuary, Belgium – The Netherlands | ND | [39] |
| | The Netherlands (surface water) | <0.3 - 0.4 | [40] |
| | Rivers in Germany | 0.1 - 5.1 | [41] |
| | Coastal area of Baltic Sea, Germany | ND - 17.9 | [42] |
| | Seine River, France | 1.0 - 4.0 | [43] |

| EDC | Sampling area | Concentration (ng/L) | References |
|---|---|---|---|
| | Ebro River, Spain | 30 - 130 | [33] |
| | Ebro River, Spain | ND | [56] |
| | Llobregat River, Spain | ND | [46] |
| | Tiber River, Italy | ND - 1.0 | [44] |
| | Venice Lagoon, Italy | <1.0 34 | [34] |
| | Thermaikos Gulf, Nothern Aegean Sea, Greece | ND | [47] |
| | Buyukcekme watershed, Istambul, Turkey | 11.7 - 14.0 | [48] |
| | Acushnet Estuary, USA | 3.01 - 4.67 | [49] |
| | South Florida, USA | NA | [50] |
| | Brazilian surface water | ND - 25 | [51] |
| | Tama River, Japan | < 0.20 | [29] |
| | Dan-Shui River, Taiwan | 7.53 - 27.4 | [30] |
| | Yellow River, China | NA | [52] |
| | Pearl rivers, South China | ND - 53.4 | [31, 32] |
| | Songhua River, Northern China | ND | [54] |
| | Yangtze River estuary, China | ND - 0.11 | [53] |

NA: Not Available. ND: Not Detected. LOD: Limit of Detection.

**Table 1.** Concentrations of oestrogens in surface waters (minimum-maximum) measured in surface waters worldwide.

### *2.1.3. Oestrogens in surface waters from the west Iberian coast (Portugal)*

Being Portugal one of the EU members that signed the commitment with the European Commission (EC) to accomplish the directives referred in the WFD document, systematic efforts have been made by our research group to develop and validate methods adequate to the measurement of EDCs in complex environmental matrices (seawater, estuarine and river waters). Also, a complementary effort has been dedicated to both gather all monitoring data and address their potential risk. In this sense, the evaluations done in Portuguese surface waters warned about risks of environmental impacts of oestrogens and can assist the competent authorities to take measures to prevent and clean up these habitats from having EDCs, either by eliminating or at least put them at concentrations below those know to be able to promote biological adverse effects.

The results revealed that the average amounts of oestrogens in Portuguese superficial waters were ≈ 6 ng/L for $E_1$ and ≈ 10 ng/L for $E_2$ and $EE_2$. These concentrations, accordingly with the *in vivo* studies referred previously (section 3.1.1.) are not only able of causing disruptive effects in aquatic animals, but also even induce negative impacts in human health [25, 57]. The findings become additionally relevant in view of the fact that these habitats are commonly used by residents and/or tourists, both for recreational and fishing purposes.

Analyzing the values of Table 2, and concerning the concentrations of all evaluated oestrogens, it concluded that habitats we studied so far have chemical quality deficiencies. Table 2 also

http://dx.doi.org/10.5772/59885

points that each analysed geographical zone had quite diverse minimum-maximal amounts. This fact corresponds to spatial differences among sampling sites, in line with the presence/absence of STPs effluents and domestic discharges in the sampled areas. The last inference is directly correlated with the data obtained in the latest national *census*, which revealed a high number of houses (over 17,000) without any sort of connection to sewers [58]. Beyond this, there is also an additional factor that is the huge number of tourists that seasonally arrive to several studied zones located in both west and south of the Iberian Peninsula [59, 60]. Due to drastic increases of the number of inhabitants, that may rise up to 50%, mainly in summer the concentration of oestrogens in surface waters raised significantly, causing seasonal damages in local biota. So, it becomes clear that the physicochemical parameters typically used to assess the quality of surface waters (i.e., temperature, pH, dissolved $O_2$, nitrites, nitrates and phosphates) are not sufficient to guarantee the protection of both environmental and human health.

Comparing the values compiled in Tables 1 and 2 it is concluded that, in general, the levels of oestrogens tend to be higher in the west Iberian Peninsula than in the rest of central/north Europe. In fact, in average, these substances in the current study area are almost similar to those measured in many Asian countries. Despite this, it is exalted the positive efforts of remediation conducted in some Portuguese environments, such as those produced in the Ave River, considered in the past as one of the most polluted of Europe [61]. There are also commendable the important efforts occurred in the Douro River estuary [62]. In fact, since our first monitoring studies in the last estuary it was possible to observe that the surface waters collected in 2005 [63] contained significantly higher amounts of oestrogens than those collected in 2009, a fact that demonstrates an important improvement of water quality [62]. Unfortunately, because there are no other data prior to 2005, with regard to the levels of $E_1$, $E_2$ and $EE_2$ in other Portuguese aquatic systems it is not possible yet to establish with certainty, trend lines relating to a progressive decrease in the concentrations of these EDCs in Portuguese surface waters. In spite of this, other important data provided by our studies demonstrate that: (*i*) several areas commonly seen as "pristine" (e.g., the Mira River) contain high levels of those oestrogens (*unpublished data*); (*ii*) there is an underestimation of the efficacy of the STPs, which at times are not adequately dimensioned, namely for coping with seasonal/touristic influxes; (*iii*) currents from both Atlantic Ocean and/or estuaries can channel pollutants, such as these oestrogens, towards protected areas (e.g., the natural reserve of the Sado River estuary) [59]. From Table 1 it is observed that also in Spain, particularly in the Ebro River for $EE_2$ [33, 56], there are efforts that seem to have been effective in reducing the environmental amounts of these EDCs.

The data repertoire summarized in Table 2 for $E_1$, $E_2$, and $EE_2$ is one of more systematic ones available in the international literature about the oestrogenic status of a particular European country. This information, which can be viewed as a benchmark for the concentrations of oestrogens in Portuguese waters, makes it possible to everybody to monitor the effectiveness of the implementation of measures that may lead to the reduction of environmental levels of those EDCs along the time.

| EDC | Sampling area | Concentration (ng/L) | References |
|---|---|---|---|
| | Lima River estuary and Atlantic coast of Viana-Castelo | 4.6 - 36.3 | [64] |
| | Ave River estuary and Atlantic coast of Vila-Conde | 0.5 - 7.2 | [61] |
| | Leça River estuary and Atlantic coast of Porto | 4.9 - 10.4 | [65] |
| | Douro River estuary | <15 - 113 | [63] |
| | Douro River estuary and Atlantic coast of Porto | 1.5 - 4.6 | [62] |
| $E_1$ | Mondego River estuary | <5.0 | [66] |
| | Mondego River and its estuary | 1.0 - 14.6 | [67] |
| | Tagus River and its estuary | ≈ 2 - ≈ 6 | *Unpublished* |
| | Sado River and its estuary | 1.0 - 9.8 | [59] |
| | Mira River and its estuary | ≈ 3 - ≈ 12 | *Unpublished* |
| | Ria Formosa | 1.0 - 2.0 | [60] |
| | Lima River estuary and Atlantic coast of Viana-Castelo | 2.4 - 24.4 | [64] |
| | Ave River estuary and Atlantic coast of Vila-Conde | 1.6 - 9.4 | [61] |
| | Leça River estuary and Atlantic coast of Porto | 3.3 - 5.9 | [65] |
| | Douro River estuary | <7.0 | [63] |
| | Douro River estuary and Atlantic coast of Porto | 5.4 - 8.5 | [62] |
| $E_2$ | Mondego River estuary | <3.0 | [66] |
| | Mondego River and its estuary | 1.5 - 18.4 | [67] |
| | Tagus River and its estuary | ≈ 3 - ≈ 20 | *Unpublished* |
| | Sado River and its estuary | 1.2 - 10.8 | [59] |
| | Mira River and its estuary | ≈ 4 - ≈ 62 | *Unpublished* |
| | Ria Formosa | 1.3 - 10.1 | [60] |
| | Lima River estuary and Atlantic coast of Viana-Castelo | 0.3 - 19.4 | [64] |
| | Ave River estuary and Atlantic coast of Vila-Conde | 0.3 - 20.4 | [61] |
| | Leça River estuary and Atlantic coast of Porto | 2.1 - 4.4 | [65] |
| | Douro River estuary | 18 - 102 | [63] |
| | Douro River estuary and Atlantic coast of Porto | <1.3 - 4.5 | [62] |
| $EE_2$ | Mondego River estuary | <12 | [66] |
| | Mondego River and its estuary | 0.3 - 11.3 | [67] |
| | Tagus River and its estuary | ≈ 4 - ≈ 20 | *Unpublished* |
| | Sado River and its estuary | 1.1 - 3.2 | [59] |
| | Mira River and its estuary | ≈ 4 - ≈ 67 | *Unpublished* |
| | Ria Formosa | 12.1 - 25.0 | [60] |

**Table 2.** Concentrations (minimum–maximum) of natural and pharmaceutical oestrogens in Portuguese surface waters.

http://dx.doi.org/10.5772/59885

## 2.2. Industrial and household products

### *2.2.1. Main characteristics and environmental origins*

There are industrial and household compounds prone to promote oestrogenic effects in wildlife and humans [68-70]. Some of these EDCs are compounds such as phenols (bisphenol A, BPA) and alkylphenols (APs) — *viz.* octylphenols (OPs) and nonylphenols (NPs) — and their ethoxylates (APEOs) (Figure 2).

| Class | Example | Chemical structure | Origin |
|---|---|---|---|
| Phenols | Bisfenol A (BPA) | 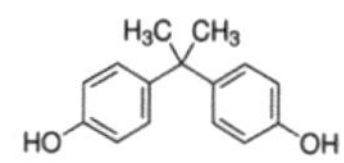 | Industrial and domestic usages [71]. |
| Alkylphenol ethoxylates (APEOs) | Octylphenol and nonylphenol ethoxylates | 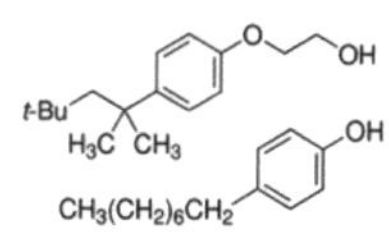 | Industrial, domestic and as pesticide additives [14, 73]. |
| | Octylphenol and nonylphenol diethoxylates | 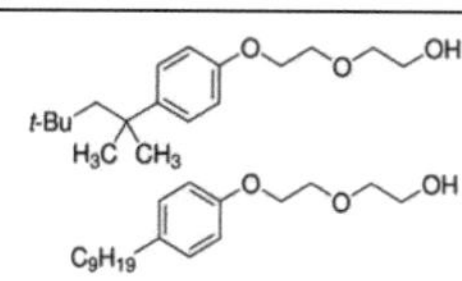 | |
| Alkylphenols (APs) | Octylphenols (OPs) | 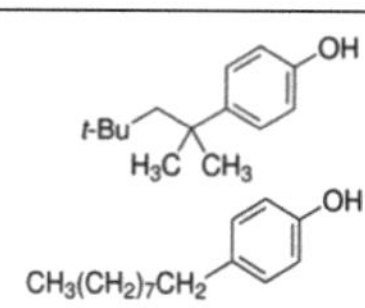 | Environmental Degradation of APEOs [73]. |
| | Nonylphenols (NPs) | 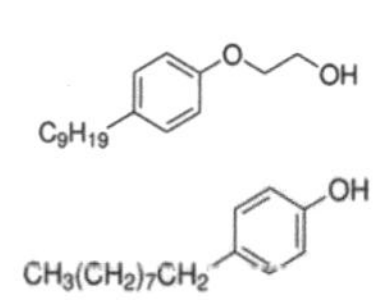 | |

**Figure 2.** Industrial and household products included in the list of compounds under surveillance by the WFD (European 2013).

Although the disruptive activity of these compounds is much lower than that of natural and synthetic oestrogens, as they may reach levels in the order of tens to hundreds of μg/L they can became harmful for aquatic fauna. Because of this, and despite great controversy between diverse agents, these compounds become subjected to strict laws that included both APs and APEOs, in the group of "priority substances in the field of water policy 2455/2001/EC" [4]. Presently, the WFD established that the concentration of NPs in surface waters should not exceed 2 μg/L [6].

BPA origin in the environment comes from the fact that it is the monomer of the polycarbonate (plastic) used in an huge variety of domestic stuffs and as an intermediate in the synthesis of epoxy resins, flame retardants and many other products [71]. In spite of its vast usage, controversial opinions do exist among those calling for its banning and those that devaluate the BPA toxic effects in realistic scenarios. The February 2007 study "Toxic Baby Bottle's", by the Environment California Research and Policy Center [72], showed that even small amounts of BPA may be one cause of diseases, including breast cancer, prostatic hyperplasia, diabetes, obesity, and hyperactivity disorders involving the immune system. Infertility and early puberty are also among the possible effects caused by BPA, and all of them are associated with the compound's ability to deregulate the endocrine system.

The APEOs sources in the environment are due to their commonly usage as non-ionic surfactant compounds and dispersants [14, 73]. Due to these properties APEOs are being used in detergents and additives of pesticide formulations. Currently, these applications are prohibited in the EU [4] as these compounds are known to readily degrade, in both aerobic and anaerobic conditions, into APs that are more toxic compounds than APEOs (Figure 3). In spite of the APs toxicity, it is known that their lifetime is not long, since they usually degrade in about 10 to 15 hours after sunlight exposure [74]. Thus, it is concluded that the ubiquitous presence of APs in surface waters implies the continuous entrance of APEOs in the environment [60].

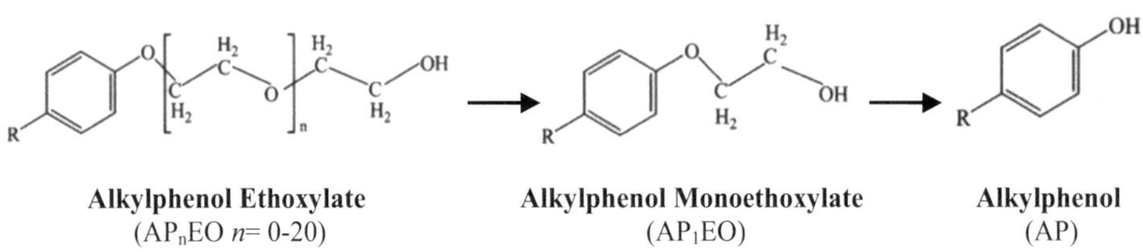


**Figure 3.** Summarized degradation mechanism of APEOs in the environment adapted from Warhurst [75].

The endocrine disrupting activity of APEOs and (especially) that of APs, whether they are octylphenols (4-OP and 4-t-OP) or nonylphenols (4-NP and 4-n-NP) is derived from the existence of similarities between the structure of these compounds and that of $E_2$ (Figure 4) [76].

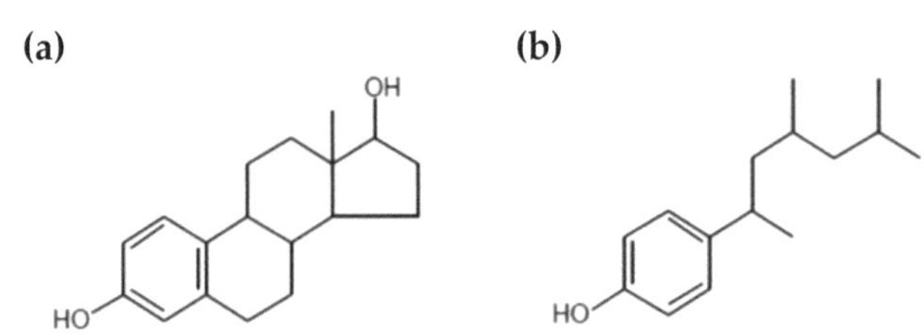


**Figure 4.** Comparison between the chemical structures of $E_2$ (**a**) and 4-NP (**b**).

As such, APs may induce oestrogenic effects using the same paths described in Section 3. These effects were proved, for example, after *in vivo* exposures of male rainbow trout (*Oncorhynchus mykiss*) to 30 µg/L of 4-OP, and of male Japanese medaka (*O. latipes*) to 30 µg/L of 4-NP, eliciting, respectively, an inhibition of the testicular growth and hermaphroditism [27, 77, 78]. Alas, as it is possible to purchase in EU countries imported products containing APEOs — see an interesting record in "APEOs Investigation Report" [79] — these EDCs continue to exist in European surface waters.

Currently, we theorize that the most likely source of APEOs in the aquatic systems is the discharge of wastewater effluents from STPs, nevertheless not neglecting the possible leaching caused by the runoff of these EDCs from landfills and agricultural areas (as APEOs are emulsifiers in some pesticide formulations).

### 2.2.2. BPA, APEOs and APs in surface waters

Table 3 shows an overview of BPA, APEOs and APs in estuaries and rivers worldwide. In line with the broad use of these EDCs it is observed that, at least up to 2005, their concentrations in surface waters were in the order of µg/L. For instance, ten years ago BPA reached concentrations of 5.0 µg/L in several German rivers [80] and the alkylphenols, 4-OP and 4-NP, levels attained 26 to 37 µg/L in several Spanish rivers and estuaries [81]. In line with these observations, it could be hypothesized that if there was not the pressure exerted by the program set out by the WFD, together with the directive 76/769/EEC [82] that established restrictions on the marketing and use of NPs and NPEOs, the current environmental content of these EDCs in European surface waters would probably be worse than that found nowadays. It is important to stress that the last directive advocates the banishment of NP and NPEOs in formulations when their levels are equal or higher than 0.1% by mass. This measure leaded to a decrease in the use of NPEOs or even their deliberate discontinuity in Europe (case of Germany) and, consequently, the number of studies that accompanied the temporal evolution of these compounds began decreasing. This aspect increases the difficulty to assess the actual amounts of APEOs and APs in European surface waters, being assumed that their usage was deprecated; a presumption that is not entirely correct, as we have been witnessing.

As shown in Table 3, the levels of APs in several EU countries continue to show potential toxicity (<0.5-37,300 ng/L). This poses obstacles to the compliance defined by WFD, since it seems impossible to achieve concentrations of ≤100 ng/L for the OPs and, ≤300 ng/L for NPs, in all EU states up to 2015. However, it is possible to observe that recent studies revealed that there is positive effort towards the reduction of the global amounts of both APs and BPA in all European countries. So, presently, and also accordingly to the compilation in Table 3, it is observed that in general the levels of APs and BPA are generally higher in Asia and South America than those measured in the EU.

In opposition, and with the exception of the two works [83, 84], before 2005 there were virtually no data about the levels of these EDCs in the west Iberian Peninsula, inc. Portuguese surface waters. These observations leaded to the creation of regular monitoring programs for these compounds, in order to make a general assessment of the situation in various locations and, when possible, monitor their evolution in time. Such temporal results are central to define if the implementation of WFD policies are being successful in the field, alone or together and correlated with biologic outputs (e.g., biomarkers data). The efforts done in the last decade for evaluating BPA, APEOs and APs pollution in Portuguese surface waters from estuaries, rivers and coastal waters are compiled in Table 4.

| EDC | Sampling area | Concentration (ng/L) | References |
|---|---|---|---|
| | Gulf of Gdansk, Poland | 26.9 - 48.1 | [85] |
| | Estuaries and rivers, The Netherlands | <8.8 - 1,000 | [40] |
| | German Rivers | 0.5 - 14 | [86] |
| | Elbe River and its tributaries, Germany | 3.8 - 92.0 | [80] |
| | Coastal area of Baltic Sea, Germany | ND - 5.7 | [42] |
| | Baden-Württemberg Rivers, Germany | <50 - 272 | [87] |
| | Glatt River, Switzerland | 9.0 - 76 | [88] |
| | Sussex River, England | <5.3 - 10 | [89] |
| | Ebro River, Spain | 10 - 20 | [33] |
| | Ebro River, Spain | ND - 61 | [56] |
| | Llobregat, Cardener, Anoia, Riera de Rubi River, Spain | <90 - 2,970 | [81] |
| | Venice Lagoon, Italy | <1.0 - 145 | [34] |
| BPA | Thermaikos Gulf, Nothern Aegean Sea, Greece | 10.6 - 52.3 | [47] |
| | New Orleans Waters,USA | 0.9 - 158 | [90] |
| | South Florida, USA | 4.8 - 32 | [50] |
| | Brazilian surface water | 25 - 84 | [51] |
| | Coastal waters of Shenzhen, China | 11.2 - 776.6 | [91] |
| | Dianchi Lake, China | 35 - 1,081 | [92] |
| | Liao River, China | 12.3 - 116.5 | [52] |
| | Songhua River, Northern China | 8.24 - 263 | [54] |
| | Pearl rivers, South China | 4.35 - 1,390 | [31, 32] |
| | Yangtze River estuary, China | 0.98 - 43.8 | [53] |
| | River waters of South Korea and seven Asian countries | 3.0 - 100 | [93] |
| | Tama River, Japan | 4.8 - 76.3 | [29] |
| | Coastal waters, Singapore | ND - 2,470 | [94] |
| | Gulf of Gdansk, Poland | <5.0 - 65.9 | [85] |
| | Estuaries and rivers, The Netherlands | <50 - 6,300 | [40] |
| OPs | German Rivers | 0.8 - 54 | [86] |
| | Baden-Württemberg River, Germany | <20 - 189 | [87] |

http://dx.doi.org/10.5772/59885

| EDC | Sampling area | Concentration (ng/L) | References |
|---|---|---|---|
| | Elbe River and its tributaries, Germany | <0.5 - 5.0 | [80] |
| | Ombrone River, Italy | 33 - 85 | [95] |
| | Glatt River, Switzerland | 6.0 - 22 | [88] |
| | Sussex River, England | 2.6 - 25 | [89] |
| | Ebro River, Spain | 20 - 70 | [33] |
| | Ebro River, Spain | 2.9 - 5.3 | [56] |
| | Llobregat, Cardener, Anoia, Riera de Rubi Spain | <90 - 21,900 | [81] |
| | Thermaikos Gulf, Nothern Aegean Sea, Greece | 1.7 - 18.2 | [47] |
| | Danube River, Hungary | 1.6 - 178 | [96] |
| | Back River, Chesapeake Bay, USA | <0.3 | [97] |
| | Brazilian surface water | ND | [51] |
| | Dianchi Lake, China | 2.0 - 73 | [92] |
| | Liao River, China | 2.3 - 13.2 | [52] |
| | Songhua River, Northern China | 1.54 - 45.8 | [54] |
| | Yellow River, China | 14.66 - 17.72 | [98] |
| | Tama River, Japan | 6.9 - 81.9 | [29] |
| | Gulf of Gdansk, Poland | 12.9 - 132.9 | [85] |
| | The Netherlands (surface water) | <110 - 4,100 | [40] |
| | Baden-Württemberg Rivers, Germany | ND - 458 | [87] |
| | Elbe River and its tributaries, Germany | 0.06 - 2,970 | [80] |
| | Rivers in Germany | 6.7 - 134 | [41] |
| | Glatt River, Switzerland | 68 - 326 | [88] |
| | Ombrone River, Italy | <2 | [95] |
| | Venice Lagoon, Italy | <0.05 - 211 | [34] |
| NPs | Ebro River, Spain | ND | [33] |
| | Ebro River, Spain | ND- 15 | [56] |
| | Llobregat, Cardener, Anoia, Riera de Rubi, Spain | <150- 37,300 | [81] |
| | Thermaikos Gulf, Nothern Aegean Sea, Greece | 22- 201 | [47] |
| | Danube River, Hungary | 8.0 - 428 | [96] |
| | Brazilian surface water | ND | [51] |
| | Back River, Chesapeake Bay, USA | 140 - 200 | [97] |
| | Buenos Aires rivers, Argentina | 100 - 7,000 | [99] |
| | Dianchi Lake, China | 5 - 57 | [92] |

| EDC | Sampling area | Concentration (ng/L) | References |
|---|---|---|---|
| | Liao River, China | 112 - 900.7 | [52] |
| | Songhua River, Northern China (4-t-NP) | 106 - 344 | [54] |
| | Songhua River, Northern China (4-n-NP) | 0.35 - 3.77 | [54] |
| | Area of Chongqing, China | 100 - 7,300 | [100] |
| | Pearl River, China | 36 - 33,000 | [31] |
| | Tama River, Japan | 51.6 - 147.0 | [29] |
| | River waters of South Korea and 7 Asian Countries | <LOD - 2,097 | [93] |
| OPEOs | The Netherlands (surface water) | <160 - 1,700 | [40] |
| | Elbe River and its tributaries, Germany | 0.6 - 9.6 | [80] |
| | Seine River, France | 55 - 63 | [101] |
| | Ombrone River, Italy (4-t-$OP_1EO$) | <94 | [95] |
| | Ombrone River, Italy (4-t-$OP_2EO$) | 6 - 34 | [95] |
| | Ebro River, Spain ($OP_2EO$) | 1.7 - 8.3 | [56] |
| | Thermaikos Gulf, Greece ($OP_1EO$) | <4 - 9.5 | [47] |
| | Thermaikos Gulf, Greece ($OP_2EO$) | <4 - 11.7 | [47] |
| | Estuaries and rivers, USA | 7 - 400 | [102] |
| | Back River, Chesapeake Bay, USA ($OP_1EO$) | <0.2 | [97] |
| | Back River, Chesapeake Bay, USA ($OP_2EO$) | <0.02 | [97] |
| NPEOs | The Netherlands (surface water) | <180 - 8,700 | [40] |
| | Elbe River and its tributaries, Germany | <0.5 - 124 | [80] |
| | Seine River, France ($NP_1EO$) | 9 - 11 | [101] |
| | Ombrone River, Italy (4-t-$NP_1EO$) | <122 | [95] |
| | Ombrone River, Italy (4-t-$NP_2EO$) | 9 - 35 | [95] |
| | Ebro River, Spain ($NP_2EO$) | 9.4 - 275 | [56] |
| | Thermaikos Gulf, Greece ($NP_1EO$) | 15.2 - 270 | [47] |
| | Thermaikos Gulf, Greece ($NP_2EO$) | 14.6 - 346 | [47] |
| | Estuaries and rivers, USA | 220 - 1,050 | [102] |
| | Back River, Chesapeake Bay, USA ($NP_1EO$) | <0.2 - 67 | [97] |
| | Back River, Chesapeake Bay, USA ($NP_2EO$) | 12 - 57 | [97] |
| | Buenos Aires, Argentina ($NP_1EO$) | 100 - 9,200 | [99] |
| | Buenos Aires, Argentina ($NP_2EO$) | 100 - 5,400 | [99] |
| | Songhua River, Northeastern China ($NP_1EO$) | 8.9 - 385 | [54] |
| | Songhua River, Northeastern China ($NP_2EO$) | 19.6 - 321 | [54] |

| EDC | Sampling area | Concentration (ng/L) | References |
|---|---|---|---|
| | Dianchi Lake, China ($NP_1EO$) | 54 - 1,942 | [92] |
| | Dianchi Lake, China ($NP_2EO$) | 98 - 2,074 | [92] |

ND: Not Detected. LOD: Limit of Detection.

**Table 3.** Concentrations (minimum–maximum) of industrial and household products in surface waters worldwide.

### *2.2.3. BPA, APEOs and APs in west Iberian Peninsula surface waters*

Recent studies revealed that surface waters taken from Portuguese aquatic environments show average concentrations of 650 ng/L for BPA, 1,000 ng/L for APEOs and 360 ng/L for APs (Table 4). Comparing such data with those reported in other countries (Table 3) it is observed that in Portugal the global amounts of these compounds are still quite high. Nevertheless, it is important to note that the values measured before/during 2005 [63, 66, 83, 84], namely for BPA and APs, are significantly higher than those measured in 2010-2011. Thus, and assuming that these results represent the wider reality of the west Iberian Peninsula, it seems that good efforts are being done to reduce the levels of industrial and household pollution (Table 4). In spite of this, Table 4 shows that APEOs exist in amounts that are still approximately one hundred fold higher than those recommended by the European legislation. These observations may be due to the presence of several textile industries and also large agricultural fields located near the sampling areas (Table 4); it should be noticed that several pesticide formulations use APEOs as dispersants. However, since similar amounts of APEOs were found in the Spanish and Greek waters [68, 69] it is possible that these EDCs are still being used, and therefore constitute a global problem of coastal areas.

| EDC | Sampling area | Concentration (ng/L) | References |
|---|---|---|---|
| BPA | Lima River estuary and Atlantic coast of Viana-Castelo | 1.9 - 35.7 | [64] |
| | Ave River estuary and Atlantic coast of Vila-Conde | 7.9 - 521.8 | [61] |
| | Leça River estuary and Atlantic coast of Porto | 30.6 - 62.4 | [65] |
| | Douro River estuary | <80 - 10,700 | [63] |
| | Douro River estuary and Atlantic coast of Porto | 20.4 - 314.0 | [62] |
| | Mondego River estuary | <6.6 - 880 | [66] |
| | Mondego River and its estuary | 8.5 - 184.6 | [67] |
| | Tagus River estuary | ≈ 13 - ≈ 320 | *Unpublished* |
| | Sado River estuary | 7.3 - 28 | [103] |
| | Sado River estuary | 12.2 - 28.9 | [59] |
| | Mira River and its estuary | ≈ 7 - ≈ 360 | *Unpublished* |
| | Ria Formosa | 6.5 - 71.7 | [60] |
| | Portuguese rivers and estuaries | 200 - 4,000 | [83] |
| | Portuguese rivers and estuaries | 0.2 - 5,000 | [84] |
| 4-OP | Lima River estuary and Atlantic coast of Viana-Castelo | 6.2 - 86.5 | [64] |

| EDC | Sampling area | Concentration (ng/L) | References |
|---|---|---|---|
| | Ave River estuary and Atlantic coast of Vila-Conde | 0.6 - 8.3 | [61] |
| | Leça River estuary and Atlantic coast of Porto | 27.0 - 68.3 | [65] |
| | Douro River estuary and Atlantic coast of Porto | < 3.5 | [62] |
| | Mondego River and its estuary | 0.7 - 1,279 | [67] |
| | Tagus River and its estuary | ≈ 6 - ≈ 150 | *Unpublished* |
| | Sado River estuary | 2.8 - 27.8 | [59] |
| | Mira River and its estuary | ≈ 6 - ≈ 28 | *Unpublished* |
| | Ria Formosa | 3.5 - 8.5 | [60] |
| | Portuguese rivers and estuaries | 0.1 - 30,000 | [84] |
| 4-t-OP | Lima River estuary and Atlantic coast of Viana-Castelo | 5.7 - 105.0 | [64] |
| | Ave River estuary and Atlantic coast of Vila-Conde | 1.3 - 25.4 | [61] |
| | Leça River estuary and Atlantic coast of Porto | 7.9 - 60.0 | [65] |
| | Douro River estuary and Atlantic coast of Porto | 5.1 - 30.6 | [62] |
| | Mondego River and its estuary | 30 - 27,502 | [67] |
| | Tagus River and its estuary | ≈ 2 - ≈ 71 | *Unpublished* |
| | Sado River and its estuary | 11.4 - 22.0 | [59] |
| | Mira River and its estuary | ≈ 4 - ≈ 27 | *Unpublished* |
| | Ria Formosa | 4.3 - 40.9 | [60] |
| 4-n-NP | Lima River estuary and Atlantic coast of V. Castelo | 3.0 - 35.4 | [64] |
| | Ave River estuary and Atlantic coast of V. Conde | 0.3 - 16.8 | [61] |
| | Leça River estuary and Atlantic coast of Porto (north) | 28.8 - 63.5 | [65] |
| | Douro River estuary and Atlantic coast of Porto | 3.3 - 116.0 | [62] |
| | Mondego River and its estuary | 20.8 - 2,770 | [67] |
| | Tagus River and its estuary | ≈ 1 - ≈ 41 | *Unpublished* |
| | Sado River estuary | 2.6 - 27.3 | [59] |
| | Mira River and its estuary | ≈ 2 - ≈ 33 | *Unpublished* |
| | Ria Formosa | 3.4 - 14.6 | [60] |
| 4-NP | Lima River estuary and Atlantic coast of Viana-Castelo | 3.9 - 649.8 | [64] |
| | Ave River estuary and Atlantic coast of Vila-Conde | 43.3 - 154.9 | [61] |
| | Douro River estuary and Atlantic coast of Porto | 88.2 - 170.0 | [62] |
| | Mondego River and its estuary | 80.6 - 1,003 | [67] |
| | Tagus River and its estuary | ≈ 200 - ≈ 1,600 | *Unpublished* |
| | Sado River estuary | 129.2 - 239.9 | [59] |
| | Mira River and its estuary | ≈ 52 - ≈ 289 | *Unpublished* |
| | Ria Formosa | 12.2 - 546.6 | [60] |
| | Portuguese rivers and estuaries | 200 - 30,000 | [83] |
| | Portuguese rivers and estuaries | 0.3 - 25,000 | [84] |

| EDC | Sampling area | Concentration (ng/L) | References |
|---|---|---|---|
| | Lima River estuary and Atlantic coast of Viana-Castelo | 8.8 - 125.0 | [64] |
| | Ave River estuary and Atlantic coast of Vila-Conde | 2.3 - 31.7 | [61] |
| | Leça River estuary and Atlantic coast of Porto | 20.8 - 72.9 | [65] |
| | Douro River estuary and Atlantic coast of Porto | 33.0 - 60.0 | [62] |
| $OP_1EO$ | Mondego River and its estuary | 10.7 - 2,337 | [67] |
| | Tagus River and its estuary | ≈ 6 - ≈ 142 | *Unpublished* |
| | Sado River estuary | 13.0 - 109.4 | [59] |
| | Mira River and its estuary | ≈ 9 - ≈ 63 | *Unpublished* |
| | Ria Formosa | 6.9 - 35.6 | [60] |
| | Lima River estuary and Atlantic coast of Viana-Castelo | 21.5 - 374.0 | [64] |
| | Ave River estuary and Atlantic coast of Vila-Conde | 44.1 - 208.7 | [61] |
| | Leça River estuary and Atlantic coast of Porto | 29.7 - 213.2 | [65] |
| | Douro River estuary and Atlantic coast of Porto | 100.0 - 424.0 | [62] |
| $OP_2EO$ | Mondego River and its estuary | 21.5 - 2,330 | [67] |
| | Tagus River and its estuary | ≈ 4 - ≈ 67 | *Unpublished* |
| | Sado River and its estuary | 60.0 - 384.2 | [59] |
| | Mira River and its estuary | ≈ 4 - ≈ 43 | *Unpublished* |
| | Ria Formosa | 46.5 - 182.1 | [60] |
| | Lima River estuary and Atlantic coast of Viana-Castelo | 44.9 - 259.1 | [64] |
| | Ave River estuary and Atlantic coast of Vila-Conde | 29.9 - 227.8 | [61] |
| | Leça River estuary and Atlantic coast of Porto | 115.6 - 923.3 | [65] |
| | Douro River estuary and Atlantic coast of Porto | 101.0 - 354.0 | [62] |
| $NP_1EO$ | Mondego River and its estuary | 95.4 - 7,794 | [67] |
| | Tagus River and its estuary | ≈ 15 - ≈ 340 | *Unpublished* |
| | Sado River and its estuary | 60.0 - 311.4 | [59] |
| | Mira River and its estuary | ≈ 14 - ≈ 816 | *Unpublished* |
| | Ria Formosa | 41.4 - 278.9 | [60] |
| | Lima River estuary and Atlantic coast of Viana-Castelo | 47.3 - 467.0 | [64] |
| | Ave River estuary and Atlantic coast of Vila-Conde | 142.6 - 750.6 | [61] |
| | Leça River estuary and Atlantic coast of Porto | 723.1 - 2,132 | [65] |
| | Douro River estuary and Atlantic coast of Porto | 212.0 - 1,148 | [62] |
| $NP_2EO$ | Mondego River and its estuary | 118.5 - 18,327 | [67] |
| | Tagus River and its estuary | ≈ 40 - ≈ 300 | *Unpublished* |
| | Sado River and its estuary | 167.0 - 1,096 | [59] |
| | Mira River and its estuary | ≈ 111 - ≈ 3,600 | *Unpublished* |
| | Ria Formosa | 49.1 - 779.7 | [60] |

**Table 4.** Concentrations (minimum–maximum) of industrial and household products in Portuguese surface waters.

## 2.3. Naturally occurring compounds present in plants

### *2.3.1. Phytoestrogens, characteristics and their environmental origin*

Accordingly to the U.S. Food Standards Agency [104], phytoestrogens are "any compound of vegetable origin, or their(s) metabolite(s) with structural similarities to $E_2$, which results in their ability to mimic or block the action of the endogenous sexual hormone in Man". Phytoestrogens fall into two classes: (*i*) flavonoids; and (*ii*) non-flavonoids. The flavonoids are subdivided into the three subclasses: (*i*) isoflavones (Figure 5); (*ii*) coumestans; and (*iii*) prenylflavonoids. The non-flavonoids include the lignans [104].

| Isoflavone | Chemical structure | Origin |
|---|---|---|
| Daizein (DAID) | 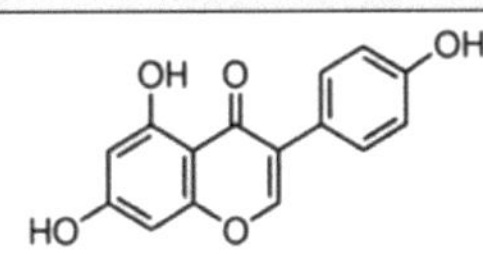 | |
| Genistein (GEN) | 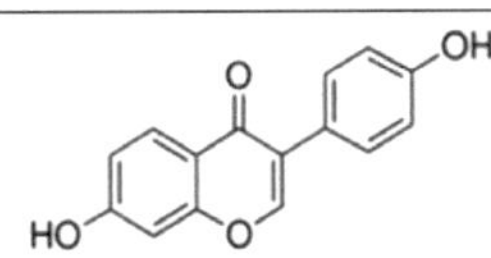 | Natural: Leachates from the decomposition of vascular plants (either living in the margins or in the waters of rivers, estuaries or coastal areas) [14, 15]. Industrial: Debris from industrial processes [105]. |
| Biochanin A (BIO-A) | 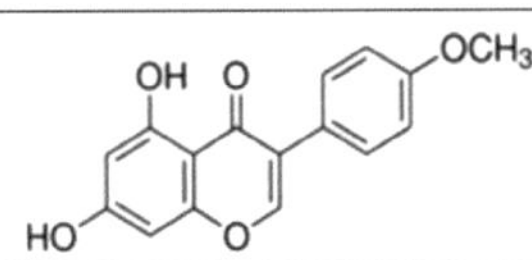 | |
| Formononetin (FORM) | 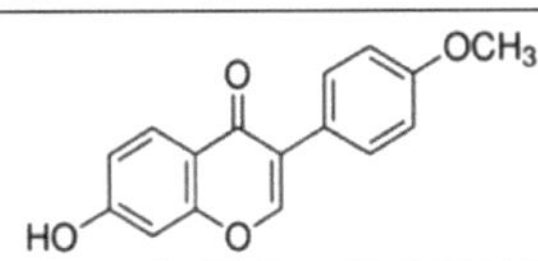 | |

**Figure 5.** Phytoestrogens with potential oestrogenic activity.

In this Chapter it is focused the group of isoflavones, which include compounds such as daidzein (DAID), genistein (GEN), biochanin A (BIO-A) and formononetin (FORM), due to their structural resemblance with $E_2$. Although not steroids, isoflavones exhibit high affinity for oestrogen receptors. In fact, both *in vivo* and *in vitro* studies have demonstrated their ability to induce abnormal liver synthesis of vitellogenin in male goldfish (*Carassius auratus*) and in rainbow trout (*O. mykiss*) [106-108], and the triggering of hermaphroditism in fish, such as the Japanese medaka (*O. latipes*) exposed to 1,000 μg/L of GEN [15]. Thus, although these compounds have not been included yet in the list of substances under the supervision by the WFD, but because their global levels in superficial waters can easily reach levels 1,000 times higher than those of $E_2$, i.e., in the order of μg/L or even mg/L, it is plausible to think that phytoestrogens may induce effects equivalent to those described for $E_2$ in spite of having a much lower potency [109]. Despite this, there are not many studies dedicated to the evaluation of these EDCs in surface waters. Also, little information exists about their origins and persistence. Presently, the main source of phytoestrogens in the aquatic environment is attributed either to the presence of the seagrass *Zostera noltii*, and/or to the leaching from the margins where plants rich in these compounds may exist, e.g., *Typha* spp., *Phragmites communis*, *Juncus acutus*, *Fuirena pubescens*, *Carex riparia* and *Carex hispida*, *Cladium mariscus*, *Callitriche stagnalis* and *Potamogeton* spp., *Trifolium* spp. and *Papilionaceae* [110-112].

Other equally important source of phytoestrogens in surface waters is their disposal as a result of industrial processes — especially in food processing industries and paper mills [105]. So, as the water levels of these compounds can quickly mount up to mg/L, it is possible that they exert in the wilderness the disruptive biological effects attributed to them [112-114]. Nonetheless, if the levels of these EDCs do not surpass ng/L and, in the absence of other potentially stressful compounds, it is most likely that phytoestrogens are harmless [115].

### 2.3.2. *Phytoestrogens in surface waters*

Comparatively to the other EDCs, the evaluation of phytoestrogens in aquatic environments, particularly in surface waters of estuaries or rivers, in less studied than the other EDCs referred in this Chapter. This is an important gap in the current knowledge since one the possible origins of these compounds is the natural aquatic flora, which generally is very developed in areas where the organic load is high and prone for eutrophication [116], which is a banal occurrence worldwide. In Table 5 it is shown a collection of studies done in several continents, and the data reveal that the highest concentrations of DAID (42,900 ng/L) and GEN (143,000 n/L) were found in Asia, in the Japanese Kanzaki River. In contrast, the highest amounts of FORM (157 ng/L) and BIO-A (59.4 ng/L) were measured in Europe, at various locations in Switzerland.

| EDC | Sampling area | Concentration (ng/L) | References |
|---|---|---|---|
| DAID | Tiber River, Italy | 2.0 - 3.0 | [44] |
| | Glatt, Töss, Swiss Midlands, Switzerland | ND - 31.5 | [117] |
| | Surface waters, Switzerland | *Detected* | [118] |
| | Drainage waters, Switzerland | 5.0 - 30 | [118] |
| | Rhine River, Germany | < 10 | [119] |
| | Several rivers, Iowa, USA | 10.5 - 41 | [120] |
| | Lake Vadnais and Metro Plant effluent channel, USA | 1.6 - 1.8 | [115] |
| | Straight Lake, USA | ND | [115] |
| | Several Rivers, Brazil | 36.2 - 276 | [121] |
| | Waters from Mullet Creek, Australia | 3.0 - 7.0 | [122] |
| | Macquarie Rivulet River, Australia | 14 - 33 | [122] |
| | Mullet Creek water, Australia | 2.0 - 12 | [122] |
| | Toolijooa surface dam (water), Australia | ND - 120 | [122] |
| | Kanzaki River, Japan | LOD - 42,900 | [123] |
| | Zhangcun River, China | ND - 1,490 | [124] |
| GEN | Tiber River, Italy | 4.0 - 7.0 | [44] |
| | Glatt, Töss, Swiss Midlands, Switzerland | ND - 24.2 | [117] |
| | Surface waters, Switzerland | ND | [118] |
| | Drainage waters, Switzerland | *Detected* - 14 | [118] |
| | Several rivers, Iowa, USA | ND - 8.0 | [120] |

| EDC | Sampling area | Concentration (ng/L) | References |
|---|---|---|---|
| | Waters from Upper Midwest (USA) | 1.4 - 1.6 | [115] |
| | Straight Lake, USA | ND | [115] |
| | Several Rivers, Brazil | 3.96 - 336 | [122] |
| | Waters from Mullet Creek, Australia | ND - 1.0 | [122] |
| | Macquarie Rivulet River, Australia | 1.0 - 8.0 | [122] |
| | Toolijooa surface dam (water), Australia | 1.0 - 20 | [122] |
| | Yeongsan and Seomjin Rivers, Korea | ND - 0.7 | [93] |
| | Salut, Malaysia | ND | [93] |
| | Khong River, Thailand | ND | [93] |
| | Long Xuyen city, Vietnam | 1.5 - 2.4 | [93] |
| | Siem Reap, Cambodia | 4.4 | [93] |
| | Fenhe, China | 3.6 - 5.0 | [93] |
| | Zhangcun River, China | ND - 2,650 | [124] |
| | Kanzaki River (Japan) | LOD - 143,000 | [123] |
| FORM | Tiber River, Italy | ND | [44] |
| | Glatt, Töss, Swiss Midlands, Switzerland | ND - 217 | [117] |
| | Surface waters, Switzerland | *Detected* - 21 | [118] |
| | Drainage waters, Switzerland | 44 - 157 | [118] |
| | Several rivers, Iowa, USA | 5.3 - 13.5 | [120] |
| | Straight Lake, USA | ND | [115] |
| | Lake Vadnais, USA | 0.9 - 1.1 | [115] |
| | Macquarie Rivulet River, Australia | ND - 2.0 | [122] |
| | Waters from Mullet Creek, Australia | ND - 1.0 | [122] |
| | Toolijooa surface dam (water), Australia | ND - 35 | [122] |
| BIO-A | Tiber River, Italy | 1.0 - 3.0 | [44] |
| | Glatt, Töss, Swiss Midlands, Switzerland | ND - 59.4 | [117] |
| | Surface waters, Switzerland | *Detected* - 12 | [118] |
| | Drainage waters, Switzerland | 7 - 22 | [118] |
| | Several rivers, Iowa, USA | 1.7 - 5.6 | [120] |
| | Lake Vadnais and Metro Plant effluent channel, USA | ND - 1.1 | [115] |
| | Straight Lake, USA | ND | [115] |
| | Waters from Mullet Creek, Australia | ND - 0.1 | [122] |
| | Macquarie Rivulet River, Australia | ND - 1.0 | [122] |
| | Toolijooa surface dam (water), Australia | ND - 4.0 | [122] |

ND: Not Detected. LOD: Limit of Detection.

**Table 5.** Concentrations (minimum–maximum) of phytoestrogens in surface waters worldwide.

### *2.3.3. Phytoestrogens in Portuguese surface waters*

Concerning the Iberian peninsula west Atlantic coast, it was found that surface waters from the Rivers Douro (ca., 19 μg/L BIO-A), Mondego (ca., 5.5 μg/L of FORM and 12 μg/L DAID)

http://dx.doi.org/10.5772/59885

and Tagus (ca., from 10 μ/L) were those holding the higher amounts of phytoestrogens (Table 6). As in these habitats there were occasions when the concentrations of the isoflavones were more than 1,000 times higher than those measured for oestrogens (mainly in spring and summer), it is supposed that those compounds may contribute significantly to endocrine disrupting phenomena occurring in those ecosystems. So, although the phytoestrogens are much less active than oestrogens ($E_2$) their very high concentrations make them worth studying and relevant in monitoring programs.

| EDC | Sampling area | Concentration (ng/L) | References |
|---|---|---|---|
| DAID | Lima River estuary and Atlantic coast of Viana-Castelo | 2.9 - 78.5 | [64] |
| | Ave River estuary and Atlantic coast of Vila-Conde | 7.7 - 74.3 | [61] |
| | Douro River estuary | <10 - 888 | [62] |
| | Douro River estuary and Atlantic coast of Porto | 6.7 - 24.2 | [63] |
| | Mondego River estuary | <3.0 - 526 | [66] |
| | Mondego River and its estuary | 52.9 - 11,945 | [67] |
| | Tagus River estuary | ≈ 4 - ≈ 20 | *Unpublished* |
| | Sado River estuary | 8.4 - 160 | [103] |
| | Sado River and its estuary | 3.4 - 32.3 | [59] |
| | Mira River and its estuary | ≈ 5 - ≈ 40 | *Unpublished* |
| | Ria Formosa | 4.6 - 14.0 | [60] |
| GEN | Lima River estuary and Atlantic coast of Viana- Castelo | 18.5 - 120.3 | [64] |
| | Ave River estuary and Atlantic coast of Vila-Conde | 36.6 - 682.3 | [61] |
| | Douro River estuary | <3.2 - 197 | [62] |
| | Douro River estuary and Atlantic coast of Porto | 16.6 - 137.8 | [63] |
| | Mondego River estuary | <2.6 - 507 | [66] |
| | Mondego River and its estuary | 127.9 - 5,093 | [67] |
| | Tagus River and its estuary | ≈ 5 - ≈ 4,500 | *Unpublished* |
| | Sado River and its estuary | 8.6 - 100 | [103] |
| | Sado River and its estuary | 24.5 - 113.4 | [59] |
| | Mira River and its estuary | ≈ 3 - ≈ 47 | *Unpublished* |
| | Ria Formosa | 404.8 - 1,158 | [60] |
| FORM | Lima River estuary and Atlantic coast of Viana-Castelo | 90.0 - 801.0 | [64] |
| | Ave River estuary and Atlantic coast of Vila-Conde | 83.0 - 362.3 | [61] |
| | Douro River estuary and Atlantic coast of Porto | 68 - 341 | [63] |
| | Mondego River and its estuary | 25.8 - 5,495 | [67] |
| | Tagus River and its estuary | ≈ 3 - ≈ 8 | *Unpublished* |
| | Sado River and its estuary | 423.4 - 2,605 | [59] |
| | Mira River and its estuary | ≈ 3 - ≈ 91 | *Unpublished* |
| | Ria Formosa | 186.3 - 1,041 | [60] |
| BIO-A | Lima River estuary and Atlantic coast of Viana-Castelo | 23.5 - 350.0 | [64] |
| | Ave River estuary and Atlantic coast of Vila-Conde | 99.0 - 398.1 | [61] |
| | Douro River estuary | <12 - 191 | [62] |
| | Douro River estuary and Atlantic coast of Porto | 728.4 - 19,091 | [63] |

| EDC | Sampling area | Concentration (ng/L) | References |
|---|---|---|---|
| | Mondego River estuary | <8.4 - 60 | [66] |
| | Mondego River and its estuary | 50.1 - 590.0 | [67] |
| BIO-A | Tagus River and its estuary | ≈ 6 - ≈ 85 | *Unpublished* |
| | Sado River and its estuary | 10 - 30 | [103] |
| | Sado River and its estuary | 130.8 - 844.5 | [59] |
| | Mira River and its estuary | ≈ 5 - ≈ 460 | *Unpublished* |
| | Ria Formosa | 91.2 - 261.4 | [60] |

**Table 6.** Concentrations (minimum–maximum) of phytoestrogens measured in Portuguese surface waters.

# 3. Individual compounds versus total estrogenic load and its endocrine disruption potential

To better understand and predict the effect of the measured concentrations of all EDCs compiled in this Chapter, in terms of action strength and consequent endocrine disrupting effects, the oestrogenic potency of each compound was estimated relative to that of the standard reference oestrogen, the $EE_2$, the most potent environmental oestrogen at this date. Thus, the average levels of each analysed EDC at every studied area in the west of the Iberian Peninsula were all converted in $EE_2$ equivalents ($EE_{2eq}$). The use of these units facilitates the interpretation of the data. The $EE_{2eq}$ estimates of the estrogenic potential of the sixteen EDCs referred in this Chapter followed the next formula [125]:

$$EE_{2eq} = C \, x \, F$$

Here, ***C*** concerns to the measured concentration of a given EDC and ***F*** refers to the $EE_2$ equivalency factor, as determined from *in vitro* assays [125]. Although this type of interpretation is very useful, the ***C*** may vary with the assay and it does not exempt the *in vivo* testing.

Interpreting the results presented here, in light of that normalization, and joining the EDCs by groups (i.e., oestrogens, APs + BPA, APEOs and phytoestrogens) it can be deduced that before 2005 the Portuguese surface waters taken from the rivers Douro, Mondego and Sado exhibited values of $EE_{2eq}$ that "hovered" between 24 and 198 ng/L, being the Douro River estuary the habitat with the highest oestrogen load (Table 7). After 2005, possibly due to the application of some of the regulations proposed by WFD, it was observed a significant decrease of the $EE_{2eq}$ in the Douro River estuary surface waters, which displayed values that stand in 12 ng/L, even considering a larger spectrum of analysed EDCs. For the Mondego and Sado Rivers it is also observed that even analysing almost the twice number of EDCs, the data obtained from surface waters in 2005 [66, 103] had similar $EE_{2eq}$ (24 ng/L) than those observed in waters from the same sampling areas in 2010-2011. Besides, from the analysis of Table 7 it is also possible to observe which group of compounds contribute the most to the final values of $EE_{2eq}$. Thus, it is concluded that by order of importance the compounds that contribute the most for

http://dx.doi.org/10.5772/59885

the $EE_{2eq}$ values in the Portuguese surface waters were: (*i*) oestrogens; (*ii*) phytoestrogens; (*iii*) APs + BPA; and (*iv*) APEOs. So, both oestrogens and phytoestrogens are important "key points" to consider when the purpose of achieving good water quality by 2015 is the main goal of the European Environment Agency (EEA). Overall, it is proposed herein that an improvement of the sewerage system could surely promote reduction of the concentration of oestrogens and eutrophication. In addition, it is also suggested that the authorities should equate ways to reduce impacts caused by the use of products containing APEOs, e.g., by regulating their imports.

| Sampling areas | | $EE_{2eq}$ (ng/L) | | | | Total |
|---|---|---|---|---|---|---|
| | | Oestrogens | APs+BPA | APEOs | Phytoestrogens | (ng/L) |
| Lima River | [64] | 18 | 0.5 | 0.000 | 13 | 32 |
| Ave River | [61] | 9.0 | 0.4 | 0.001 | 12 | 22 |
| Leça River | [65] | 10 | 0.01 | 0.000 | *NA* | 10 |
| Douro River | [63] | 192 | 0.25 | NA | 5.1* | 198 |
| Douro River | [62] | 9.0 | 0.45 | 0.002 | 2.9 | 12 |
| Mondego River | [66] | 16 | 0.04 | NA | 9.0* | 25 |
| Mondego River | [67] | 12 | 2.0 | 0.004 | 58 | 72 |
| Tagus River | *Unpublished* | ≈ 11 | ≈ 1 | ≈ 0 | ≈ 43 | 55 |
| Sado River | [103] | 16 | 0.005 | *NA* | 8.7* | 25 |
| Sado River | [59] | 9.2 | 0.6 | 0.001 | 12 | 22 |
| Mira River | *Unpublished* | ≈ 52 | ≈ 1 | ≈ 0 | ≈ 1 | 54 |
| Ria Formosa | [60] | 24 | 0.8 | 0.001 | 28 | 52 |

Data not available (NA) or (*) summations containing different number of analysed EDCs.

**Table 7.** Estimation of the estrogenic potential of several Portuguese surface waters.

## 4. Status of waters in the European Union and in Portugal

Since the beginning of the implementation of the WFD, the EC was aware that it would not be an easy task to attain the proposed quality goals stated in all EU member states within a limited period of time — 15 years [3]. Therefore, although strict targets ought to be accomplished in all states, it was considered some temporal flexibility to completely achieve the main goals, as it was considered that each nation has its own environmental (and social) characteristics. In this vein, a 2007 report from the EC revealed that nineteen EU states still showed significant weaknesses in the implementation of the WFD and, called attention to the risk of the purposes set for 2015 may not be met. Therefore, in order to coerce the accomplishment of the WFD requirements, the EC appointed the EEA as a periodic gauge which role has been the evaluation of the water quality in each country that assumed to apply the WFD. In this context, during the last evaluation by the EEA, Portugal was identified as having not yet implemented a plan for the management of all national watersheds (Judgment from 21 June 2012 in Case C-223/11,

Portugal) [126]. As this task was considered essential for the implementation of various articles defined in the WFD, including the Article 8 that aims the implementation of standards for water monitoring, Portugal together with others (Spain, Greece and Luxembourg) were condemned by the Court of Justice of the European Community. Besides this occurrence, in 2013 the WFD published a list of other, most common, defaults recorded in many states [127]: (*i*) existence of severe gaps in the levels of chemical pollutants from anthropogenic origins in surface waters; (*ii*) 60% of groundwater resources in cities were over-exploitation; (*iii*) 25% of the groundwater was polluted; (*iv*) 47% of the surface waters showed bad ecological status; and (*v*) 50% of the wetlands showed extinction risks of indigenous species. Considering the first item of this list, it is demonstrated the need of implement chemical monitoring programs for all states involved in the implementation of the WFD. As a corollary, we do emphasize herein the relevance of the regular chemical monitoring and the implementation of strategies for reducing the levels of the EDCs referred in this Chapter.

## 5. Impact of natural and xenoestrogenic compounds in human health

Estimating with certainty the contribution of aquatic environmental pollution — namely by the above mentioned EDCs — to the burden of disease in humans is extremely difficult and consequently quite polemic [10, 128]. This fact comes from the difficulty to measure and link exposures with the health disorders that may occur in humans, as these are not in regular contact with "oestrogenic waters" as aquatic animals. However, the consumption of contaminated drinking water and/or seafood together with some other sporadic contact between humans and contaminated waters, e.g., during recreational activities either in sea or fluvial beaches [60, 64], may change some preconception about this issue. In fact, and despite the confounding variables, recent studies have linked the presence of environmental natural oestrogens, phytoestrogens and xenoestrogens with the development of a range of disorders that go from immune deficiencies, birth defects, chronic endocrine diseases to cancer (Table 8).

During the last decade researchers devoted to both environmental health and human oncology have shown an increasing interest in the environmental impacts of EDCs over human health as the chemical structures of some of these chemicals, namely those refereed in this work, resemble that of $E_2$ which is a molecule that evolution maintained conserved amongst different species [10]. This means that, alike fishes and other aquatic animals, the distribution of oestrogen receptors in mammalian/human tissues is so wide that the presence of these EDCs are able to interfere with the orchestration of an important number of pathways, some of which, are close related with the development of cancer [129-132]. Besides, in both fish and mammals high levels of oestrogens induce the production of reactive oxygen species causing hypomethylation and microsatellite instability [133, 134]; these phenomena, which is an early step in the process of carcinogenesis, cause DNA adducts and other genetic damages, seen, e.g., by the emergence of micronuclei, a fact that was observed by our group in fish caught in areas described here as having high estrogenic loads [135].

http://dx.doi.org/10.5772/59885

| EDCs | Human health disorders | References |
|---|---|---|
| $E_1$, $E_2$ and $EE_2$ | Immune deficiencies | [23, 24] |
| | Ovarian Cancer | [136] |
| | Cancer in children and adolescent | [137] |
| | Abnormal prostate development | [138] |
| BPA and APs | Breast Cancer | [10, 139] |
| | Human reproduction | [140] |
| | Reproductive development | [141] |
| | Premature puberty and endometriosis development | [142] |
| | Fetal development | [143] |
| | Defects in human male germ cells | [144] |
| Phytoestrogens | Breast cancer | [145] |
| | Hypospadias | [146] |
| | Puberty disorders | [147] |
| | Masculine infertility | [148] |
| | Endocrine modulation | [149, 150] |

**Table 8.** Examples of some disorders promoted by the EDCs focused in this Chapter.

Some epidemiologic studies also support the correlation between oestrogenic EDCs and cancer as, it was found that in Europe childhood cancer incidence is having an annual increase of 1% [137]. This worrying result it is also associated with a rising trend of other cancer types such as the soft tissue sarcoma, brain tumours, germ-cell tumours, lymphomas, renal cancers, leukaemia, breast cancer and lung cancer in women [10, 151, 152]. These occurrences are much preoccupant and alert all society to the possible risk that these compounds can pose for public health.

## 6. Conclusion and perspectives

As demonstrated in this Chapter, with regard to the xenobiotics that can act as oestrogens there is still much to do in both Portugal and other countries in order to reduce this type of chemical pollution in the surface waters from rivers, estuaries and coastal areas. Thus it would be very useful to conceive national monitoring plans, coordinated in time and space (location of the areas under evaluation), using not only chemical methods but also biological tools (e.g., via the usage of biomarkers). This type of plans, involving and networking public and private agents, would make it possible to assess risks and if measures of prevention and remediation that are being promoted on the ground produce, the desired effects, namely as required by the implementation of the WFD. With regard to research activities done in the west Iberian Peninsula, we seek to continue developing projects that allow the diagnosis of the aquatic systems, not only focusing the attention in the type of EDCs discussed here but also in others judged relevant, such as emerging pharmaceutical compounds, PAHs, PCBs and pesticides — some data are already published concerning these compounds [153-159]. Introduction of passive sampling methods should be pursued too, to get time-integrated characterizations. In parallel, we also view as utterly important to contribute with knowledge about the mechanisms of action that underlie the disruptive effects in aquatic organisms, as illustrated in works we co-authored [160-169]. At last, it is very relevant to reinforce the efforts to investigate cause-effect associations related with potential long term risks of drinking (inc. tape) waters contaminated with estrogenic compounds, both by monitoring the types and quantities of compounds [170] and by epidemiological approaches [171].

## Acknowledgements

This work was partially supported by the European Regional Development Fund (ERDF), through the COMPETE – Operational Competitiveness Programme, and by national funds, via FCT – Foundation for Science and Technology: projects PTDC/MAR/70436/2006 and PEst-C/MAR/LA0015/2013.

## Author details

Maria João Rocha[1*] and Eduardo Rocha[2]

*Address all correspondence to: mjsrocha@netcabo.pt

1 Interdisciplinary Centre for Marine and Environmental Research (CIIMAR/CIMAR), University of Porto (UPorto), Portugal. Laboratory of Histology and Embryology, Institute of Biomedical Sciences Abel Salazar (ICBAS), UPorto, Portugal

2 Interdisciplinary Centre for Marine and Environmental Research (CIIMAR/CIMAR), University of Porto (UPorto), Portugal. Laboratory of Histology and Embryology, Institute of Biomedical Sciences Abel Salazar (ICBAS), UPorto, Portugal

## References

[1] Barnett TP, Adam JC, Lettenmaier DP. Potential Impacts of a Warming Climate on Water Availability in Snow-Dominated Regions. Nature 2005; 438(7066) 303-309.

[2] Commission E. The Eu Biodiversity Strategy to 2020. Publications Office of the European Union 2011.

[3] WFD. Directive 2000/60/Ec of the European Parliament and of the Council, in, Official Journal of the European Communities, 2000.

[4] WFD. Decision No 2455/2001/Ec of the European Parliament and of the Council of 20 November 2001 Establishing the List of Priority Substances in the Field of Water Policy and Amending Directive 2000/60/Ec, in, Official Journal of the European Communities, 2001.

[5] WFD. Directive 2008/105/Ec of the European Parliament and of the Council of 16 December 2008 on Environmental Quality Standards in the Field of Water Policy, Amending and Subsequently Repealing Council Directives 82/176/Eec, 83/513/Eec, 84/156/Eec, 84/491/Eec, 86/280/Eec and Amending Directive 2000/60/Ec of the European Parliament and of the Council in, Official Journal of the European Union, 2008.

[6] WFD. Directive 2013/39/Eu of the European Parliament and of the Council of 12 August 2013 Amending Directives 2000/60/Ec and 2008/105/Ec as Regards Priority Substances in the Field of Water Policy, in, Official Journal of the European Union, 2013.

[7] NIH. Endocrine Disruptors, in, National Institutes of Health U.S. Department of Health and Human Services, 2010.

[8] Kordon C, Gaillard RC. Hormones and the Brain. Research and Perspectives in Endocrine Interactions. In: Springer-Verlag Berlin Heidelberg New York; 2006. p

[9] Tierney KB, Farrell AP, Brauner CJ, (Eds.). Fish Physiology: Organic Chemical Toxicology of Fishes, Academic Press; 2013.

[10] Fucic A, Gamulin M, Ferencic Z, Katic J, Krayer von Krauss M, Bartonova A, Merlo D. Environmental Exposure to Xenoestrogens and Oestrogen Related Cancers: Reproductive System, Breast, Lung, Kidney, Pancreas, and Brain. Environmental Health 2012; 11(Suppl 1) S8.

[11] Ferreira M, Antunes P, Gil O, Vale C, Reis-Henriques MA. Organochlorine Contaminants in Flounder (*Platichthys flesus*) and Mullet (*Mugil cephalus*) from Douro Estuary, and Their Use as Sentinel Species for Environmental Monitoring. Aquatic Toxicology 2004; 69(4) 347-357.

[12] Mills LJ, Chichester C. Review of Evidence: Are Endocrine-Disrupting Chemicals in the Aquatic Environment Impacting Fish Populations? Science of the Total Environment 2005; 343(1-3) 1-34.

[13] Ying GG, Kookana RS, Chen ZL. On-Line Solid-Phase Extraction and Fluorescence Detection of Selected Endocrine Disrupting Chemicals in Water by High-Performance Liquid Chromatography. Journal of Environmental Science and Health Part B-Pesticides Food Contaminants and Agricultural Wastes 2002; 37(3) 225-234.

[14] Lintelmann J, Katayama A, Kurihara N, Shore L, Wenzel A. Endocrine Disruptors in the Environment - (Iupac Technical Report). Pure and Applied Chemistry 2003; 75(5) 631-681.

[15] Kiparissis Y, Hughes R, Metcalfe C, Ternes T. Identification of the Isoflavonoid Genistein in Bleached Kraft Mill Effluent. Environmental Science and Technology 2001; 35(12) 2423-2427.

[16] Gutendorf B, Westendorf J. Comparison of an Array of *in Vitro* Assays for the Assessment of the Estrogenic Potential of Natural and Synthetic Estrogens, Phytoestrogens and Xenoestrogens. Toxicology 2001; 166(1–2) 79-89.

[17] Sumpter JP. Endocrine Disrupters in the Aquatic Environment: An Overview. Acta Hydrochimica et Hydrobiologica 2005; 33(1) 9-16.

[18] McLachlan JA, Simpson E, Martin M. Endocrine Disrupters and Female Reproductive Health. Best Practice & Research Clinical Endocrinology & Metabolism 2006; 20(1) 63-75.

[19] Milnes MR, Bermudez DS, Bryan TA, Edwards TM, Gunderson MP, Larkin ILV, Moore BC, Guillette LJ. Contaminant-Induced Feminization and Demasculinization of Nonmammalian Vertebrate Males in Aquatic Environments. Environmental Research 2006; 100(1) 3-17.

[20] Scott AP, Sanders M, Stentiford GD, Reese RA, Katsiadaki I. Evidence for Estrogenic Endocrine Disruption in an Offshore Flatfish, the Dab (*Limanda limanda* L.). Marine Environmental Research 2007; 64(2) 128-148.

[21] Hotchkiss AK, Lambright CS, Ostby JS, Parks-Saldutti L, Vandenbergh JG, Gray LE, Jr. Prenatal Testosterone Exposure Permanently Masculinizes Anogenital Distance, Nipple Development, and Reproductive Tract Morphology in Female Sprague-Dawley Rats. Toxicological Sciences 2007; 96(2) 335-345.

[22] Matthiessen P. An Assessment of Endocrine Disruption in Mollusks and the Potential for Developing Internationally Standardized Mollusk Life Cycle Test Guidelines. Integrated environmental assessment and management 2008; 4(3) 274-284.

[23] Ansar Ahmed S. The Immune System as a Potential Target for Environmental Estrogens (Endocrine Disrupters): A New Emerging Field. Toxicology 2000; 150(1–3) 191-206.

[24] Chalubinski M, Kowalski ML. Endocrine Disrupters - Potential Modulators of the Immune System and Allergic Response. Allergy 2006; 61(11) 1326-1335.

[25] Waring RH, Harris RM. Endocrine Disrupters: A Human Risk? Molecular and Cellular Endocrinology 2005; 244(1-2) 2-9.

[26] Belfroid AC, Van der Horst A, Vethaak AD, Schafer AJ, Rijs GBJ, Wegener J, Cofino WP. Analysis and Occurrence of Estrogenic Hormones and Their Glucuronides in Surface Water and Waste Water in the Netherlands. Science of the Total Environment 1999; 225(1-2) 101-108.

[27] Metcalfe CD, Metcalfe TL, Kiparissis Y, Koenig BG, Khan C, Hughes RJ, Croley TR, March RE, Potter T. Estrogenic Potency of Chemicals Detected in Sewage Treatment

http://dx.doi.org/10.5772/59885

Plant Effluents as Determined by in Vivo Assays with Japanese Medaka (*Oryzias latipes*). Environmental Toxicology and Chemistry 2001; 20(2) 297-308.

[28] Peters REM, Courtenay SC, Cagampan S, Hewitt ML, MacLatchy DL. Effects on Reproductive Potential and Endocrine Status in the Mummichog (*Fundulus leteroclitus*) after Exposure to 17 Alpha-Ethynylestradiol in a Short-Term Reproductive Bioassay. Aquatic Toxicology 2007; 85(2) 154-166.

[29] Furuichi T, Kannan K, Glesy JP, Masunaga S. Contribution of Known Endocrine Disrupting Substances to the Estrogenic Activity in Tama River Water Samples from Japan Using Instrumental Analysis and *in Vitro* Reporter Gene Assay. Water Research 2004; 38(20) 4491-4501.

[30] Chen CY, Wen TY, Wang GS, Cheng HW, Lin YH, Lien GW. Determining Estrogenic Steroids in Taipei Waters and Removal in Drinking Water Treatment Using High-Flow Solid-Phase Extraction and Liquid Chromatography/Tandem Mass Spectrometry. Science of the Total Environment 2007; 378(3) 352-365.

[31] Peng X, Yu Y, Tang C, Tan J, Huang Q, Wang Z. Occurrence of Steroid Estrogens, Endocrine-Disrupting Phenols, and Acid Pharmaceutical Residues in Urban Riverine Water of the Pearl River Delta, South China. Science of the Total Environment 2008; 397(1–3) 158-166.

[32] Zhao JL, Ying GG, Chen F, Liu YS, Wang L, Yang B, Liu S, Tao R. Estrogenic Activity Profiles and Risks in Surface Waters and Sediments of the Pearl River System in South China Assessed by Chemical Analysis and *in Vitro* Bioassay. Journal of Environmental Monitoring 2011; 13(4) 813-821.

[33] Brossa L, Marcé RM, Borrull F, Pocurull E. Occurrence of Twenty-Six Endocrine-Disrupting Compounds in Environmental Water Samples from Catalonia, Spain. Environmental Toxicology and Chemistry 2005; 24(2) 261-267.

[34] Pojana G, Gomiero A, Jonkers N, Marcomini A. Natural and Synthetic Endocrine Disrupting Compounds (Edcs) in Water, Sediment and Biota of a Coastal Lagoon. Environment International 2007; 33(7) 929-936.

[35] Jobling S, Beresford N, Nolan M, Rodgers-Gray T, Brighty GC, Sumpter JP, Tyler CR. Altered Sexual Maturation and Gamete Production in Wild Roach (*Rutilus rutilus*) Living in Rivers That Receive Treated Sewage Effluents. Biology of Reproduction 2002; 66(2) 272-281.

[36] Lange A, Paull GC, Hamilton PB, Iguchi T, Tyler CR. Implications of Persistent Exposure to Treated Wastewater Effluent for Breeding in Wild Roach (*Rutilus rutilus*) Populations. Environmental Science & Technology 2011; 45(4) 1673-1679.

[37] Tyler CR, Lange A, Paull GC, Katsu Y, Iguchi T. The Roach (*Rutilus rutilus*) as a Sentinel for Assessing Endocrine Disruption. Environmental Sciences 2007; 14(5) 235-253.

[38] van Aerle R, Nolan M, Jobling S, Christiansen LB, Sumpter JP, Tyler CR. Sexual Disruption in a Second Species of Wild Cyprinid Fish (the Gudgeon, *Gobio gobio*) in United Kingdom Freshwaters. Environmental Toxicology and Chemistry 2001; 20(12) 2841-2847.

[39] Noppe H, Verslycke T, De Wulf E, Verheyden K, Monteyne E, Van Caeter P, Janssen CR, De brabander HF. Occurrence of Estrogens in the Scheldt Estuary: A 2-Year Survey. Ecotoxicology and Environmental Safety 2007; 66(1) 1-8.

[40] Vethaak AD, Lahr J, Schrap SM, Belfroid AC, Rijs GBJ, Gerritsen A, de Boer J, Bulder AS, Grinwis GCM, Kuiper RV, Legler J, Murk TAJ, Peijnenburg W, Verhaar HJM, de Voogt P. An Integrated Assessment of Estrogenic Contamination and Biological Effects in the Aquatic Environment of the Netherlands. Chemosphere 2005; 59(4) 511-524.

[41] Kuch HM, Ballschmiter K. Determination of Endocrine-Disrupting Phenolic Compounds and Estrogens in Surface and Drinking Water by Hrgc-(Nci)-Ms in the Picogram Per Liter Range. Environmental Science & Technology 2001; 35(15) 3201-3206.

[42] Beck IC, Bruhn R, Gandrass J, Ruck W. Liquid Chromatography-Tandem Mass Spectrometry Analysis of Estrogenic Compounds in Coastal Surface Water of the Baltic Sea. Journal of Chromatography A 2005; 1090(1-2) 98-106.

[43] Cargouet M, Perdiz D, Mouatassim-Souali A, Tamisier-Karolak S, Levi Y. Assessment of River Contamination by Estrogenic Compounds in Paris Area (France). Science of the Total Environment 2004; 324(1-3) 55-66.

[44] Lagana A, Bacaloni A, De Leva I, Faberi A, Fago G, Marino A. Analytical Methodologies for Determining the Occurrence of Endocrine Disrupting Chemicals in Sewage Treatment Plants and Natural Waters. Analytica Chimica Acta 2004; 501(1) 79-88.

[45] Rodriguez-Mozaz S, López de Alda MJ, Barceló D. Monitoring of Estrogens, Pesticides and Bisphenol a in Natural Waters and Drinking Water Treatment Plants by Solid-Phase Extraction–Liquid Chromatography–Mass Spectrometry. Journal of Chromatography A 2004; 1045(1–2) 85-92.

[46] López-Roldán R, de Alda ML, Gros M, Petrovic M, Martín-Alonso J, Barceló D. Advanced Monitoring of Pharmaceuticals and Estrogens in the Llobregat River Basin (Spain) by Liquid Chromatography–Triple Quadrupole-Tandem Mass Spectrometry in Combination with Ultra Performance Liquid Chromatography–Time of Flight-Mass Spectrometry. Chemosphere 2010; 80(11) 1337-1344.

[47] Arditsoglou A, Voutsa D. Occurrence and Partitioning of Endocrine-Disrupting Compounds in the Marine Environment of Thermaikos Gulf, Northern Aegean Sea, Greece. Marine Pollution Bulletin 2012; 64(11) 2443-2452.

[48] Aydin E, Talinli I. Analysis, Occurrence and Fate of Commonly Used Pharmaceuticals and Hormones in the Buyukcekmece Watershed, Turkey. Chemosphere 2013; 90(6) 2004-2012.

[49] Zuo Y, Zhang K, Deng Y. Occurrence and Photochemical Degradation of 17α-Ethinylestradiol in Acushnet River Estuary. Chemosphere 2006; 63(9) 1583-1590.

[50] Singh S, Azua A, Chaudhary A, Khan S, Willett K, Gardinali P. Occurrence and Distribution of Steroids, Hormones and Selected Pharmaceuticals in South Florida Coastal Environments. Ecotoxicology 2010; 19(2) 338-350.

[51] Sodré FF, Pescara IC, Montagner CC, Jardim WF. Assessing Selected Estrogens and Xenoestrogens in Brazilian Surface Waters by Liquid Chromatography–Tandem Mass Spectrometry. Microchemical Journal 2010; 96(1) 92-98.

[52] Wang L, Ying GG, Zhao JL, Liu S, Yang B, Zhou LJ, Tao R, Su HC. Assessing Estrogenic Activity in Surface Water and Sediment of the Liao River System in Northeast China Using Combined Chemical and Biological Tools. Environmental Pollution 2011; 159(1) 148-156.

[53] Shi J, Liu X, Chen Q, Zhang H. Spatial and Seasonal Distributions of Estrogens and Bisphenol a in the Yangtze River Estuary and the Adjacent East China Sea. Chemosphere 2014; 111(0) 336-343.

[54] Zhang Z, Ren N, Kannan K, Nan J, Liu L, Ma W, Qi H, Li Y. Occurrence of Endocrine-Disrupting Phenols and Estrogens in Water and Sediment of the Songhua River, Northeastern China. Archives of Environmental Contamination and Toxicology 2014; 66(3) 361-369.

[55] Isobe T, Shiraishi H, Yasuda M, Shinoda A, Suzuki H, Morita M. Determination of Estrogens and Their Conjugates in Water Using Solid-Phase Extraction Followed by Liquid Chromatography-Tandem Mass Spectrometry. Journal of Chromatography A 2003; 984(2) 195-202.

[56] Gorga M, Petrovic M, Barceló D. Multi-Residue Analytical Method for the Determination of Endocrine Disruptors and Related Compounds in River and Waste Water Using Dual Column Liquid Chromatography Switching System Coupled to Mass Spectrometry. Journal of Chromatography A 2013; 1295(0) 57-66.

[57] Safe SH. Endocrine Disruptors and Human Health - Is There a Problem? An Update. Environmental Health Perspectives 2000; 108(6) 487-493.

[58] Census. Resultados Definitivos - Portugal, in: I.N.d. Estatística, (Ed.), Lisboa, 2011.

[59] Rocha MJ, Cruzeiro C, Reis M, Rocha E, Pardal MA. Determination of 17 Endocrine Disruptor Compounds and Their Spatial and Seasonal Distribution in the Sado River Estuary (Portugal). Toxicological & Environmental Chemistry 2013; 95(2) 237-253.

[60] Rocha M, Cruzeiro C, Reis M, Rocha E, Pardal M. Determination of Seventeen Endocrine Disruptor Compounds and Their Spatial and Seasonal Distribution in Ria For-

mosa Lagoon (Portugal). Environmental Monitoring and Assessment 2013; 185(10) 8215-8226.

[61] Rocha MJ, Cruzeiro C, Rocha E. Quantification of 17 Endocrine Disruptor Compounds and Their Spatial and Seasonal Distribution in the Iberian Ave River and Its Coastline. Toxicological & Environmental Chemistry 2013; 95(3) 386-399.

[62] Rocha MJ, Cruzeiro C, Rocha E. Development and Validation of a Gc-Ms Method for the Evaluation of 17 Endocrine Disruptor Compounds, Including Phytoestrogens and Sitosterol, in Coastal Waters - Their Spatial and Seasonal Levels in Porto Costal Region (Portugal). Journal of Water & Health 2013; 11(2) 281-296.

[63] Ribeiro C, Tiritan M, Rocha E, Rocha M. Seasonal and Spatial Distribution of Several Endocrine-Disrupting Compounds in the Douro River Estuary, Portugal. Archives of Environmental Contamination and Toxicology 2009; 56(1) 1-11.

[64] Rocha M, Cruzeiro C, Peixoto C, Rocha E. Annual Fluctuations of Endocrine-Disrupting Compounds at the Lower End of the Lima River, Portugal, and in Adjacent Coastal Waters. Archives of Environmental Contamination and Toxicology 2014; 67(3) 389-401.

[65] Rocha MJ, Ribeiro M, Ribeiro C, Couto C, Cruzeiro C, Rocha E. Endocrine Disruptors in the Leça River and Nearby Porto Coast (Nw Portugal): Presence of Estrogenic Compounds and Hypoxic Conditions. Toxicological & Environmental Chemistry 2012; 94(2) 262-274.

[66] Ribeiro C, Pardal M, Martinho F, Margalho R, Tiritan M, Rocha E, Rocha M. Distribution of Endocrine Disruptors in the Mondego River Estuary, Portugal. Environmental Monitoring and Assessment 2009; 149(1-4) 183-193.

[67] Rocha M, Cruzeiro C, Reis M, Pardal M, Rocha E. Spatial and Seasonal Distribution of 17 Endocrine Disruptor Compounds in an Urban Estuary (Mondego River, Portugal): Evaluation of the Estrogenic Load of the Area. Environmental Monitoring and Assessment 2014; 186(6) 3337-3350.

[68] Arditsoglou A, Voutsa D. Passive Sampling of Selected Endocrine Disrupting Compounds Using Polar Organic Chemical Integrative Samplers. Environmental Pollution 2008; 156(2) 316-324.

[69] David A, Fenet H, Gomez E. Alkylphenols in Marine Environments: Distribution Monitoring Strategies and Detection Considerations. Marine Pollution Bulletin 2009; 58(7) 953-960.

[70] Knez J. Endocrine-Disrupting Chemicals and Male Reproductive Health. Reproductive BioMedicine Online 2013; 26(5) 440-448.

[71] Rochester JR. Bisphenol a and Human Health: A Review of the Literature. Reproductive Toxicology 2013; 42(0) 132-155.

[72] Gibson RL. Toxic Baby Bottles. Scientific Finds Leaching Chemicals in Clear Plastic Baby Bottles, in, Environment California Research and Policy Center, 2007, pp. 1-36.

[73] Ying G-G, Williams B, Kookana R. Environmental Fate of Alkylphenols and Alkylphenol Ethoxylates—a Review. Environment International 2002; 28(3) 215-226.

[74] Ahel M, Schaffner C, Giger W. Behaviour of Alkylphenol Polyethoxylates Surfactants in the Aquatic Environment - III. Occurrence and Elimination of Their Persistent Metabolites During Infiltration of River Water to Groundwater. Water Research 1996; 30(1) 37-46.

[75] Warhurst AM. An Environmental Assessment of Alkylphenol Ethoxylates and Alkylphenols, in, 1995.

[76] Wang SL, Chang YC, Chao HR, Li CM, Li LA, Lin LY, Papke O. Body Burdens of Polychlorinated Dibenzo-P-Dioxins, Dibenzofurans, and Biphenyls and Their Relations to Estrogen Metabolism in Pregnant Women. Environmental Health Perspectives 2006; 114(5) 740-745.

[77] Jobling S, Sheahan D, Osborne JA, Matthiessen P, Sumpter JP. Inhibition of Testicular Growth in Rainbow Trout (*Oncorhynchus mykiss*) Exposed to Estrogenic Alkylphenolic Chemicals. Environmental Toxicology and Chemistry 1996; 15(2) 194-202.

[78] Balch G, Metcalfe C. Developmental Effects in Japanese Medaka (*Oryzias latipes*) Exposed to Nonylphenol Ethoxylates and Their Degradation Products. Chemosphere 2006; 62 (8) 1214-1223.

[79] Group B. Apeos Investigation Report as of July 2013, in, 2013.

[80] Stachel B, Ehrhorn U, Heemken O-P, Lepom P, Reincke H, Sawal G, Theobald N. Xenoestrogens in the River Elbe and Its Tributaries. Environmental Pollution 2003; 124(3) 497-507.

[81] Céspedes R, Lacorte S, Raldúa D, Ginebreda A, Barceló D, Piña B. Distribution of Endocrine Disruptors in the Llobregat River Basin (Catalonia, NE Spain). Chemosphere 2005; 61(11) 1710-1719.

[82] EEC. Coucil Directive of 27 July 1976 on the Approximation of the Laws, Regulations and Administrative Provisions of the Member States Relating to Restrictions on the Marketing and Use of Certain Dangerous Substances and Preparations (76/769/Eec), in, 1976.

[83] Azevedo DA, Lacorte S, Viana P, Barceló D. Occurrence of Nonylphenol and Bisphenol-a in Surface Waters from Portugal. Journal of the Brazilian Chemical Society 2001; 12(4) 532-537.

[84] Quirós L, Céspedes R, Lacorte S, Viana P, Raldúa D, Barcelò D, Piña B. Detection and Evaluation of Endocrine-Disruption Activity in Water Samples from Portuguese Rivers. Environmental Toxicology and Chemistry 2005; 24(2) 389-395.

[85] Staniszewska M, Falkowska L, Grabowski P, Kwasniak J, Mudrak-Cegiolka S, Reindl AR, Sokolowski A, Szumilo E, Zgrundo A. Bisphenol A, 4-Tert-Octylphenol, and 4-Nonylphenol in the Gulf of Gdansk (Southern Baltic). Archives of Environmental Contamination and Toxicology 2014; 67(3) 335-347.

[86] Kuch HM, Ballschmiter K. Determination of Endocrine-Disrupting Phenolic Compounds and Estrogens in Surface and Drinking Water by Hrgc–(Nci)–Ms in the Picogram Per Liter Range. Environmental Science & Technology 2001; 35(15) 3201-3206.

[87] Bolz U, Hagenmaier H, Körner W. Phenolic Xenoestrogens in Surface Water, Sediments, and Sewage Sludge from Baden-Württemberg, South-West Germany. Environmental Pollution 2001; 115(2) 291-301.

[88] Voutsa D, Hartmann P, Schaffner C, Giger W. Benzotriazoles, Alkylphenols and Bisphenol A in Municipal Wastewaters and in the Glatt River, Switzerland. Environmental Science and Pollution Research 2006; 13(5) 333-341.

[89] Liu Y, Zhou JL, Wilding A. Simultaneous Determination of Endocrine Disrupting Phenolic Compounds and Steroids in Water by Solid-Phase Extraction-Gas Chromatography-Mass Spectrometry. Journal of Chromatography A 2004; 1022(1-2) 179-189.

[90] Boyd GR, Palmeri JM, Zhang SY, Grimm DA. Pharmaceuticals and Personal Care Products (Ppcps) and Endocrine Disrupting Chemicals (Edcs) in Stormwater Canals and Bayou St. John in New Orleans, Louisiana, USA. Science of the Total Environment 2004; 333(1-3) 137-148.

[91] Liu Y, Guan Y, Tam N, Mizuno T, Tsuno H, Zhu W. Influence of Rainfall and Basic Water Quality Parameters on the Distribution of Endocrine-Disrupting Chemicals in Coastal Area. Water, Air, & Soil Pollution 2010; 209(1-4) 333-343.

[92] Wang B, Huang B, Jin W, Zhao S, Li F, Hu P, Pan X. Occurrence, Distribution, and Sources of Six Phenolic Endocrine Disrupting Chemicals in the 22 River Estuaries around Dianchi Lake in China. Environmental Science and Pollution Research 2013; 20(5) 3185-3194.

[93] Duong CN, Ra JS, Cho J, Kim SD, Choi HK, Park J-H, Kim KW, Inam E, Kim SD. Estrogenic Chemicals and Estrogenicity in River Waters of South Korea and Seven Asian Countries. Chemosphere 2010; 78(3) 286-293.

[94] Basheer C, Lee HK, Tan KS. Endocrine Disrupting Alkylphenols and Bisphenol-a in Coastal Waters and Supermarket Seafood from Singapore. Marine Pollution Bulletin 2004; 48(11–12) 1161-1167.

[95] Ciofi L, Ancillotti C, Chiuminatto U, Fibbi D, Checchini L, Orlandini S, Del Bubba M. Liquid Chromatographic–Tandem Mass Spectrometric Method for the Simultaneous Determination of Alkylphenols Polyethoxylates, Alkylphenoxy Carboxylates and Alkylphenols in Wastewater and Surface-Water. Journal of Chromatography A 2014; 1362(0) 75-88.

[96] Nagy P, Fekete J, Sharma VK. Octylphenol and Nonylphenol in Surface Water of Ráckevei-Soroksári Danube Branch, Hungary. Journal of Environmental Science and Health, Part A 2005; 40(9) 1679-1688.

[97] Loyo-Rosales JE, Schmitz-Afonso I, Rice CP, Torrents A. Analysis of Octyl- and Nonylphenol and Their Ethoxylates in Water and Sediments by Liquid Chromatography/Tandem Mass Spectrometry. Analytical Chemistry 2003; 75(18) 4811-4817.

[98] Yang X, Liu M, Wang Z, Li Q, Zhang Z. Determination of 4-Tert-Octylphenol in Surface Water Samples of Jinan in China by Solid Phase Extraction Coupled with GC-MS. Journal of Environmental Sciences 2013; 25(8) 1712-1717.

[99] Babay PA, Itria RF, Ale EER, Becquart ET, Gautier EA. Ubiquity of Endocrine Disruptors Nonylphenol and Its Mono- and Di-Ethoxylates in Freshwater, Sediments, and Biosolids Associated with High and Low Density Populations of Buenos Aires, Argentina. Clean-Soil Air Water 2014; 42(6) 731-737.

[100] Shao B, Hu J, Yang M, An W, Tao S. Nonylphenol and Nonylphenol Ethoxylates in River Water, Drinking Water,and Fish Tissues in the Area of Chongqing, China. Archives of Environmental Contamination and Toxicology 2005; 48(4) 467-473.

[101] Cladière M, Bonhomme C, Vilmin L, Gasperi J, Flipo N, Tassin B. Modelling the Fate of Nonylphenolic Compounds in the Seine River — Part 1: Determination of in-Situ Attenuation Rate Constants. Science of the Total Environment 2014; 468–469(0) 1050-1058.

[102] Ferguson PL, Iden CR, Brownawell BJ. Distribution and Fate of Neutral Alkylphenol Ethoxylate Metabolites in a Sewage-Impacted Urban Estuary. Environmental Science & Technology 2001; 35(12) 2428-2435.

[103] Ribeiro C, Pardal M, Tiritan M, Rocha E, Margalho R, Rocha M. Spatial Distribution and Quantification of Endocrine-Disrupting Chemicals in Sado River Estuary, Portugal. Environmental Monitoring and Assessment 2009; 159(1-4) 415-427.

[104] FSA. Food Standards Agency, Working Group on Phytoestrogens and Health of the Committee of Toxicology of Chemicals in Food, Consumer Products and the Environment: Phytoestrogens and Health, in: C. Copyright, (Ed.), COT Report 2003.

[105] Kelly MM, Fleischhacker NT, Rearick DC, Arnold WA, Schoenfuss HL, Novak PJ. Phytoestrogens in the Environment, Ii: Microbiological Degradation of Phytoestrogens and the Response of Fathead Minnows to Degradate Exposure. Environmental Toxicology and Chemistry 2014; 33(3) 560-566.

[106] Ishibashi H, Kobayashi M, Koshiishi T, Moriwaki T, Tachibana K, Tsuchimoto M, Soyano K, Iguchi T, Mori C, Arizono K. Induction of Plasma Vitellogenin Synthesis by the Commercial Fish Diets in Male Goldfish (*Carassius auratus*) and Dietary Phytoestrogens. Journal of Health Science 2002; 48(5) 427-434.

[107] Latonnelle K, Fostier A, Le Menn F, Bennetau-Pelissero C. Binding Affinities of Hepatic Nuclear Estrogen Receptors for Phytoestrogens in Rainbow Trout (*Oncorhynchus*

*mykiss*) and Siberian Sturgeon (*Acipenser baeri*). General and Comparative Endocrinology 2002; 129(2) 69-79.

[108] Latonnelle K, Le Menn F, Kaushik SJ, Bennetau-Pelissero C. Effects of Dietary Phytoestrogens *in Vivo* and *in Vitro* in Rainbow Trout and Siberian Sturgeon: Interests and Limits of the *in Vitro* Studies of Interspecies Differences. General and Comparative Endocrinology 2002; 126(1) 39-51.

[109] Hoerger CC, Wettstein FE, Hungerbühler K, Bucheli TD. Occurrence and Origin of Estrogenic Isoflavones in Swiss River Waters. Environmental Science & Technology 2009; 43(16) 6151-6157.

[110] Mackova Z, Koblovska R, Lapcik O. Distribution of Isoflavonoids in Non-Leguminous Taxa – an Update. Phytochemistry 2006; 67(9) 849-855.

[111] Booth NL, Overk CR, Yao P, Totura S, Deng Y, Hedayat AS, Bolton JL, Pauli GF, Farnsworth NR. Seasonal Variation of Red Clover (Trifolium Pratense L., Fabaceae) Isoflavones and Estrogenic Activity. Journal of Agricultural and Food Chemistry 2006; 54(4) 1277-1282.

[112] Benassayag C, Perrot-Applanat M, Ferre F. Phytoestrogens as Modulators of Steroid Action in Target Cells. Journal of Chromatography B 2002; 777(1–2) 233-248.

[113] Clotfelter ED, Rodriguez AC. Behavioral Changes in Fish Exposed to Phytoestrogens. Environmental Pollution 2006; 144(3) 833-839.

[114] Cheshenko K, Pakdel F, Segner H, Kah O, Eggen RIL. Interference of Endocrine Disrupting Chemicals with Aromatase Cyp19 Expression or Activity, and Consequences for Reproduction of Teleost Fish. General and Comparative Endocrinology 2008; 155(1) 31-62.

[115] Rearick DC, Fleischhacker NT, Kelly MM, Arnold WA, Novak PJ, Schoenfuss HL. Phytoestrogens in the Environment, I: Occurrence and Exposure Effects on Fathead Minnows. Environmental Toxicology and Chemistry. 2014; 3(33) 553-559.

[116] Dolbeth M, Cardoso P, Pardal M. Impact of Eutrophication on the Seagrass Assemblages of the Mondego Estuary (Portugal). In: A.A. Ansari, S. Singh Gill, G.R. Lanza, W. Rast (eds.) Eutrophication: Causes, Consequences and Control. Springer Netherlands; 2011. p225-246.

[117] Hoerger CC, Wettstein FE, Hungerbuehler K, Bucheli TD. Occurrence and Origin of Estrogenic Isoflavones in Swiss River Waters. Environmental Science & Technology 2009; 43(16) 6151-6157.

[118] Erbs M, Hoerger CC, Hartmann N, Bucheli TD. Quantification of Six Phytoestrogens at the Nanogram Per Liter Level in Aqueous Environmental Samples Using $^{13}c_3$-Labeled Internal Standards. Journal of Agricultural and Food Chemistry 2007; 55(21) 8339-8345.

[119] Pawlowski S, Ternes T, Bonerz M, Kluczka T, van der Burg B, Nau H, Erdinger L, Braunbeck T. Combined in Situ and *in Vitro* Assessment of the Estrogenic Activity of Sewage and Surface Water Samples. Toxicological Sciences 2003; 75(1) 57-65.

[120] Kolpin DW, Hoerger CC, Meyer MT, Wettstein FE, Hubbard LE, Bucheli TD. Phytoestrogens and Mycotoxins in Iowa Streams: An Examination of Underinvestigated Compounds in Agricultural Basins. Journal of Environmental Quality 2010; 39(6) 2089-2099.

[121] Kuster M, Azevedo DA, de Alda MJL, Neto FRA, Barcelo D. Analysis of Phytoestrogens, Progestogens and Estrogens in Environmental Waters from Rio de Janeiro (Brazil). Environment International 2009; 35(7) 997-1003.

[122] Kang J, Price WE, Hick LA. Simultaneous Determination of Isoflavones and Lignans at Trace Levels in Natural Waters and Wastewater Samples Using Liquid Chromatography/Electrospray Ionization Ion Trap Mass Spectrometry. Rapid Communications in Mass Spectrometry 2006; 20(16) 2411-2418.

[123] Kawanishi M, Takamura-Enya T, Ermawati R, Shimohara C, Sakamoto M, Matsukawa K, Matsuda T, Murahashi T, Matsui S, Wakabayashi K, Watanabe T, Tashiro Y, Yagi T. Detection of Genistein as an Estrogenic Contaminant of River Water in Osaka. Environmental Science & Technology 2004; 38(23) 6424-6429.

[124] Wang C, Wang L, Zhao QS, Chen JH, Zheng L, Zheng MG, Zhang RT, Wang ZJ. Cloud Point Extraction Coupled with Hplc-Dad for the Determination of Genistein and Daidzein in River Water. Analytical Methods 2013; 5(15) 3688-3692.

[125] Beck I-C, Bruhn R, Gandrass J. Analysis of Estrogenic Activity in Coastal Surface Waters of the Baltic Sea Using the Yeast Estrogen Screen. Chemosphere 2006; 63(11) 1870-1878.

[126] EUR-Lex. Case C-223/11: Judgment of the Court (Fifth Chamber) of 21 June 2012 — European Commission V Portuguese Republic (Failure of a Member State to Fulfil Obligations — Environment — Directive 2000/60/Ec — European Union Water Policy — River Basin District Management Plans — Publication and Notification to the Commission — None — Information and Consultation of the Public on the Envisaged Management Plans — None), in, 2012.

[127] EC. European Comission - a Water Blueprint for Europe, in, Blueprint, 2013.

[128] Briggs D. Environmental Pollution and the Global Burden of Disease. British Medical Bulletin 2003; 68(1-24.

[129] Chen G, Zeng Q, Tse G. Estrogen and Its Receptors in Cancer. Medicinal Research Reviews 2008; 28(6) 954-974.

[130] Gonzales R, Ansar S, Duckles S, Krause D. Androgenic/Estrogenic Balance in the Male Rat Cerebral Circulation: Metabolic Enzymes and Sex Steroid Receptors. J Cereb Blood Flow Metab 2007; 27(11) 1841-1852.

[131] Lemmen J, Arends R, van Boxtel A, van der Saag P, van der Burg B. Tissue and Time Dependent Estrogen Receptor Activation in Estrogen Reporter Mice. Journal of Molecular Endocrinology 2004; 32(3) 689-701.

[132] Roy D, Liehr J. Estrogen DNA Damage and Mutations. Mutation Research 1999; 424((1-2) 107-115.

[133] Cavalieri E, Stack D, Devanesan P. Molecular Origin of Cancer: Catechol Estrogen-3,4-Quinones as Endogenous Tumor Initiators. Proc Nat Acad Sci USA 1997; 94(20) 10937 - 10942.

[134] Liehr J. Genotoxicity of the Steroidal Oestrogens Oestrone and Oestradiol:Possible Mechanism of Uterine and Mammary Cancer Development. Human Reproduction Update 2001; 7(3) 273-281.

[135] Carrola J, Santos N, Rocha M, Fontainhas-Fernandes A, Pardal M, Monteiro RF, Rocha E. Frequency of Micronuclei and of Other Nuclear Abnormalities in Erythrocytes of the Grey Mullet from the Mondego, Douro and Ave Estuaries—Portugal. Environmental Science and Pollution Research 2014; 21(9) 6057-6068.

[136] Ganmaa D, Sato A. The Possible Role of Female Sex Hormones in Milk from Pregnant Cows in the Development of Breast, Ovarian and Corpus Uteri Cancers. Medical Hypotheses 2005; 65(6) 1028-1037.

[137] Pritchard-Jones K, Kaatsch P, Steliarova-Foucher E, Stiller C, Coebergh J. Cancer in Children and Adolescence in Europe: Developments over 20 Years and Future Challenges. European Journal of Cancer 2006; 42(13) 2183-2190.

[138] Taylor JA, Richter CA, Ruhlen RL, Saal FSV. Estrogenic Environmental Chemicals and Drugs: Mechanisms for Effects on the Developing Male Urogenital System. Journal of Steroid Biochemistry and Molecular Biology 2011; 127(1-2) 83-95.

[139] Kim EJ, Lee D, Chung BC, Pyo H, Lee J. Association between Urinary Levels of Bisphenol-A and Estrogen Metabolism in Korean Adults. Science of the Total Environment 2014; 470 1401-1407.

[140] Sugiura-Ogasawara M, Ozaki Y, Sonta SI, Makino T, Suzumori K. Exposure to Bisphenol A Is Associated with Recurrent Miscarriage. Human Reproduction 2005; 20(8) 2325-2329.

[141] Caserta D, Di Segni N, Mallozzi M, Giovanale V, Mantovani A, Marci R, Moscarini M. Bisphenol A and the Female Reproductive Tract: An Overview of Recent Laboratory Evidence and Epidemiological Studies. Reproductive Biology and Endocrinology 2014; 12 37

[142] Dhaini HR, Nassif RM. Exposure Assessment of Endocrine Disruptors in Bottled Drinking Water of Lebanon. Environmental Monitoring and Assessment 2014; 186(9) 5655-5662.

[143] Lee BE, Park H, Hong YC, Ha M, Kim Y, Chang N, Kim BN, Kim YJ, Yu SD, Ha EH. Prenatal Bisphenol a and Birth Outcomes: Moceh (Mothers and Children's Environmental Health) Study. International Journal of Hygiene and Environmental Health 2014; 217(2-3) 328-334.

[144] Rouiller-Fabre V, Habert R, Livera G. Effects of Endocrine Disruptors on the Human Fetal Testis. Annales d'Endocrinologie 2014; 75(2) 54-57.

[145] Albini A, Rosano C, Angelini G, Amaro A, Esposito AI, Maramotti S, Noonan DM, Pfeffer U. Exogenous Hormonal Regulation in Breast Cancer Cells by Phytoestrogens and Endocrine Disruptors. Current Medicinal Chemistry 2014; 21(9) 1129-1145.

[146] Carmichael SL, Cogswell ME, Ma C, Gonzalez-Feliciano A, Olney RS, Correa A, Shaw GM, Natl Birth Defects P. Hypospadias and Maternal Intake of Phytoestrogens. American Journal of Epidemiology 2013; 178(3) 434-440.

[147] Patisaul HB. Effects of Environmental Endocrine Disruptors and Phytoestrogens on the Kisspeptin System. In: A.S. Kauffman, J.T. Smith (eds.) Kisspeptin Signaling in Reproductive Biology. New York: Springer; 2013. p455-479.

[148] Eustache F, Mondon F, Canivenc-Lavier MC, Lesaffre C, Fulla Y, Berges R, Cravedi JP, Vaiman D, Auger J. Chronic Dietary Exposure to a Low-Dose Mixture of Genistein and Vinclozolin Modifies the Reproductive Axis, Testis Transcriptome, and Fertility. Environmental Health Perspectives 2009; 117(8) 1272-1279.

[149] Vollmer G, Starcke S, Wober J, Zierau O. Endocrine Modulation and the Fragile Balance of Homeostasis - an Overview. Neuroendocrinology Letters 2002; 23(2) 37-42.

[150] Patisaul HB, Jefferson W. The Pros and Cons of Phytoestrogens. Frontiers in neuroendocrinology 2010; 31(4) 400-419.

[151] Ferlay J, Autier P, Boniol M, Heaune M, Colombet M, Boyle P. Estimates of the Incidence and Mortality in Europe in 2006. Annals of Oncology 2007; 18(3) 581-592.

[152] Giannandrea F, Paoli D, Figà-Talamanca I, Lombardo F, Lenzi A, Gandini L. Effect of Endogenous and Exogenous Hormones on Testicular Cancer: The Epidemiological Evidence. The International Journal Of Developmental Biology 2013; 57(2-4) 255-263.

[153] Madureira TV, Barreiro JC, Rocha MJ, Cass QB, Tiritan ME. Pharmaceutical Trace Analysis in Aqueous Environmental Matrices by Liquid Chromatography-Ion Trap Tandem Mass Spectrometry. Journal of Chromatography A 2009; 1216(42) 7033-7042.

[154] Madureira TV, Rocha MJ, Cass QB, Tiritan ME. Development and Optimization of a Hplc-Dad Method for the Determination of Diverse Pharmaceuticals in Estuarine Surface Waters. Journal of Chromatographic Science 2010; 48(3) 176-182.

[155] Madureira TV, Barreiro JC, Rocha MJ, Rocha E, Cass QB, Tiritan ME. Spatiotemporal Distribution of Pharmaceuticals in the Douro River Estuary (Portugal). Science of the Total Environment 2010; 408(22) 5513-5520.

[156] Rocha MJ, Ferreira PC, Reis PA, Cruzeiro C, Rocha E. Determination of Polycyclic Aromatic Hydrocarbons in Coastal Sediments from the Porto Region (Portugal) by Microwave-Assisted Extraction, Followed by Spme and Gc-Ms. Journal of Chromatographic Science 2011; 49(9) 695-701.

[157] Rocha MJ, Ribeiro MFT, Cruzeiro C, Figueiredo F, Rocha E. Development and Validation of a Gc-Ms Method for Determination of 39 Common Pesticides in Estuarine Water - Targeting Hazardous Amounts in the Douro River Estuary. International Journal of Environmental Analytical Chemistry 2012; 92(14) 1587-1608.

[158] Madureira TV, Rocha MJ, Cruzeiro C, Rodrigues I, Monteiro RAF, Rocha E. The Toxicity Potential of Pharmaceuticals Found in the Douro River Estuary (Portugal): Evaluation of Impacts on Fish Liver, by Histopathology, Stereology, Vitellogenin and Cyp1a Immunohistochemistry, after Sub-Acute Exposures of the Zebrafish Model. Environmental Toxicology and Pharmacology 2012; 34(1) 34-45.

[159] Madureira TV, Velhote S, Santos C, Cruzeiro C, Rocha E, Rocha MJ. A Step Forward Using Quechers (Quick, Easy, Cheap, Effective, Rugged, and Safe) Based Extraction and Gas Chromatography-Tandem Mass Spectrometry-Levels of Priority Polycyclic Aromatic Hydrocarbons in Wild and Commercial Mussels. Environmental Science and Pollution Research 2014; 21(9) 6089-6098.

[160] Rocha MJ, ReisHenriques MA. Plasma and Urine Levels of $C_{-18}$, $C_{-19}$ and $C_{-21}$ Steroids in an Asynchronous Fish, the Tilapia *Oreochromis mossambicus* (Teleostei, Cichlidae). Comparative Biochemistry and Physiology C-Pharmacology Toxicology & Endocrinology 1996; 115(3) 257-264.

[161] Rocha MJ, Reis-Henriques MA. Plasma Levels of $C_{-18}$-, $C_{-19}$- and $C_{-21}$-Steroids in Captive and Feral Female Sea Bass. Journal of Fish Biology 1999; 55(1) 26-34.

[162] Rocha MJ, Reis-Henriques MA. Steroid Metabolism by Ovarian Follicles of the Sea Bass *Dicentrarchus labrax*. Comparative Biochemistry and Physiology C-Pharmacology Toxicology & Endocrinology 2000; 125(1) 85-91.

[163] Rocha MJ, Reis-Henriques MA. Steroid Metabolism by Ovarian Follicles of the Tilapia *Oreochromis mossambicus* (Teleostei, Cichlidae). Comparative Biochemistry and Physiology B-Biochemistry & Molecular Biology 1998; 121(1) 85-90.

[164] Castro LFC, Rocha MJ, Lobo-da-Cunha A, Batista-Pinto C, Machado A, Rocha E. The 17 Beta-Hydroxysteroid Dehydrogenase 4: Gender-Specific and Seasonal Gene Expression in the Liver of Brown Trout (*Salmo trutta* f. *fario*). Comparative Biochemistry and Physiology B-Biochemistry & Molecular Biology 2009; 153(2) 157-164.

[165] Ribeiro C, Urbatzka R, Castro LFC, Carrola J, Fontainhas-Fernandes A, Monteiro RAF, Rocha E, Rocha MJ. *In Vitro* Exposure of Nile Tilapia (*Oreochromis niloticus*) Testis to Estrogenic Endocrine Disrupting Chemicals: mRNA Expression of Genes Encoding Steroidogenic Enzymes. Toxicology Mechanisms and Methods 2012; 22(1) 47-53.

http://dx.doi.org/10.5772/59885

[166] Urbatzka R, Rocha E, Reis B, Cruzeiro C, Monteiro RAF, Rocha MJ. Effects of Ethinylestradiol and of an Environmentally Relevant Mixture of Xenoestrogens on Steroidogenic Gene Expression and Specific Transcription Factors in Zebrafish. Environmental Pollution 2012; 164 28-35.

[167] Castro LFC, Lobo-da-Cunha A, Rocha MJ, Urbatzka R, Rocha E. Pex11 Alpha in Brown Trout (*Salmo trutta* f. *fario*): Expression Dynamics During the Reproductive Cycle Reveals Sex-Specific Seasonal Patterns. Comparative Biochemistry and Physiology A-Molecular & Integrative Physiology 2013; 164(1) 207-214.

[168] Silva P, Rocha MJ, Cruzeiro C, Malhao F, Reis B, Urbatzka R, Monteiro RAF, Rocha E. Testing the Effects of Ethinylestradiol and of an Environmentally Relevant Mixture of Xenoestrogens as Found in the Douro River (Portugal) on the Maturation of Fish Gonads - A Stereological Study Using the Zebrafish (*Danio rerio*) as Model. Aquatic Toxicology 2012; 124 1-10.

[169] Sousa ML, Silva A, Malhao F, Rocha MJ, Rocha E, Urbatzka R. Viability Analysis of Oocyte-Follicle Complexes and Gonadal Fragments of Zebrafish as Baseline for Toxicity Testing. Toxicology Mechanisms and Methods 2014; 24(1) 42-49.

[170] Esteban S, Gorga M, González-Alonso S, Petrovic M, Barceló D, Valcárcel Y. Monitoring endocrine disrupting compounds and estrogenic activity in tap water from Central Spain. Environmental Science and Pollution Research 2014; 21(15) 9297-9310.

[171] Brody JG, Aschengrau A, McKelvey W, Swartz CH, Kennedy T, Rudel RA. Breast cancer risk and drinking water contaminated by wastewater: a case control study. Environmental Health 2006; 5:28.

Chapter 8

# Impact of Pesticides on Environmental and Human Health

Mariana Furio Franco Bernardes, Murilo Pazin,
Lilian Cristina Pereira and Daniel Junqueira Dorta

Additional information is available at the end of the chapter

http://dx.doi.org/10.5772/59710

## 1. Introduction

Pesticides constitute any substance or mixture of substances intended for preventing, destroying, repelling, or mitigating any pest. They can also serve as plant regulators, defoliants, or dessicants [1].

Chemicals have long been used to control pests. Sumerians already employed sulfur compounds to control insects and mites 4500 years ago. Pyrethrum, a compound derived from the dried flowers of *Chrysanthemum cinerariaefolium*, has been applied as an insecticide for over 2000 years. Salt or sea water has been used to control weeds. Inorganic substances, such as sodium chlorate and sulfuric acid, or organic chemicals derived from natural sources were widely employed in pest control until the 1940s [2].

During World War II (1939-1945), the development of pesticides increased, because it was urgent to enhance food production and to find potential chemical warfare agents [3]. Consequently, the1940s witnessed a marked growth in synthetic pesticides like DDT, aldrin, dieldrin, endrin, parathion, and 2,4-D. In the 1950s, the application of pesticides in agriculture was considered advantageous, and no concern about the potential risks of these chemicals to the environment and the human health existed [2].

In 1962, Rachel Carson published the book "Silent Spring", in which she mentioned problems that could arise from the indiscriminate use of pesticides. This book inspired widespread concern about the impact of pesticides on the human health and the environment. In 1967, Ratcliffe [4] noted increased incidence of raptor nests with broken eggs in the United Kingdom. This author showed that the sharp decline in eggshell thickness coincided with the beginning of the widespread use of DDT in agriculture (1945–1946). In the 1970s, pest resistance emerged which, combined with influence of the book "Silent Spring", and accumulated evidence on the effects of pesticides, culminated in banning of the use of DDT in the United States in 1972. Thereafter, other countries discontinued the use of DDT, as well [5].

The 1970s and 1980s saw the introduction of more selective pesticides. In the 1990s, research activities concentrated on finding new members of existing pesticides that were even more selective. Besides, pesticides with new chemical groups emerged. During this period, safer chemicals arose. In addition, Integrated Pest Management (IPM) systems, came into play – these systems used crop production methods that attracted predators or parasites that attacked pests and timed pesticide applications to coincide with the most susceptible period of the pest's life cycle, thereby reducing the amount of applied pesticides [2].

However, IPM or related methods did not eliminate the need for pesticides. These chemicals ensure the production of adequate quantities of high quality pest-free crops, which is important for food supply, prevents human diseases transmitted by insect or rodent vectors, and positively impacts public health [6].

The best pesticide policies need to reconcile environmental concerns with economic realities – pest management is mandatory, and farmers must survive economically. A number of studies have described the problems that not using pesticides would cause. Without pesticides, food production would be lower, and larger cultivated farm areas would be necessary to produce the same amount of food, which would impact the wildlife habitat. More frequent cultivation of the fields would be increase soil loss due to erosion, too. Knutson et al. [7] have pictured the U.S. society without pesticides: agricultural production would decrease, food prices would rise, farmers would be less competitive in global markets, and U.S. exports would drop, leading to many job losses [8].

Despite their benefits, pesticides can be hazardous to both humans and the environment. Countless chemicals are environmentally stable, prone to bioaccumulation, and toxic [6]. Because some pesticides can persist in the environment, they can remain there for years. Environmental contamination or occupational use can expose the general population to pesticides residues, including physical and biological degradation products present in the air, water, and food [9].

Less than 1% of the total amount of pesticides applied for weed and pest control reach the target pests. A large quantity of pesticides is lost via spray drift, off-target deposition, run-off, and photodegradation, for instance, which can have undesirable effects on some species, communities, or ecosystems as a whole, as well as on the humans [10]. Another relevant factor is that low concentrations of many chemicals may not elicit acute detectable effects in organisms, but they may induce other damage, like genetic disorders and physiological alterations, which reduce life span in the long run [11].

There are various ways to group pesticides, including classification based on the pests they control. Some example, insecticides combat insect growth or survival, herbicides act against plants, weeds, and grasses, rodenticides tight against rats and other rodents, avicides act against bird populations, fungicides attack fungi, and nematicides combat nematodes [12]. The global pesticide market divided according to the type of pesticide is as follows: 42.48% herbicides, 25.57% insecticides, 24.19% fungicides, and 7.76% other types of pesticides [13].

Pesticides grouping can also rely on their chemical structure. Organophosphorus (chlorpyrifos and diazinon), carbamates (carbaryl and aldicarb), organochlorine (DDT and aldrin), pyrethrins and pyrethroids (cyfluthrin and cypermethrin), benzoic acids (dicamba), triazines (atrazine and simazine), phenoxyacetic derivatives (2,4-D), dipyridyl derivatives (diquat and paraquat), glycine derivatives (glyphosate), and dithiocarbamates (maneb and ziram) [12].

Pesticides that bear similar chemical structures exhibit similar mechanism of toxicity and physicochemical properties, as well as comparable fate and transport properties. This chapter will deal with pesticides according to their chemical group. Pesticides belonging to different chemical classes but which have similar toxic effects, such as the ability to induce oxidative stress and act as endocrine disrupters will be treated as well.

## 2. Physical and chemical properties and stages of intoxication

### 2.1. Organophosphorus

Organic compounds containing phosphorus, the so called organophosphorus compounds (OP), have found application as pesticides and war gases since their synthesis, in 1937 [14]. OP contain carbon and derive from phosphorous acid. Their primary structure may vary depending on whether they bear sulfur (S) or oxygen (O) double binds. X is a group of the general structure that separates when the compound binds to acetylcholinesterase (AChE). On the basis of the variations in their general structure, it is possible to subdivide these compounds into phosphates, phosphorothioates, phosphoramidates, and phosphonate, for example. The structural difference between these compounds results in peculiar characteristics regarding OP metabolism and toxicity. Some representatives of this class of pesticides are Diazinon, Malathion, and Paration [15].

The skin, conjunctiva, gastrointestinal tract, and lungs rapidly absorb most OP compounds. Cytochrome $P_{450}$ isozymes metabolize these chemicals in the liver, which sometimes generates metabolites that are more toxic than the parent compounds [16]. One example is the oxon form, which may bind to cholinesterase or undergo hydrolysis to a dialkyl phosphate and a hydrolyzed organic moiety specific to the pesticide [14]. Most OP are polar and hence water soluble. Their metabolites arise 12 to 48 h after exposure. However, a few compounds, such as dichlofenthion, possess high partition coefficients, which culminates in long-lasting symptoms [17].

These pesticides can reversibly or irreversibly stablish covalent bonds with the serine residue in the active site of acetyl cholinesterase, to prevent the natural function of this enzyme in the catabolism of neurotransmitters [14]. The formation of complexes between acetylcholinesterase enzymes and organophosphates leads to phosphorylation and deactivation, and the neurotransmitter acetylcholine consequently accumulates in the synaptic cleft. The accumulation of large amounts of acetylcholine stimulates and exhausts cholinergic synapses due to the excessive cholinergic activity produced by these agents [18]. The cholinesterase-bound phosphate group can lose the o,o-dialkyl groups or undergo hydrolysis, to regenerate the active enzyme. This process occurs not only in insects, but also in humans and the wildlife [14].

The main symptoms of pesticides intoxication can be differentiated into syndromes like the muscarinic syndrome, in which the action of acetylcholine on the smooth muscle, heart, and exocrine glands increases bronchial secretion, tearing, and sweating; disrupts the gastrointestinal tone to cause nausea, vomiting, and diarrhea; and elicits urinary incontinence, bronchospasm, miosis, and bradycardia. Another example is the nicotine syndrome, in which acetylcholine accumulates at the motor nerve endings in the autonomic ganglia and causes tremors, spasms, hypertonicity, hyperreflexia, paralysis, or muscle weakness and stimulates the sympathetic autonomic ganglia, to promote tachycardia, pallor, hyperglycemia, and hypertension. Additional effects on the central nervous system (CNS) include anxiety, headache, dizziness, ataxia, sleep and memory disorders seizures, tremors, respiratory depression, and coma. Some OP still have teratogenic potential and mutagenic effects. Laboratory diagnosis of this syndrome involves determination of cholinesterase activity [19].

To treat poisoning with OP, it is necessary to maintain vital functions and assess cholinesterase levels in the red cells and pseudocholinesterase levels in the plasma, before therapy. It is important to avoid the use of parasympathomimetic agents, which may increase the anticholinesterase activity. Treatment should start with atropine, which acts as a competitive muscarinic anticholinergic agent, together with pralidoxime, until complete control of the symptoms. After atropinization, administration of furosemide prevents pulmonary congestion, whereas administration of benzodiazepines controls seizures [20].

### 2.2. Carbamates

Carbamates insecticides produce clinical signs and symptoms of cholinergic excess that resemble the signs elicited by organophosphate toxicity, except that the effects are more reversible and less severe [14]. The mechanisms underlying carbamates poisoning involve carbamylation of the active site of acetylcholinesterase, which inactivate this essential enzyme in the nervous system of humans and other animal species [21]. The reaction of carbamates with acetylcholinesterase is similar to the reaction of OP with the same enzyme. However, reactivation of the carbamylated enzyme by hydrolysis is faster as compared with reactivation of the phosphorylated enzyme, with reversal of inhibition typically occurring half an hour or less after exposure [22]. Nevertheless, reports on cases of neuropathy after poisoning exist [23].

Organisms readily absorb carbamates through the lungs, gastrointestinal tract, and skin. Fortunately, carbamates poorly penetrate the blood-brain barrier. Therefore, they affect brain cholinesterases activity minimally and promote fewer CNS symptoms as compared with organophosphates. In addition, the spontaneous in vivo hydrolysis of the carbamate-cholinesterase complex contributes to less severe and less enduring symptoms.

The main symptoms of carbamates intoxication are miosis, salivation, sweating, tearing, rhinorrhea, behavioral change, abdominal pain, vomiting, diarrhea, urinary incontinence, bronchospasm, dyspnea, hypoxemia, bradycardia, bronchial secretions, pulmonary edema,

http://dx.doi.org/10.5772/59710

respiratory failure, drop in body temperature, incoordination, lip tingling, tremors, and seizures. Less common symptoms include muscle spasms, twitching, muscle weakness (including respiratory muscles), paralysis, tachycardia, and hypertension [24].

The treatment of carbamates intoxication includes maintenance of vital functions. It is crucial to avoid the use of parasympathomimetic agents, because they may increase the anticholinesterase activity. Treatment should start with atropine, followed by administration of furosemide, only if necessary. If poisoning is due to pure carbamates only, it is not necessary to administrate pralidoxime, except in cases that these carbamates are associated with OPs [15].

### 2.3. Organochlorines

Organochlorine is used mainly as insecticides. Human body burden due to organochlorine pesticides results from the universal presence of these contaminants in the environment. This constitutes a major public health concern; indeed, organochlorines have been linked with cancer, asthma, diabetes, and growth disorders in children [25]. Organochlorine pesticides include cyclodienes, hexachlorocyclohexane isomers, and DDT and its analogues (e.g., DDE, methoxyclor, and dicofol) [14].

Exposure to organochlorines occurs via ingestion of contaminated food or water, inhalation of vapor, and absorption through the skin. Occupational and other domiciliary exposures are also possible. Dietary exposure results in bioaccumulation of these chemicals in the human body [26].

Organochlorines have similar structure – they all contain a cyclodiene ring. The lungs, gastrointestinal tract, and skin can absorb all these compounds. In addition, although the organism absorbs approximately 10% of the applied dose, lipid solvents increase dermal penetration [15], thereby raising the risk of intoxication in the case of workers who apply these products in crops without proper protective equipment.

The accumulation of organochlorine compounds is a result of their chemical structure and their physical properties such as polarity and solubility. These fat-soluble compounds persist in both the body and the environment. Consequently, researchers and regulatory agencies have banned several organochlorines [14].

The main symptoms of organichlorines intoxication are dizziness, headache, anorexia, nausea, vomiting, malaise, dermatitis, diarrhea, apprehension, excitement, irritability, gait disorders, excessive sweating, altered reflexes, muscle weakness, tremors, spasms, mental confusion, anxiety, seizures, coma, and death. The carcinogenicity of this class of compound is assigned to polychlorocyclodiene compounds that form epoxides during their biotransformation. Because organochlorines have long half-life, these levels in the serum constitute a marker of exposure to these pesticides [15].

To treat organochlorines intoxication, it is necessary to maintain the vital functions, administer diazepam and phenobarbital by slow injection, to control seizures, and to monitor the airways closely. Lorazepam constitutes an alternative to diazepam. Ion exchange resins can also be administered orally. Arrhythmias that damage the myocardium rarely occur. Lidocaine is the treatment of choice [27].

### 2.4. Pyrethrins and pyrethroids

Pyrethrins and pyrethroids function mainly as iseticides. Pyrethrins are natural compounds originating from the plant *Chrysanthemum cinerariaefolium*. They comprise active agents (pyrethrins I-VI), but pyrethrins I and II are the most active. These compounds decompose rapidly in the presence of light, but synthetic production of pyrethroids around 1950 overcame some disadvantages of natural pyrethrins [15].

Crude pyrethrum is a dermal and respiratory allergen, probably due it is to non-insecticidal ingredients. Contact dermatitis and allergic respiratory reactions (rhinitis and asthma) have occurred after exposure to this compound [28].

Both pyrethrins and pyrethroids bear an acid moiety, a central ester bond, and an alcohol moiety in their structure. This class of compounds typically exists as stereoisomers (*trans* and *cis*) for a total of eight different stereoenantiomers. In adittion, they comprise two main groups, Type I and Type II, which bear a cyano group in the alpha position or not, respectively [29].

After absorption, rapid pyrethroids distribution occurs in the organism. Therein, these compounds undergo biotransformation via two mechanisms: hydrolysis of the ester linkage by carboxylesterases and oxidation of the alcohol moiety by cytochromes $P_{450}$ [30]. Pyrethroids exert the same mechanism of action in insects and mammals. Both pyrethrins and pyrethroids have insecticide potential because they can disrupt the muscular system and alter the normal functioning of voltage-dependent sodium channels. Sodium channels play an important role in the cell-to-cell communication, which is vital for the function of more excitable cells involved in the action potential that the excitable cells can propagate in the CNS. Pyrethroids bind to the $\alpha$-subunit of the sodium channel that is left open for a longer time, to increase membrane permeability to sodium. Consequently, these compounds cause paralysis, especially in flying insects, known as knockdown. The specific interaction of pyrethroids with the sodium channel shows both the activation and inactivation properties of the sodium channel, making the hyperexcited cells [31]. After interaction of moderate levels of pyrethroids with the sodium channel, the cell can continue to operate in an abnormal state of hyperexcitability. The amplitude of the sodium current remains unchanged until the level of hyperexcitability overwhelms the maintenance of the activity of the sodium channel. This culminates in depolarization and blocks conduction of the action potential until the situation in the cell becomes unsustainable [31].

The toxicodynamics of pyrethroids may also include other mechanisms such as antagonism of gamma-aminobutyric acid (GABA), stimulation of chloride channels modulated by protein kinase, modulation of nicotinic cholinergic transmission, increased release of noradrenaline, and deregulation of calcium homeostasis. Authors have also proposed that pyrethroids act on the voltage-sensitive chloride channels as well as on the voltage-dependent calcium channels [31].

Diagnosis can be difficult because acute pyrethroid poisoning can be mistaken for OP intoxication. Pyrethroid poisoning symptoms are: tremors, spasms, incoordination, prostration, drooling, irregular movements of the limbs, tonic and clonic convulsions, and hypersensitivity to stimuli. It can also cause skin irritation and tingling due to hyperactivity of cutaneous sensory nerve fibers. Eye miosis also occurs due to exposure [32].

Because exposure to pyrethroids does not usually prompt systemic effects, most patients only require decontamination of the skin and eyes, besides basic maintenance of the vital functions. Paresthesia usually subsides within 12-24 h, which dismisses direct treatment. If severe skin irritation occurs, application of DL-α-tocopherol acetate (Vitamin E) should alternate this problem. Gastric lavage is discarded in case of ingestion, because solvents present in many formulations may increase the risk of aspiration pneumonia. Ingestion of a potentially toxic amount requires administration of activated charcoal within one hour of the event [32].

### 2.5. Triazines

Triazines are effective and inexpensive compounds that have found application as herbicides. They combat a wide spectrum of weeds by inhibiting photosynthesis and the electron transport chain in plants. Physiological and molecular changes due to accumulation of these compounds in organisms remain unclear. Human exposure to triazines has been associated with carcinogenicity and endocrine disruption, but these effects are still debatable [33]. The chemical structures of triazine herbicides correspond to permutations of the alkyl substituted 2,4-diamines of chlorotriazine [14].

After absorption, these compounds undergo conjugation with glutathione or simply dealkylation. The chlorine group of the triazine structure is replaced with the free-SH group of glutathione, the terminal peptide is cleaved, and the cysteine moiety is N-acetylated. The mercapturate residues and the dealkylation metabolites are subsequently excreted in the urine [14]. Triazines have low acute oral and dermal toxicity. Chronic toxicity studies have primarily indicated reduced body weight gain [16].

Atrazine is the often most studied triazine herbicide. Authors have investigated their carcinogenic potential in mice and rats. Tumor incidence did not augment in mice, whereas atrazine appeared to increase the incidence of mammary carcinoma in Sprague-Dawley rats [34, 35].

Reports of human poisoning by this class of compounds are rare. When they happen, irritation at the site of contamination such as the skin, eyes, nose, and TGI occurs. Triazines may be carcinogenic and teratogenic, but there is still no evidence that this is really the case. Contamination with atrazine may also cause sensory motor polyneuropathy [15, 33].

Because exposure to triazines usually causes local irritation, in most cases it is only necessary to decontaminate the site exposed to the substance, besides offering basic life support [15].

### 2.6. Phenoxy derivatives

The structures of phenoxy derivatives bear an aliphatic carboxylic acid moiety attached to a chloride or methyl-substituted aromatic ring. The commonest phenoxy herbicides are 2,4-dichlorophenoxyacetic acid (2,4-D) and 2,4,5-trichlorophenoxyacetic acid (2,4,5-T). A combination of these two herbicides in equal proportions affords Agent Orange, a product applied in the jungles of Vietnam, Laos, and Cambodia during the Vietnam War. Manufacture of phenoxy herbicides often requires co-formulation with ioxynil and/or bromoxynil, which are generally more toxic than the herbicides. Moreover, other more toxic substances can emerge during the fabrication of some of these herbicides at excessively high temperatures, such as at chlorinated dibenzo dioxin and chlorinated dibenzo furan [36]. Because 2,4,5-T contains the highly toxic and persistent 2,3,7,8-tetrachlorodibenzeno-*p*-dioxin along with other chlorinated dioxins and furans, regulatory agencies have banned it for most applications [14].

Phenoxy salts and esters rapidly dissociate or hydrolyze in vivo, so the toxicity of the derivative will depend mainly on the acid form of the pesticide. Individuals and species vary substantially in terms of phenoxy herbicides elimination. The biological half-life of herbicides in humans reportedly varies from 12 to 72 h [36], but long half-lives occur at large doses and after prolonged exposure [28].

The gastrointestinal tract absorbs phenoxy derivatives. The lungs absorb them less, their cutaneous absorption is minimal, and fat does not store them. Phenoxy derivatives exhibit a variety of mechanisms of toxicity including dose-dependent cell membrane damage, uncoupling of oxidative phosphorylation, and disruption of acetylcoenzyme A metabolism [36]. Phenoxy acids and esters are moderately irritating to the skin, eyes, and the respiratory, gastrointestinal, and mucous membranes. Their toxicity on the CNS is dose-dependent. These derivatives disrupt the blood-brain barrier and the neuronal membrane transport mechanisms, and damage to the intracellular membrane results in uncoupling of oxidative phosphorylation [36]. In addition, prolonged inhalation of these herbicides may cause burning sensation in the nasopharynx and dizziness. Some recent studies have examined female exposure to herbicides and assessed effects such as spontaneous abortion, birth defects, and infertility, among others [28].

Intoxication by this class of compounds is uncommon, but when they occur they can cause serious sequelae. The main symptoms are nausea, dizziness, vomiting, burning in the mouth, constipation, abdominal pain, numbness, diarrhea, gastrointestinal bleeding, gastrointestinal fluid loss, vasodilation and/or direct toxicity due to grafting hypotension, ECG alterations like ventricular or supraventricular tachycardia and, on rare occasions, sinus bradycardia. In more severe cases, agitation, confusion, weakness, paralysis, coma, and death by ventricular fibrillation can occur, and chances of survival are small. Other disrupted functions comprise changes in the NCS [36]. Some compounds of this class (e.g., 2,4,5-T) can also produce carcinogenic and teratogenic effects as well as hepatotoxicity. As for metabolic acidosis, clinical signs such as hyperthermia (due to uncoupling of oxidative phosphorylation), renal failure, increased aspartate aminotransferase and alanine and lactate dehydrogenase, thrombocytopenia, hemolytic anemia, and hypocalcemia activities can arise [36].

In general, treatment of phenoxy derivatives poisoning includes maintenance of the vital functions. If the poisoning is due to ingestion, administration of activated charcoal is necessary for adsorption of the compounds, provided that intoxication occurred within an hour. Systemic poisoning calls for hemodialysis, but other effective purification methods exist, like alkalinization of the urine flow and increase of urine volume to facilitate excretion. To control seizures, administration of benzodiazepines is mandatory [36].

http://dx.doi.org/10.5772/59710

### 2.7. Dipyridyl derivatives

The dipyridyl compounds paraquat and diquat are non-selective contact herbicides that have found wide application in agriculture and industries. They help to control weeds. However, these compounds are highly toxic and managing poisoning with these substances requires a great skill and knowledge of proper management procedures [28].

Paraquat (1,1′-dimethyl-4,4′-dipyridylium) is a dipyridylium quaternary ammonium compound related to diquat and morfamquat. The latter product is the least toxic but also the least effective herbicide [15]. Their biotransformation produces free radicals, with consequent lipid peroxidation and cell injury [37].

Paraquat causes aggressive tissue damage in the lungs, kidney, and liver. The major target organ of paraquat poisoning is the lung, which consists of the most lethal and the least treatable manifestation of toxicity. Reactive oxygen species (ROS) play a crucial role in paraquat induced pulmonary injury, characterized by edema hemorrhage and hypoxemia, as well as infiltration of inflammatory cells [28, 38].

The other representative of this class is diquat (1,1′-ethylene-2,2′-bipyridilium), which causes fewer poisoning events than paraquat, the reason why reports on human toxicity and animal experimental data are less extensive for diquat than paraquat. The mechanisms of paraquat and diquat toxicity are similar: radicals destroy lipid membranes. After absorption, diquat does not selectively concentrate in the lung tissue, but it exerts severe toxic effects on the CNS, an event that is not typical in the case of paraquat [28]. The kidney is the main excretory pathway for absorbed diquat. Renal damage is therefore an important feature of diquat poisoning [15, 28].

A very interesting action against poisoning by diquat and paraquat is the addition of an emetic agent in their formulations, wherein the additive acts rapidly in the body and causes the individual to regurgitate the pesticide before it performs its toxic action [38 - 40]. The main poisoning symptoms are dehydration resulting from vomiting. The high oxidative stress elicited by these herbicides causes necrosis in the gastrointestinal tract, kidney tubules, liver, and lung; in the latter case, respiratory failure and pulmonary fibrosis may occur. Ingestion of large amounts of these compounds leads to death within two to three weeks, a result of acute renal failure, hepatitis, and especially respiratory failure caused by pulmonary inflammation and fibrosis. In addition to the systemic effects, these compounds are very harmful to the skin and may cause severe burns [38, 41].

The treatment of poisoning with dipyridyl derivatives includes maintenance of the vital functions, minimization of the absorption of the compound more cathartic (activated charcoal), acceleration of excretion (forced diuresis, hemodialysis, or hemoperfusion), abatement of the effects on the affected tissue, and fluid replacement. Topical lesions should be treated with topical silver sulfadiazine, combined with systemic antibiotics [41]. An addition method to recognize paraquat poisoning is to test the urine with sodium dithionite [42].

### 2.8. Glycine derivatives

Two representatives of this class are glyphosate (N-phosphonomethyl glycine) and glufosinate (N-phosphonomethyl homoalanine), marketed primarily as the isopropylamine salt (glyphosate) or ammonium salt (glufosinate). Both substances are broad-spectrum nonselective systemic herbicides with application in for post-emergent control of annual and perennial plants. Although both compounds contain a P=O moiety, they are not organophosphates, but organophosphonates, and they do not inhibit AChE [36].

Glyphosate, which contains phosphorus, is a herbicide used in 75% of all the genetically modified crops (GMCs), which tolerate high concentrations of this compound [36, 43]. Glyphosate inhibits an enzyme in the biosynthesis of tryptophan, phenylalanine, and tyrosine, present in plants, fungi, and bacteria, but not in animals or humans. [44]. However, according to literature reports, glyphosate can enter living organisms, including humans, where it exerts various toxic effects [45].

One pathway of glyphosate metabolism involves formation of aminomethylphosphonic acid (AMPA) by action of glyphosate oxidoreductase; AMPA is also the metabolite that emerges in humans [36]. Knowledge of the toxicokinetics of glyphosate derives mainly from animal studies and the similar patterns of absorption, metabolism, and eliminations in humans [46]. Rats absorb only 30% glyphosate after oral administration [36]. Glyphosate plasma concentrations peak at 1-2 h, and declined thereafter, with distributions to the intestine, colon, kidney, and bones [47].

The mechanisms of toxicity of glyphosate formulations are complicated [36]. The most widely used glyphosate product is Roundup®, formulated as a concentrate containing 41% glyphosate [16]. Some in vitro studies have suggested that, at high concentrations of glyphosate, its metabolites and impurities may reduce acetylcholinesterase (AChE) activity [48], although no evidence for significant AChE inhibition in mammals in vivo exists [36]. A study published in the *Archives of Toxicology* by Koller and colleagues showed increased in nuclear aberrations after exposure to glyphosate concentrations between 10 and 20 mg/L, which indicated DNA damage [49]. In adition, in vitro tests using isolated rat liver mitochondria showed that glyphosate uncoupled the electron transport chain [50].

Glufosinate inhibits the synthesis of glutamine in plants, and plant death occurs as a consequence of the increased ammonia levels [16]. Glufosinate supress the activity of glutamine synthetase and glutamate decarboxylase, reducing glutamic acid levels and elicits various types of moderate-to-severe CNS toxicities [51]. Given the differences in the biochemical and metabolic pathways of plants and mammals, glufosinate ammonium formulations are minimally toxic to humans [52]. However, ingestion of the undiluted form can cause grave outcomes such as seizures, respiratory arrest, coma, and disturbance of consciousness, which appear after a latent period of 4 – 60 h [53]. No work has reported that this compound induces genotoxic or carcinogenic effects or that impacts reproduction and fertilization [16].

The effects of this class of compounds range from irritation upon local contact (skin, GI), to hypotension, development of acute renal failure with oliguria, and severe hypoxia and death [54].

http://dx.doi.org/10.5772/59710

The treatment of glycine derivatives poisoning includes maintenance of the vital functions. Hemodialysis is crucial to reduce the amount of toxins normally excreted by the kidney, thereby preventing the impacts on this organ [54].

### 2.9. Dithiocarbamates

Dithiocarbamates comprise two groups: [1] dimethyldithiocarbamate and [2] ethylenebisdithiocarbamate, depending on which metal cation is present in the chemical structure. The nomenclature of various compounds of this class is related to the association of the metal cations; e. g., maneb (manganese), and zineb and ziram (zinc) [16, 50].

The slow absorption of these compounds means that they have low acute oral and dermal toxicity. On the other hand, chronic exposure to dithiocarbamates leads to adverse effects due to contact with dithiocarbamate acid or metal ligand [16].

The metabolite that arises from dithiocarbamates biotransformation is ethylenethiourea (ETU), which induces thyroid cancer and modifies thyroid hormones. Moreover, dithiocarbamates and disulfiram have similar structures, and both can inhibit acetaldehyde dehydrogenase, the enzyme that converts acetaldehyde into acetic acid [55].

Although these products are little toxicity to humans, they are potential precursors of ethylenethiourea, which has carcinogenic and teratogenic action.

There is no specific treatment for poisoning with this class of compounds, so only maintenance of vital functions and minimization of their absorption (activated charcoal) are necessary.

### 2.10. Others

Others classes of pesticides exist, including the chloroacetanilide commonly used in agriculture. A number of chloroacetanilides, like alachlor, acetochlor, metolachlor, and propachlor are carcinogenic [56]. The metabolism of chloroacetanilides most likely proceeds via conjugation with glutathione, as judged from the amount of glutathione-related metabolites in the urine of rats treated with these herbicides. [57]. However, the predicted differences between humans and rats in terms of disposition together with the lower rates of alachlor metabolism in human nasal microsomes have led scientists to question the human relevance of chloroacetanilide olfactory carcinogenicity [58].

Benzimidazoles are another important class of pesticides. They are commonly used as veterinary medicines (anthelmintics) and pesticides. They inhibit microtubule formation when they bind to free β-tubulin monomers at the colchicine-binding site [59].

Regarding new technologies, nanopesticides or nanoplant protection products represent an emerging technological development. In relation to pesticide use, these technologies could offer a range of benefits including increased efficacy and durability, and they use of smaller amounts of active ingredients [60]. Nanopesticides "involve either very small particles of a pesticide active ingredient (ai) or other small engineered structures with useful pesticidal properties" [61]. Nanoformulations combine several surfactants, polymers (organic), and metal nanoparticles (inorganic) in the nanometer size range [62].

| | Physical and Chemical Properties | Exposition | Toxicokinetics | Toxicodynamics | Signs and Symptoms | Treatment |
|---|---|---|---|---|---|---|
| **Organophosphorus** | Organic compounds containing phosphorus[15]. The properties vary with the size and structure. In general are more soluble in organic solvents [65]. | Skin, conjunctiva, gastrointestinal tract, and lungs[16]. | Rapidly absorbed and metabolized by P450 isozymes in oxom form, more toxic than the parent compounds[16]. | Covalent bonds with the serine residue in the active site of acetyl cholinesterase (reversibly or irreversibly)[14]. | Muscarinic syndrome and nicotine syndrome, resulting of excess acetylcholine in the synaptic cleft[19]. | Maintenance of vital functions and cholinesterase levels. It is important to avoid the use of parasympathomimetic agents[20]. |
| **Carbamates** | The carbamate is an ester derivative[14]. A wide range of melting points (50 to 150°C) is found for these compounds and the majority have low vapor pressures and poor volatiliry at usual temperatures [21]. | Lungs, gastrointestinal tract, and skin[22]. | Readily absorbed by organisms with exception the blood-brain barrier[22]. | Carbamylation of the active site of acetylcholinesterase[22]. | Miosis, salivation, sweating, tearing, rhinorrhea, behavioral change, abdominal pain, vomiting, diarrhea[24]. | Maintenance of vital functions and cholinesterase levels. It is important to avoid the use of parasympathomimetic agents[24]. |
| **Organochlorines** | They all contain a cyclodiene ring. Fat-soluble compounds persist in both the body and the environment[15]. The majority of organochlorines are sparingly soluble and semivolatile [66]. | Lungs, gastrointestinal tract, and skin[26]. | The organism absorbs approximately 10% of the applied dose, but the lipid solvents increase the accumulation[15]. | Endocrine disrupters and growth disorders in children[25]. | Dizziness, headache, anorexia, nausea, vomiting, malaise, dermatitis, diarrhea, muscle weakness, tremors, spasms, mental confusion, anxiety[15]. | Maintenance of vital functions and administer diazepam and phenobarbital to control seizures, and to monitor the airways closely[27]. |
| Pyrethrins and Pyrethroids | Both bear an acid moiety, a central ester bond, and an alcohol moiety in their structure[29]. Generally, have been low vapor pressures, low Henry's law constants, and large octanol/ | Skin, lungs and gastrointestinal[28]. | After absorption, are rapidly distributed in the organism and undergo biotransformation by | They can disrupt the muscular system and alter the normal functioning of voltage-dependent sodium channels. This interaction | Tremors, spasms, incoordination, prostration, drooling, irregular movements of the limbs, tonic and clonic convulsions, and | Decontamination of the skin and eyes, besides basic maintenance of the vital functions[32]. |

http://dx.doi.org/10.5772/59710

| | Physical and Chemical Properties | Exposition | Toxicokinetics | Toxicodynamics | Signs and Symptoms | Treatment |
|---|---|---|---|---|---|---|
| | water coefficients (Kow), and are not very soluble in water [67,68]. | | hydrolysis or oxidation by P450 isozymes[30]. | shows the hyperexcited cells[31]. | hypersensitivity to stimuli[32]. | |
| **Triazines** | Permutations of the alkyl substituted 2,4-diamines of chlorotriazine[14]. The retention in soils can varies as a function of the alkyl chain-length, such as the melting point varies between (133 – 177 °C) [69]. | Skin, eyes, nose, and gastrointestinal[16]. | Undergo conjugation with glutathione or dealkylation[14]. | Mechanism not defined[34, 35]. | Irritation at the site of contamination. Carcinogenic and teratogenic evidences[15, 33]. | It is necessary to decontaminate the site exposed to the substance[15]. |
| **Phenoxy Derivatives** | An aliphatic carboxylic acid moiety attached to a chloride or methyl-substituted aromatic ring[36]. It's adsorption coefficient (Koc) varied by four-fold, from 76 to 315 L kg(-1) [70] and the main compound has melting point is around 140 °C [71]. | Gastrointestinal and Lungs[36]. | They rapidly dissociate or hydrolyze in vivo, and fat does not store them[36]. | Cell membrane damage, uncoupling of oxidative phosphorylation and and esters are irritating to the skin, eyes, and the respiratory, gastrointestinal, and mucous membranes[36, 28]. | Nausea, dizziness, vomiting. As for metabolic acidosis, clinical signs such as hyperthermia (due to uncoupling of oxidative phosphorylation), renal failure, increased aspartate aminotransferase and alanine and lactate dehydrogenase[36]. | Maintenance of the vital functions, decrease the adsorption of the compounds[36]. |
| **Dipyridyl Derivatives** | Are a dipyridylium quaternary ammonium[28]. Diquat for example it is practically nonvolatile with a vapour pressure of <0,013 mPa and very soluble in water [21]. | Skin, eyes, lungs, and gastrointestinal[28, 38]. | Their biotransformation produces free radicals, with consequent lipid | Tissue damage in the lungs, kidney, and liver as consequence to lipid peroxidation[37, 38]. | Dehydration resulting from vomiting. The high oxidative stress causes necrosis in the gastrointestinal tract, | Minimization of the absorption of the compound more cathartic, acceleration of excretion, abatement of the effects on the affected tissue, and fluid |

| | Physical and Chemical Properties | Exposition | Toxicokinetics | Toxicodynamics | Signs and Symptoms | Treatment |
|---|---|---|---|---|---|---|
| | | | peroxidation and cell injury[37]. | | kidney tubules, liver, and lung[38, 41]. | replacement[41, 42]. |
| **Glycine Derivatives** | Marketed primarily as the isopropylamine salt (glyphosate) or ammonium salt (glufosinate). Although compounds contain a P=O moiety they do not inhibit AChE such as organophosphates[36]. Glyphosate is a relatively strong acid with a pH of 2 in 1% aqueous solution[21]. | Skin, gastrointestinal[36]. | Formation of aminomethylphosphonic acid (AMPA) by action of glyphosate oxidoreductase[36]. | DNA damage and uncoupling the electron transport chain[49,50]. | Seizures, respiratory arrest, coma, and disturbance of consciousness and irritation upon local contact[33]. | Maintenance of the vital functions[54]. |
| **Dithiocarbamates** | Maneb and Zineb, for example, are identical in structure with exception the cátion. Maneb is moderately water soluble and stable under normal conditions, while Zineb are slightly soluble in water and unstable in light[21]. | They show slow absorption by oral and dermal contact [16]. | Biotransformation of dithiocarbamates form ethylenethiourea (ETU) [55]. | Your metabolic induces thyroid cancer, modifies thyroid hormones and can inhibit acetaldehyde dehydrogenase[55]. | Carcinogenic and teratogenic action and thyroid problems[55]. | There is no specific treatment for poisoning[55]. |

**Table 1.** Summary of the physicochemical properties and phase of the intoxication of different classes of pesticides

Recently, some studies have reported on the nanomaterial-induced perturbation of different cell death pathways. In the majority of the cases, the key to understanding the toxicity of nanomaterials is that their smaller size as compared with cells and cellular organelles allows them to penetrate these basic biological structures and disrupt their normal function [63]. Thus, advances in research into the mechanism of action of nanopesticides will allow better prediction of the consequences of human exposure to these materials.

All these compounds are among more than 1000 active ingredients that are marketed as insecticide, herbicide, and fungicide. However, with the news pest resistance and need to hygienic controls the quantities of the formulations have been increased constantly [64].

Ass seen above, pesticides currently used over the world are numerous and have various chemical and physico-chemical properties [21]. Nevertheless, is already known that long-term contact to pesticides can harm human life and can disturb the function of different organs in the body, including nervous, endocrine, immune, reproductive, renal, cardiovascular, respiratory systems, and chronic diseases, including cancer, Parkinson, Alzheimer, multiple sclerosis, diabetes [64].

## 3. Pesticides and oxidative stress

Interest in the toxicological aspects of oxidative stress has grown in recent years. Many researchers have focused on the mechanistic aspect of oxidative damage and cellular responses in biological systems, mainly in the case of pesticides, because oxidative stress is a condition that stems from exposure to various classes of these compounds.

Oxidative stress occurs when the rate of reactive species production exceeds the rate of reactive species decomposition in antioxidant systems, which culminates in increased oxidative damage in different cellular targets [72]. Reactive species comprise substances that do not necessarily have unpaired electrons but are very reactive due to their instability [73]. Free radicals are atoms, molecules, or ions with unpaired electrons on an otherwise open shell configuration are examples of reactive species. Their electrons are usually highly reactive [74].

Oxygen and nitrogen free radicals play an essential role in the physiological control of cell function in biological systems. Living cells continuously produce these radicals [73]. In aerobic organisms, several basic cellular metabolic processes induce production of reactive oxygen species (ROS) within cells. Cellular respiration involves reduction of molecular oxygen ($O_2$) to water during oxidative phosphorylation in the electron transport chain, to generate reactive, partially reduced intermediates such as the superoxide anion radical ($\cdot O2^{-}$), hydrogen peroxide ($H_2O_2$), and the hydroxyl radical ($HO\cdot$) [75]. Around 5% of these ROS originate from electron transport chain processes and can damage cellular components [76]. Moreover, several enzymes produce ROS, thereby constituting a second source of ROS synthesis in cells [77].

Regulated ROS production is higher in organisms, and maintenance of redox homeostasis is essential for the physiological health [78]. Living organisms have developed adequate enzymatic and nonenzymatic antioxidant mechanisms to protect cellular components from oxidative damage [79].

Exposure to some xenobiotics, especially toxic chemical pollutants, such as pesticides, may produce an imbalance between endogenous antioxidants and ROS, with subsequent decrease in antioxidant defenses to trigger oxidative stress in biological systems, damage to tissues, inflammation, degenerative diseases, and aging [79]. As mentioned previously, many classes of pesticides induce oxidative stress, through several different mechanisms. They may affect the redox cycle by donating electrons to or withdrawing electrons from cell components. During metabolism, they may deplete glutathione (endogenous antioxidant) or even inactivate other endogenous antioxidants [74]. In short, oxidative stress can take place either through overproduction of free radicals or alteration in antioxidant mechanisms [80]. Increased concentration of plasma and red blood cell thiobarbituric acid reactive substances (TBARs), changes in the antioxidant status, and altered activities of cellular enzymes such as superoxide dismutase (SOD) and catalase (CAT) indicated higher oxidative stress in pesticides sprayers. Hence, many researchers have associated exposure to pesticides with oxidative stress [81].

Several works have described oxidative stress induction after exposure to organophosphorus insecticides. The stress is a result of intracellular $Ca^{+2}$ influx, which leads to cholinergic hyperactivity and activates proteolytic enzymes and nitric oxide synthase, which in turn generates free radicals [74]. Fenitrothion, a phosphorothioate, has been linked to histopathological effects on the liver and kidneys and cytotoxic effects on the lungs. These effects originate from ROS generation via pesticide metabolism by P450 or via high-energy consumption coupled with inhibition of oxidative phosphorylation [82]. Moreover, hydrocarbon insecticides chlorinated like DDT can induce oxidative stress after metabolic activation by $CYP_{450}$ [80].

Synthetic pyrethroids are less persistent and less toxic to mammals and birds. Deltamethrin is one of the pyrethroids that has found wide acceptability. Nevertheless, this pyrethroid has effects on the nervous, respiratory, and hematological systems in fish, and it displays tumorigenicity in rodents [80]. All these effects are due to oxidative stress; they impact various antioxidants [83].

A classic example of oxidative stress induction among pesticides is the action of dipyridyls such as paraquat. This compound enters the redox cycle and constantly generates ROS such as the superoxide anion and the hydroxyl and peroxyl radicals [74]. ROS play a crucial role in the development of paraquat-induced pulmonary injury [38]. The basic mechanism of oxidative stress in this class is simple: the dipyridyl initiates a cyclic oxidation/reduction process. First, they undergo one-electron reduction by NADPH to form free radicals. The latter donate their electron to $O_2$, to give a superoxide radical. Upon NADPH exhaustion, to superoxides react to produce hydroxyl free radicals and other reactive species that lead to oxidative stress and consequent cell death [80]. The free radicals react with lipids in cell membranes, to start a destructive process known as lipid peroxidation. The lung is the organ that is mostly involved in this case [38]. Other compounds, like dithiocarbamates mainly inhibit antioxidant enzymes, such as SOD and catalase [84].

http://dx.doi.org/10.5772/59710

Pesticides can induce free radical formation by altering the way that cell organelles, like mitochondria operate. Rotenone, an insecticide of the class of rotenoids, strengthens the case for complex I inhibition – rotenone specifically binds to complex I, to inhibit the electron flow through the respiratory chain. Deficiencies in the mitochondrial respiratory chain diminish ATP synthesis and produce ROS, which culminates in oxidative stress, mitochondrial depolarization, and initiation of cell death processes [16, 75].

In this context, many studies in human or animals have evidenced that pesticides exert their toxic action in the body via oxidative stress induction both upon acute and chronic exposure.

## 4. Pesticides and endocrine disruption

The endocrine system refers to glands located in several areas of the body. Glands release some hormones that enter the circulation and act on specific "target" organs. If an event disrupts the endocrine system, some organs will not receive the correct amount of hormones and might not function properly or even function wrongly. In this context, low levels of some pesticides in the environment can impair the endocrine system [85].

Besides their primary action as pesticides, organophosphorus, carbamates, and organochlorines can act as endocrine disruptors and affect the function of hormones by blocking, mimicking, displacing, or acting to subvert their natural roles in living species. DDT and its metabolites are among the most famous endocrine disruptors. DDT was widely used in the 1950s and 1960s, and it is still allowed in some countries. Its proven estrogenic action can affect the reproductive system of mammals and birds [86].

In vitro and in vivo studies have shown that pyretroids also act as endocrine disruptors, but their effects only arise at relatively high levels [87]. Atrazine, a triazine herbicide, may also exert endocrine-disrupting effects on amphibians [5].

## 5. Pesticides and human health

Many workers and residents, especially in the rural sector, are in contact with pesticides on a daily basis, so they are at high risk of poisoning by these compounds. This exposure can cause neuropsychiatric sequelae (mood disorders, depression, and anxiety), because many pesticides underlie changes in the function (e.g., cholinergic crisis) of the central, peripheral, and autonomic nervous system, which are often followed by suicide attempts. In addition to being causative agents of neuropsychiatric disorders that might culminate in suicide, these effects may lead to the use of pesticides as a weapon [88].

According to data released by the World Health Organization (WHO) [89], suicide by pesticides is common in many Asian and Latin American countries. Pesticides are often poorly controlled and widely available, particularly in countries of low and middle income [42]. The first epidemiological reports of suicides involving pesticides appeared in the beginning of the

1990s. Currently, homicides and suicides involving pesticides have raised the concern of many organizations and governments as, depression and suicide clearly correlate with high exposure to pesticides. This concern has motivated and still motivates many studies into how and why exposure to pesticide occurs; researchers have also caught methods to solve this serious social problem [88].

Detoxification measures after poisoning are crucial, no matter whether exposure was intentional, accidental, or occupational. Recognition of poisoning is easy when the patient knows which pesticide he/she was exposed to or when symptoms are typical. However, poisoning may be unclear if the patient has generalized symptoms. Therefore, along with the procedures to terminate contamination, an investigation with family members and the people present at the time of contamination, and information on patient care should exist. These individual will be questioned, about the way in which the patient was exposed to the contaminant and about the possibility of simultaneous intoxication with other poisons [27]. Along with these recognition steps the analytical detection of pesticides is mandatory.

Decontamination methods must be combined with care and maintenance of vital signs and administration of antidotes. It is important to bear in mind that new cases of contamination may appear. Furthermore, professionals as well as other patients staying in the same ward as the contaminated individuals must wear protective equipment until decontamination and treatment are complete [27].

Methods exist to decontaminate patients poisoned via gastrointestinal tract. Gastric lavage is extremely invasive and aggressive to the body, so it is indicated only in potentially fatal cases. The cathartic method, which elicits bowel movement to force excretion of the pesticide, is not suitable when poisoning induces diarrhea. Administration of adsorbents is an alternative – adsorbents can bind to the toxic agent, to form a stable compound. This compound is not absorbed by the gastrointestinal tract and is subsequently excreted with the feces. This method is commonly performed in conjunction with the cathartic method. The most usual adsorbent is activated charcoal, but it does not adsorb all pesticides. Finally, the syrup ipeac, a medicinal plant, can help to induce vomit. However, this procedure is contraindicated in the case of ingestion of hydrocarbons or corrosive substances [27, 28].

In the case of dermal exposure, it is necessary to start the decontamination process by placing the patient under a shower and using soap and water to remove the chemicals from the skin, hair, nails, ear canals, and other possibly contaminated body parts. If contact occurs by the ocular route, it is essential to rinse the eyes with plenty of clean water. All the materials and clothes used by the patient at the time of intoxication, like clothes and shoes, should be removed. In cases of large contamination, it is crucial to consider the need to decontaminate all the people who work in the emergency system [27, 28].

Because hundreds of pesticides compositions exist, we will focus on the clinical profile and treatment of pesticides that cause major poisoning, in terms of quantity and severity of cases. In general, treatment aims to override the mechanism of action of the toxic pesticides, and many possibilities exist (Table 2).

http://dx.doi.org/10.5772/59710

| |
|---|
| Pharmacological antagonism - competes with pesticides for the target site |
| Physiological antagonism - reversal of a physiological effect of the pesticide |
| Changing distribution to tissues – e.g., competition with membrane pumps |
| Modification of biochemical pathways - interferes with the biochemical response of the pesticide |
| Chelation of a pesticide to disable it |
| Treatment of pathological response to tissue injury caused by pesticides |

**Table 2.** Methods used to override the mechanism of toxic action of pesticides [39].

An example of suicide attempt has been the case of a man aged 22 who tried to kill himself by drinking a solution of paraquat (50 mL). He underwent gastric lavage and received activated charcoal. Later, he was discharged. However, the treatment did not suffice – four days later, the man returned to the hospital with sore throat, dysphagia, retrosternal pain, hemoptysis, and blistering and ulceration of the mouth and tongue. Biochemical tests revealed elevated creatinine levels, leukocytosis, hyponatremia, and metabolic acidosis. Because the effect had become systemic, the patient had to undergo hemodialysis and immunosuppressive therapy (cyclophosphamide, methylprednisolone, and dexamethasone). The patient did not improve and presented hemoptysis. Examination of the thoracic region detected localized alveolar infiltrate, pulmonary opacities, pneumomediastinum, pneumothorax, and subcutaneous emphysema. The patient's condition worsened, and he -underwent the same immunosuppressive therapy again. The patient recovered gradually; he was discharged after four weeks. After four months, he was working again. His lungs did not return to perfect condition – the man still this place crackles in the lower lung fields, universally distributed wheezing and pleural friction in the right hemithorax, and dyspnea after physical exertion [40].

An example of homicide involving pesticides is the case of a 52-year-old entrepreneur that was killed by injections of poison in his abdomen, conducted by their business rivals. Soon after he was attacked, the man was taken to a private clinic to receive primary treatment, and later he was taken to a hospital, where hours later he was pronounced dead. The body was sent to the morgue for post-mortem examination. Necropsy revealed distended abdomen and two punctures by needles in this region; necrotic changes appeared in the tissue around these two holes. Analysis of the organs revealed congested and edematous brain and lungs, as well as congested stomach with hemorrhagic spots. The toxicological analysis report described the presence of organochlorine pesticides in the region of the piercings and all viscera. This suggested that the man died due to cerebral and pulmonary edema after organochlorine poisoning [90].

Apart from intentional exposure to pesticides, cases of accidental poisoning occur frequently. A Latin American man (66 years old), who had a history of diabetes mellitus (type 2), hypertension, and alcohol abuse, was admitted to the emergency department unconscious, reaching a score of 5 in the Glasgow Coma Scale; he also presented hypotension (blood pressure 87/45 mmHg), sweating, and hypoxia. On the basis of reports by his wife, she had accidentally mixed

Roundap in his alcohol, and he had ingested between 350 and 500 mL of rum Roundup. About two hours after ingestion, she found him with altered mental status, non-bilious vomiting, and difficulty to wake, but he did not present bleeding. Biochemical analysis revealed high hypoxia and lactic acidosis as well as AG and high osmolar gap. First care included intubation, ventilation, and fluid bolus with 2 L of normal saline and 1 L of sodium bicarbonate. His condition worsened, and he rapidly went into shock (blood pressure 66/43 mmHg), with acute renal failure, hyperkalemia, leukocytosis, and worsening lactic acidosis. On the basis of these results, health professionals administered high dose of Levophed (Hospira, Lake Forest, Illinois) and vasopressin to provide pressure support and continuous veno-venous hemofiltration. After 24 h, the patient's conditions improved. Treatment was discontinued, and renal and cerebral functions were fully recovered [91].

Finally, cases of poisoning due to occupational exposure exist. Some pesticides can cause topical damage when they come in contact with the skin, as in the case of two farm workers admitted to the hospital in great pain due to extensive chemical burns in the perineal and scrotal regions, caused by Ducatalon (a dipyridyl herbicide containing a mixture of diquat and paraquat). The men suffered burns due to a leak in the equipment they used to spray the herbicide. Lesions reduced upon topical treatment with silver sulfadiazine associated with systemic administration of antibiotics. Fortunately, in a few days, the damaged skin recovered without scars. After replacement of the faulty equipment, no more injuries occurred [41].

## 6. Pesticides and environmental health

Pesticides reach the environment primarily during preparation and application. Application can take place via different techniques, depending on factors such as the formulation type, the controlled pest and, the application timing. In agriculture, it is possible to apply pesticides to the crop or to the soil. Liquids sprays are commonly used in crops; for example, boom sprayers, tunnel sprayers, or aerial application. Systemic pesticides can also be employed. As for soils, pesticides can be applied as granules, injected as a fumigant, or sprayed onto the soil surface, which is possibly followed by pesticide incorporation into the soil top layer. Seeds are sometimes treated with pesticides prior to planting. [92].

After application, pesticides can be taken up by target organisms, degraded, or transported to the groundwater; they can also enter the surface water bodies, volatilize to atmosphere, or reach non-target organisms by ingestion, for example. The physical and chemical properties of the pesticide, soil, site conditions, and management practices influence the behavior and fate of pesticides [93].

Concerning the physical and chemical properties of pesticides, their solubility determines their transport in surface runoff and their leaching to groundwater. The higher the solubility, the greater the carrying and leaching. The partition coefficient also affects the behavior of pesticides, and many chemicals do not leach because soil particles adsorb them.

Adsorption depends on the chemical and also on the soil type. The volatility of pesticides indicates their tendency to become a gas; the higher the volatility (high vapor pressure), the larger their loss to the atmosphere. Environmental conditions such as temperature and humidity impact volatility, which can occur from soil, plants, or surface water, and may continue for several days or weeks after pesticide application. In the atmosphere, the chemicals can be transported over long distances. Subsequent atmospheric deposition can contribute to surface water pollution. Finally, the degradation of pesticides that also determines the behavior and fate of these compounds in the environment. Degradation (their brake down into other chemical forms) can occur by photodecomposition, microorganisms, and a variety of chemical and physical reactions. Pesticides with low biodegradation are called persistent, they can remain in the environment for a long time [94, 95].

Soil properties can also affect the movement of pesticides. In relation to the soil texture, coarse-textured sands and gravels have high infiltration capacities, and water tends to percolate through the soil and reach groundwater. Fine-textured soils such as clays generally have low infiltration capacities, so water tends to run off, reaching streams and lakes. Moreover, soil containing more clay in its composition bears larger surface area to adsorb pesticides. Regarding permeability, highly permeable soils allow water to more easily. This water may contain dissolved pesticides, which will reach groundwater. Texture influences soil permeability. Ultimately, soils with high organic matter content can adsorb pesticides and retain water with dissolved chemicals. Moreover, these soils possess a larger population of microorganisms that can degrade the pesticides [93, 94].

The site conditions that can determine pesticide behavior in the environment are depth until the groundwater, geological conditions, topography, and climate. In the case of shallow groundwater, the soil filters smaller amount of water with chemicals and adsorbs and degrades lower quantities of pesticides, so contamination is a major concern. Regarding the geological conditions, the presence of wells, sinkholes, and highly permeable materials, such as gravel deposits, facilitates groundwater contamination. On the other hand, the existence of drainage ditches, streams, ponds, and lakes increases the probability that rainfall or irrigation runoff will contaminate surface water. In relation to topography, flat landscapes, areas with closed drainage systems where water drains toward the center of a basin, and especially sinkhole areas, are more susceptible to groundwater contamination. As for climate, large rainfall or irrigation may culminate in large amounts of water percolating through the soil, to reach groundwater. Rainfall can also carry pesticides to surface waters, contaminating rivers, lakes, and seas, and taking these chemicals to distant places [94].

Finally, management practices can affect the movement of pesticides. With respect to the application methods, pesticides injected or incorporated into the soil are more available for leaching and reaching groundwater, whereas pesticides sprayed onto crops are more susceptible to volatilization and surface runoff, reaching surface waters and the atmosphere. Concerning the application rates and timing, the use of larger amounts of a pesticide during are rainfall or irrigation facilitates the assess of the chemical to groundwater. With respect to handling practices, correct storage and disposal of the pesticides containers impact environmental contamination [94].

The fact that a contaminant is present in the environment does not necessarily mean that it will reach an organism. The contaminant and the organism must overlap in time and space for exposure to occur. Contact can be dermal or oral or even via inhalation, gills, and, more rarely, injection [5].

Once pesticides reach non-target organisms, they may undergo biotransformation via reactions like hydrolysis, oxidation, reduction, or conjugation catalyzed by liver enzymes. Biotransformation is an effort of the organism to detoxify and eliminate xenobiotics, but this process can also produce metabolites that are more toxic than their parent compound, a phenomenon called bioactivation. An example of bioactivation is the biotransformation of DDT, which is not highly toxic to birds, into DDE, which causes thinning of eggshells because it disrupts calcium metabolism [5].

In organisms, the absorption of a pesticide with high lipid solubility and low elimination rate can lead to bioaccumulation of this chemical in the fatty tissue, and the final concentration of the chemical in the organism will be higher than its concentration in the environment [96]. When the bioaccumulated chemical passes from lower to higher trophic levels through the food chain, successively greater pesticide concentrations emerge in animals of higher trophic level. This phenomena is called biomagnification. The offspring of top predators can also become contaminated, mainly in the case of marine mammals, because they can consume milk with extremely high fat and pesticides content [5].

Application of pesticide involves not only the active ingredient but also the whole formulation. Therefore, the environment and the human are exposed to both the active and inert ingredients. Although inert ingredients have no pesticidal activity, facilitate application of the pesticides – they enhance the active compound penetration into the target organism as well as the toxic action. Hence, the inert ingredients raise the formulation toxicity even in non-target organisms [35]. One example is the formulation of glyphosate, which is an active ingredient. It contributes a little to the total toxicity of the formulated product, particularly in the case of aquatic organisms, which are more sensitive to surface-active substances [97].

The categorization of pesticides commonly relies on their persistence in the environment. Organochlorine pesticides are persistent, whereas organophosphates, carbamates, phenoxyacid derivatives, chloroacetanilides, pyrethroids, and others are non-persistent. Compared with persistent pesticides, non-persistent chemicals have much shorter environmental half-lives and do not tend to bioaccumulate. Nevertheless, because of the heavy agricultural use of these chemicals, exists concern about their presence in the environment [14].

The non-persistent pesticides organophosphorus and carbamates act on acetylcholinesterase. The presence of this enzyme in insects, birds, fish, and all mammals allows these pesticides to reach both target and non-target organisms. [98]. Pesticides such as organophosphorus and carbamates can affect numerous teleost behaviors [99]. The pesticides that inhibit acetylcholinesterase are polar and water soluble. Moreover, their metabolism in the body is fast, and their degradation in the environment is relatively rapid. Therefore, organophosphorus and carbamates do not tend to bioaccumulate in aquatic species. However, the accumulation of these compounds in fish and invertebrates was reported long ago [100].

Organophosphorus compounds do not persist in the environment. However, their large-scale use and their decomposition rates in the environment cause these compounds to accumulate in soils, from where they subsequently enter groundwater and rivers [101]. A recent study detected the organothiophosphate insecticide chlorpyrifos in air and seawater in the Arctic, which demonstrated the long-range transport of this chemical [102]. Diazinon, another organophosphorus compound, frequently occurs in point sources (wastewater treatment plant effuent) and non-point sources (storm water runoff) in urban and agricultural areas. This pesticide is extremely toxic to birds and the aquatic life [103].

Organophosphorus compounds are acutely toxic, broad-spectrum pesticides. In the environment, secondary poisoning can occur when predators consume animals poisoned by these chemicals. Examples of contamination by organophosphorus are numerous. In Argentina in 1995–1996, approximately 6000 wintering Swainson's hawks (*Buteo swainsoni*) became poisoned after they fed on grasshoppers sprayed with the organophosphorus insecticide monocrotophos [5].

An example of carbamate contamination occurred with the pesticide, aldicarb, which polluted groundwater in the United States. Other carbamates such as carbaryl and its degradation product 1-naphthol have emerged in surface waters. The metabolite 1-naphtol is more toxic than its parent compound, and it has arisen in India [104].Methomyl, carbaryl and carbofuran, commonly used carbamates, have appeared in the aquatic environment [105].Carbofuran has commonly been associated with wildlife pesticide poisoning events when applied in the granular form. Apparently, birds mistake them for seeds [5].

Organochlorines have long environmental half-lives and tend to bioaccumulate and biomagnify in organisms. A series of evaporation and deposition steps as well as migration of animals containing bioaccumulated organochlorines can transport these compounds through the environment, carrying it to animals in higher levels of the food chain. These persistent chemicals thus occur thousands of miles away from their origin [14]. The properties of organochlorines like aldrin and dieldrin result in direct mortality of predatory birds, such as sparrow hawks and kestrels [5]. These chemicals have intensive use in agricultural and industrial activities, so they emerge across the world, including the deserted plateau and the polar zone [106]. The organochlorine chlorothalonil is a fungicide that has arisen in seawater and air in the Arctic as well as in snow cores in Arctic Canada. Endolsulfan, an organochlorine insecticide, has appeared in animals from Greenland like marine fish and mammals [102].

Despite the ban on many organochlorine compounds in the 1970s, some countries still fabricate and use chemicals such as DDT to control vector disease [98]. Other countries have replaced organochlorines with the less persistent and more effective organophosphorus compounds [107].

Pyrethrins and Pyrethroids are non-persistent pesticides used worldwide as insecticides in agriculture, forestry, households, public health and stored products [108]. Therefore, urban and peri-urban populations are potentially chronically exposed to these compounds [87].

Pyrethrins and Pyrethroids act on sodium channels in the nervous system of numerous phyla, such as arthropods and chordates [87]. Pyrethrins and Pyrethroids present low acute toxicity to mammals and birds and constitute one of the safest insecticides to man. However, at low concentrations these chemicals are acutely toxic to a wide range of aquatic organisms and insects [108].

Pyrethrins are natural compounds extracted from chrysanthemum flowers; pyrethroids are synthetic compounds whose structure resembles the structure of pyrethrins [87]. Light degrades these chemicals. Modification of pyrethroids over the years has enhanced their insecticidal activity and persistence in the environment [109]. Compared with pyrethrins, pyrethroids are more stable under light [108], which incurs increased environmental risks associated with their use [5]. Pyrethrins and Pyrethroids display high selectivity and easy degradability in the environment as compared with other pesticides, been a favored replacement for organophosphorus compounds [110].

Pyrethroids strongly adsorb to soil particles, but they can move in runoff with soil particles and reach sediments, consequently entering aquatic ecosystems and affecting aquatic organisms like invertebrates and fish [108]. Fish are highly sensitive to pyrethrin and pyrethroid products, and contamination of lakes, streams, ponds, or any aquatic habitat is a concern [109]. Moreover, some formulations contain additional insecticides, insect repellents, and solvents such as alcohol and petroleum, which increase pesticide toxicity [109].

Triazines basically consist of herbicide compounds, are relatively persistent and migrate easily through the soil into surface and ground waters [111]. In soil, they undergo degradation mainly in a microbial action, but the role of photodegradation is still significant [112]. Residues of triazines have emerged in soil, surface waters, and groundwater in areas where the application of agrochemicals has taken place [111].

Herbicides are often benign with regard to impacts on animals; however, these compounds can have toxic effects at concentrations found in the environment [5]. Furthermore, indiscriminate use of this herbicide, careless handling, accidental spillage, or discharge of untreated effluents into natural water ways can harm the fish population and other aquatic organisms and may contribute to long-term effects in the environment. Atrazine, a triazine herbicide, is one of the most often detected pesticides in streams, rivers, ponds, reservoirs, and groundwater [113].

Phenoxy derivatives basically consist of compounds with herbicide action. They are soluble in water and can pollute surface and ground waters. Phenoxy derivatives display moderate toxicity, but some chlorinated metabolites can be toxic to human and aquatic organisms [114]. In addition, the metabolites may have mutagenic and carcinogenic properties. 2,4-D and MCPA, which are also phenoxy herbicides, can undergo degradation by biotic and abiotic mechanisms. However, these processes may not suffice to reduce the concentrations of chlorinated phenoxy derivatives on many sites [115].

Regarding dipyridyl derivatives, the best-known compounds are diquat and paraquat, developed as herbicides and desiccants. Diquat is water soluble and persistent in the aquatic system. However, it can bind to soil, which reduces its mobility in the environment. Although herbicides are usually little toxic to animals, diquat is toxic to some aquatic organisms [116]. Soil adsorbs paraquat, which presents its leaching to ground water; soil microorganisms and photolysis degrade this herbicide [117]. The herbicide glyophosate bears glycine, which adsorbs to soil, undergoes degradation by bacteria, and has low potential for runoff. However, is it highly water soluble and emerges in surface waters. Glyphosate is little toxic to mammals, but the surfactants present in some formulations rise the toxicity of this chemical. Hence, some formulations, mainly those intended for aquatic vegetation control, can kill amphibians [5]. Many authors have demonstrated that glyphosate formulations can cause genetic damage in fish [97].

Dithiocarbamates (DTC) function mainly as fungicides that protect crops, but they also work as rodent repellents [118]. The intensive use of dithiocarbamates in agriculture often contaminates water bodies [119]. Ziram, one of the best-known dithiocarbamates, is toxic to aquatic organisms [120].

Other examples of chemical classes of pesticides exist. Alachlor and metolachlor belong to the group of chloroacetanilides. These herbicides and their degradation products have arisen in surface and groundwater [121]. Diuron, a urea derivative, can pollute freshwaters by leaching through the soil. It has appeared in marinas and coastal areas [122]. Additionally, trifluralin, a dinitroanilin, has emerged in Arctic air and seawater [102].

Therefore, a huge amount and variety of pesticides exist in the environment. Many chemicals that exist at low concentrations may not cause acute detectable effects in organisms, but they may induce other kinds of damage, like genetic disorders and physiological alterations that, in the long run, reduce the organisms life span [11].

## 7. Methods to detect pesticides

A wide range of methodologies exist to identify possible exposure to pesticides. When identification is necessary due to poisoning of a patient attended in the clinic, the general procedures include anamnesis, physical examination, evaluation of clinical signs, and diagnostic and toxicological analysis. If the investigation aims to qualify and/or quantify a possible pesticide, it is generally necessary to collect a sample and analyze it for the presence of pesticides and/or metabolites in biological samples (blood, liver, stomach contents) and/or the environment (air, water, ground). Selection of the test will depend on the purpose of the analysis. It is also essential to consider the financial costs of a method. Simpler tests are still important, – apart from been inexpensive, many offer high sensitivity, specificity, precision, and accuracy, all of which are factors that are crucial for reliable analysis [123, 124].

Prior to analyzes pesticides samples analysts have to go through similar steps: definitions of the analytical problem (target analyte and its properties), choice of detection methods (immunoassays spectrometry), sampling (how to collect and store the sample), sample preparation (solubilization, extraction, concentration, and separation), calibration (qualification and/or quantification of the analyte), calculation and evaluation of the results, and actions to complete the analysis [125].

Sample storage for long periods should ensure that no sample degradation or external contamination occurs. Well-sealed containers stored under refrigeration and protected from light are mandatory. To avoid any type of external interference during analysis, none of the employed materials should modify or degrade the pesticide in the sample. The analysis of pesticides, mainly in water, ambient air, and soil sediments, often requires a purification step to clean the sample and pre-concentrate the analytes, to improve the quality of the analytical results. The extraction process is a key analytical step – it extracts the desirable compounds for further separation and characterization. Liquid-liquid extraction, and pre-concentration procedures, such as solid-phase extraction and solid-phase microextraction, are the most commonly used methods, but other extraction methods are also applicable depending on the objective [126]. Extraction of residues from the sample matrix demands appropriate solvents for maximum extraction efficiency and minimal co-extraction of interfering substances. The extraction solvents must be highly pure. Blank tests help to prove that the matrix does not interfere in the analyzes. After extraction, a purification step removes the interfering substance with minimal loss of the analyte. The final solution should include an appropriate solvent for analyte determination by the selected method [127].

Below is a didactic description of the main separations and detection methods.

### 7.1. Physicochemical methods

Gas chromatography (GC), Liquid Chromatography (LC), and Capillary Electrophoresis (CE) constitute physicochemical separation methods.

When the analyzed pesticide is volatile or semi-volatile, GC still is the method of choice: it offers higher resolution and lower detection limits. GC is usually associated with multiple detectors whose choice will depend on the characteristics of the target analytes. GC is based on sample volatilization and introduction into a chromatographic column coated or packed with a solid or liquid stationary phase. A gaseous mobile phase elutes the analyte; this phase is inert, and does not interact with the analyte. The carrier gases should be pure and chemically inert, too, and the choice will depend on the detector. The commonest carrier gases are helium, argon, nitrogen, carbon dioxide, and hydrogen [128].

LC has emerged as a great separation tool. It allows for effective separation of nonvolatile and thermally unstable pesticides that are incompatible with GC. During LC, extracts pass through multiple adsorbent columns that can discriminate between the components of the matrix and target analyte. The degree of selectivity will vary according to the adsorbent present in the column (alumina, silica gel, or Florisil), mesh size, and activity levels. Columns can be used separately or in combination [129].

CE is a powerful tool to separate and identify a wide range of molecules. EC provides high resolution, and large separation efficiency. It requires small sample size and low solvent consumption analyzes is faster and operational coats are low [130].

An ideal detector should ensure adequate sensitivity, good stability and reproducibility, and linear response to various concentrations of the analytes. It should also operate in a wide range of temperature, have reduced response time (independent of the flow), and be easy to handle.

http://dx.doi.org/10.5772/59710

The detector response should be equivalent for all the analytes or selective to certain classes of compounds. Ultimately, the detector should not destroy the sample. Unfortunately, a switch that exhibits all these characteristics does not exist, so it is necessary to select the detector according to the desired goal [128].

Several types of detectors are commercially available. They can come coupled to the separation device. These detectors use photometric or fluorimetric methods, thermal conductivity, diode array detection, electrons capture, atomic absorption, or pesticides mass/charge evaluation. The latter method is currently in evidence due because it is highly sensitive, offers autonomy, and performs a variety of functions. Electron capture and mass spectrometry are the most often used to detect pesticides.

The electron capture detector (ECD) is usually employed to search for organic pesticides, because it is highly sensitive and selective toward molecules containing electronegative functional groups. It also detects masses in the order of pictograms and can analyze traces of pesticides. However, ED cannot detect compounds with low electron affinity. Its excellent properties are useful for analysis of pesticides in both the environmental area and hospitals. A detector called μECD is also available in the market. It is advantageous over ECD in term of sensitivity, stability, and robustness [131].

Mass spectrometry (MS) is based on the ionization, acceleration, and separation of the generated molecules and ions according their mass/charge (m/z) ratio. This Provides a typical spectrum that gives the relative mass abundance of the different ionic species as a function of m/z so, which permits unambiguous identification of molecules. Mass spectrometry is a confirmation technique that is less subject to misunderstanding. Nevertheless, it has a drawback – it destroys the analyte [132].

As mentioned previously, the choice of method will depend on the case. LC-MS and GC-MS are the methods that generally separate and detect pesticides most suitable. These methods play a very important role in the analysis of pesticides and related compounds and are applicable in several areas like environmental analysis, food safety, and occupational toxicology, among others. Because they can serve various purposes, these methods also help to detect compounds in different samples, such as water, soil, sediment, sludge, vegetables and fruits, and animals and humans tissues and fluids [124, 126]. Obviously, method will based on the needs and characteristics of the target pesticide, and each sample will have their own features, which will depend on their physicochemical properties.

### 7.2. Biological

Chemical analysis of isolated compounds is commonly used to monitor environmental pollution, but such analyses can be limited and expensive and cannot indicate the biological effects. In contrast, biological tests indicate the toxicity of a ride range of compounds or environmental samples, and are therefore essential to determine the environmental impacts of the presence of these chemicals [133]. Immunoassays and biosensors are methods related to the biological factor. Immunoassays are a powerful tool in clinical laboratories and one of the most widely applied analytical techniques.

The reagents kits and the equipment necessary to perform immunoassays are commercially available and rely on fluorescent, chemiluminescent or other detection methods. Immunoassays can detect a wide range of compounds including drugs, proteins, and hormones; they can also identify and quantify the presence of pesticides residues in various samples such as natural water, food, and blood, among others [129].

Regarding biosensors, organisms such as *Drosophila melanogaster* fly species may aid the detection of pesticides in food samples and other matrixes such as water, soil, plants, and animal tissue. This test model is advantageous, because these insects have low tolerance to toxic substances with insecticidal character, besides being experimental models of easy creation, manipulation, and maintenance. In addition, they require few financial resources and can remain under laboratory conditions. However, this method only serves to detect the presence of pesticides, but it cannot identify the detected compound. Therefore, after using this probe, the analyst has to employ a chromatographic, for example, to identify the group of pesticides in that sample [123].

## 8. Summary of important points and perspectives

The chapter begins with an introduction about pesticides, citing the Second World War and the publication of the book "Silent Spring" by Rachel Carson. Even in the introduction, it is mentioned the Integrated Pest Management (IPM) and the risks and benefits of pesticides use.

Subsequently, the chapter presents the topic "physicochemical properties and stages of intoxication." This topic cites the physicochemical properties, the exposure, toxicokinetic, toxicodynamic and clinical phase of organophosphorous, carbamates, organochlorines, pyrethrins and pyrethroids, triazines, phenoxy derivatives, dipyridyl derivatives, glycine derivatives, dithiocarbamates, and others. In the latter group, the nanopesticides are mentioned.

The chapter also discusses the pesticides as inducers of oxidative stress and endocrine disruptors action of two important issues. Beyond, adress three topics differences: pestidas and human health, pesticides and environmental health, and methods of detection of these compounds. In the first, there are examples of intoxication from occupational, accidental and intentional exposure, besides decontamination methods. The second topic shows how a pesticide reaches the environment, and how it behaves. In other words, if hits the water, soil, and / or are biodegraded. Finally, the third topic addresses methods of detection of pesticides. Gas chromatography (GC), Liquid Chromatography (LC), and Capillary Electrophoresis (CE) constitute physicochemical methods. Immunoassays and biosensors are methods related to the biological factor.

Currently, there is a pursuit of a sustainable society, generating huge concern for human health just like the environment, this occurs due to action/persistence of pesticides in the environment, as well as its toxic effects to humans and other living beings. This pursuit for a healthier society tries to combat the toxic effects of pesticides, as they have caused a large reduction in biodiversity (mainly insects pollinators), and affect humans causing genetic mutations, Mutagenicity and carcinogenicity, reproductive damages as well as disturbances behavioral (depression and suicides). Faced with this problem, many governments have sought to measures to limit access to these compounds, aimed at protecting human and environmental health, such as work done by the governments of India, Western Samoa and Finland, which restricted access to pesticides and reduced cases of suicides in their countries [42, 134].

This concern can also be viewed on the growing interest of researchers and regulatory agencies regarding research related to biopesticides and biological control of pests, also seeking the quality of environmental and human health mainly in the near future [135].

## Author details

Mariana Furio Franco Bernardes[1], Murilo Pazin[1], Lilian Cristina Pereira[1] and Daniel Junqueira Dorta[2]

1 Faculdade de Ciências Farmacêuticas de Ribeirão Preto - FCFRP, Universidade de São Paulo- USP, Brazil

2 Departamento de Química, Faculdade Filosofia, Ciências e Letras de Ribeirão Preto-FFCLRP, Universidade de São Paulo – USP, Brazil

## References

[1] USEPA - United States of Environmental Protection Agengy. About pesticides. U.S. EPA. http://www.epa.gov/pesticides/about/index.htm (Accessed 27 August 2014).

[2] Unsworth 2010 - History of pesticide use. International Union of pure and applied chemistry (IUPAC). 2010. http://agrochemicals.iupac.org/index.php?option=com_sobi2&sobi2Task=sobi2Details&catid=3&sobi2Id=31 (Accessed 2 September 2014).

[3] Gupta PK. Toxicity of herbicides. In: GUPTA, R. C. (Ed) Veterinary toxicology: Basic and clinic principles. USA: Elsevier. 2007. p.567-586.

[4] Ratcliffe D. Decreases in eggshell weight in certain birds of prey. Nature 1967; 215: 208-210.

[5] Levengood JM, Beasley VR. Principles of ecotoxicology. In: Gupta RC (ed.) Veterinary toxicology: basic and clinical principles. Academic press, Amterdan. 2007. p. 689-708.

[6] Fenik J, Tankiewicz M, Biziuk M. Properties and determination of pesticides in fruits and vegetables. Trends in Analytical Chemistry 2011; 30 [6]: 814-826.

[7] Knutson RD, Taylor CR, Penson JB, Smith EG. Economic impacts of reduced chemical use. Knutson and Associates, College Station, Texas. 1990.

[8] Delaplane K S. Pesticide Usage in the United States: History, Benefits, Risks, and Trends. The University of Georgia, Athens, Georgia 1996. http://ipm.ncsu.edu/safety/factsheets/pestuse.pdf (Accessed 20 August 2014).

[9] Mostafalou S, Abdollahi M. Pesticides and human chronic diseases: Evidences, mechanisms, and perspectives. Toxicology and Applied Pharmacology 2013; 268: 157-177.

[10] Hernández AF, Parrón T, Tsatsakis AM, Requena M, Alarcón R, López-Guarnido O. Toxic effects of pesticide mixtures at a molecular level: Their relevance to human Health. Toxicology 2013; 307: 136-145.

[11] Poletta GL, Larriera A, Kleinsorge E, Mudry MD. Genotoxicity of the herbicide formulation Roundup® (glyphosate) in broad-snouted caiman (Caiman latirostris) evidenced by the Comet assay and the Micronucleus test. Mutation Research 2009; 672: 95-102.

[12] EPA - Environmental Protection Agency. Overview of the Ecological Risk Assessment Processin the Office of Pesticide Programs,U.S., Environmental Protection Agency. 2004. http://www.epa.gov/espp/consultation/ecorisk-overview.pdf (Acessed 13 August 2014).

[13] Matthews G, Bateman R, Miller P. Book Pesticide application methods. John Wiley & Sons. 2008. Available from http://onlinelibrary.wiley.com/book/10.1002/9780470760130 (Accessed 4 September 2014).

[14] Barr D B, Needham LL. Analytical methods for biological monitoring of exposure to pesticides: a review. Journal of Chromatography B 2002; 778: 5-29.

[15] Ellenhorn MJ, Barceloux DG. Medical Toxicology. Diagnosis and Treatment of Human Poisoning. Ed. Elsevier, New York, 1988. 1512p.

[16] Costa LG. Toxic Effects of Pesticides. In: Klaassen CD. (ed). Cassarett and Doull's Toxicology *The Basic Science of Poisons*. 7 Ed, McGraw-Hill, New York, 2008. p. 883-930.

[17] Davies JE, Barquet A, Freed VH, Haque R, Morgade C, Sonneborn RE, Vaclavek C. Human pesticide poisonings by a fat soluble organophosphate insecticide. Archives of Environmental Health 1975; 30: 608-613.

[18] Ho IK, Fernando JC, Sivam SP, Hoskins B. Roles of Dopamine and GABA in neurotoxicity of organophosphorous cholinesterase inhibitors. Proceedings of the Western Pharmacoly Society 1984; 27: 177-180.

[19] Paudyal BP. Organophosphorus poisoning. Journal of Nepal Medical Association 2008; 47(172): 251-258.

[20] Thiermann H, Worek F, Kehe K. Limitations and challenges in treatment of acute chemical warfare agent poisoning. Chemico Biological Interactions 2013; 206[3]: 435-43.

[21] Ecobichon DJ. Carbamate insecticides. In: Krieger R (ed). Handbook of Pesticide Toxicology. San Diego, CA: Academic Press; 2001. p.1087-1106.

[22] Jokanovic M. Medical treatment of acute poisoning with organophosphorus and carbamate pesticides, Toxicology Letters 2009; 190: 107-115.

[23] Marrs TC, Maynard RL. Neurotransmission system as targets for toxicants: a review. Cell Biology and Toxicology 2013; 29: 381-396.

[24] Rosman Y, Makarovsky I, Bentur Y, Shrot S, Dushnistky T, Krivoy A. Carbamate poisoning: treatment recommendations in the setting of a mass casualties event. American Journal of Emergence Medicine 2009; 27[9]:1117-1124.

[25] Lee DH, Lee IK, Song K, Steffes M, Toscano W, Baker BA, Jacobs DR. A strong dose-response relation between serum concentrations of persistent organic pollutants and diabetes. Diabetes Care 2006; 29: 1638-1644.

[26] Snedeker S. Pesticides and breast cancer risk: a review of DDT, DDE and dieldrin. Environmental Health Perspectives 2001; 109 (suppl 1): 35-47.

[27] Simpson WM Jr, Schuman SH. Recognition and management of acute pesticide poisoning. American Family Physician. 2002; 65: 1599-1604.

[28] Reigart JR, Roberts JR. Recognition and Management of Pesticide Poisonings. 5ª Ed. United States Environmental Protection Agency, 1999. http://www.epa.gov/oppfead1/safety/healthcare/handbook/handbook.pdf (Accessed 4 September 2014).

[29] Zhang Q, Zhang W, Wang X, Li P. Immunoassay Development for the Class-Specific Assay for Types I and II Pyrethroid Insecticides in Water Samples. Molecules 2010; 15: 164-177.

[30] Sogorb MA, Vilanova E. Enzymes involved in the detoxification of organophosphorus, carbamate and pyrethroid insecticides through hydrolysis. Toxicology Letters 2002; 128: 215-228.

[31] Ray DE, Fry JR. A reassessment of the neurotoxicity of pyrethroid insecticides. Pharmacology & Therapeutics 2006; 111[1]: 174-193.

[32] Bradberry SM, Cage SA, Proudfoot AT, Vale JA. Poisoning due to Pyrethroids. Toxicology Reviews 2005; 24 [2]: 93-106.

[33] Sathiakumar N, MacLennan PA, Mandel J, Delzell E. A review of epidemiologic studies of triazine herbicides and cancer. Critical Review in Toxicology 2011; 41: 1-34.

[34] Mayhew DA, Taylor GD, Smith SH, Banas DA. Twenty-four month combined chronic oral toxicity and oncogencity study in rats utilizing atrazine technical grade. Lab

Study No.: 410-1102, Accession No. 262714-262727, American Biogenics Corp., Decatur, 1986. p. 2-6.

[35] Zeljezic D, Garaj-Vrhovac, V, Perkovic P. Evaluation of DNA damage induced by atrazine and atrazine-based herbicide in human lymphocytes in vitro using a comet and DNA diffusion assay. Toxicology in vitro 2006; 20: 923-935.

[36] Bradberry SM, Proudfoot AT, Vale A. Glyphosate Poisoning. Toxicology Reviews 2004; 23: 159-167.

[37] Honore P, Hantson P, Fauville JP, Peeters, A. Manieu, P. Paraquat poisoning: State of the art. Acta Clinica Belgica 1994; 49:220-8.

[38] Toygar M, Aydin I, Agilli M, Aydin FN, Oztosun M, Gul H, Macit E, Karslioglu Y, Topal T, Uysal B, Honca M. The relation between oxidative stress, inflammation, and neopterin in the paraquat-induced lung toxicity. Human and Experimental Toxicity, 2014. *In press*. Ver volume ou colocar link.

[39] Bateman DN. Pharmacological treatments of paraquat poisoning. Human Toxicology 1987; 6[1]: 57-62.

[40] Neves FF, Sousa RB, Pazin-Filho A, Cupo P, Elias Júnior J, Nogueira-Barbosa MH. Severe paraquat poisoning: clinical and radiological findings in a survivor. Jornal Brasileiro de Pneumologia 2010; 36[4]: 513-516.

[41] Ronnen M, Klin B, Suster S. Mixed diquat/paraquat-induced burns. International Journal of Dermatology 1995; 34[1]: 23-5.

[42] Sarchiapone M, Mandelli L, Iosue M, Andrisano C, Roy A. Controlling access to suicide means. International Journal of Environmental Research and Public Health. 2011; 8: 4550-4562.

[43] Kwiatkowska M, Nowacha-Krukowska H, Bukowska B. The effects of glyphosate, its metabolites and impurities on erythrocyte acetylcholinesterase activity. Environmental Toxicology and Pharmacology 2014; 37: 1101-1108.

[44] Campbell AW. Glyphosate: its effects on humans. Alternatives Therapies in Health and Medicine 2014; 20: 9-11.

[45] de Liz Oliveira Cavalli VL, Cattani D, Heinz Rieg CE, Pierozan P, Zanatta L, Benedetti Parisotto E, Wilhelm Filho D, Mena Barreto Silva FR, Pessoa-Pureur R, Zamoner A. Roundup disrupted male reproductive functions by triggering calcium-mediated cell death in rat testis and Sertoli cells. Free Radicals Biology and Medicine 2013; 65: 335-346.

[46] Williams GM, Kroes R, Munro IC. Safety evaluation and risk assessment of the herbicide Roundup and its active ingredient, glyphosate, for humans. Regulatory Toxicology and Pharmacology 2000; 31: 117-65.

[47] Chan PC, Mahler JF. NTP technical report on the toxicity studies of glyphosate (CAS no. 1071-83-6) administered in dosed feed to F344/N rats and B6C3F$_1$ mice. Toxicity Reports Series 1992; 16: 1-D3.

[48] Sandrini JZ, Rola RC, Lopes FM, Buffon HF, Freitas MM, Martins Cde M, da Rosa CE. Effects of glyphosate on cholinesterase activity of the mussel Perna perna and the fish Danio rerio and Jenynsia multidentata: in vitro studies. Aquatic Toxicology. 2013; 130-131:171-173.

[49] Koller VJ, Furhacker M, Nersesyan A, Mišik M, Eisenbauer M, Knasmueller S. Cytotoxic and DNA-damaging properties of glyphosate and Roundup in humanderived buccal epithelial cells. Archieves of Toxicology 2012; 86[5]:805-813.

[50] Alonzo HGA, Corrêa CL. Praguicidas. In: Oga S, Camargo MMA, Batistuzzo JA. (eds) Fundamentos de Toxicologia. 4ª. Ed. Editora Atheneu, São Paulo; 2014. p. 323-341.

[51] Inoue Y, Onodera M, Fujita T, Fujino Y, Kikuchi S, Endo S. Factors associated with severe effects following acute glufosinate poisoning. Clinical Toxicology 2013; 51: 846-849.

[52] Park JS, Kwak SJ, Gil HW, Kim SY, Hong SY. Glufosinate Herbicide Intoxication Causing Unconsciousness, Convulsion, and 6th Cranial Nerve Palsy. Journal of Korean Medical Science 2013; 28: 1687-1689.

[53] Hori Y, Tanaka T, Fujisawa M, Shimada K. Toxicokinetics of DL-glufosinate enantiomer in human BASTA poisoning. Biological and Pharmaceutical Bulletin 2003; 26: 540-543.

[54] Sampogna RV, Cunard R. Roundup intoxication and a rationale for treatment. Clinical Nephrolpgy 2007; 68[3]: 190-6.

[55] Belpoggi F, Soffritti M, Guarino M, Lambertini L, Cevolani D, Maltoni C. Results of Long-Term Experimental Studies on the Carcinogenicity of Ethylene-bis- Dithiocarbamate (Mancozeb) in Rats. Annals of the New York Academy of Sciences 2006; 982: 123-136.

[56] Dearfield KL, McCarroll NE, Protzel A, Stack HF, Jackson MA, Waters M.D. A survey of EPA/OPP and open literature on selected pesticide chemicals. II. Mutagenicity and carcinogenicity of selected chloroacetanilides and related compounds. Mutatation Research 1999; 443: 183-221.

[57] Ashby J, Kier L, Wilson AG, Green T, Lefevre PA, Tinwell H, Willis GA, Heydens WF, Clapp MJ. Evaluation of the potential carcinogenicity and genetic toxicity to humans of the herbicide acetochlor. Human & Experimental Toxicology 1996; 15: 702-735.

[58] Heydens WF, Lamb IC, Wilson AGE. Chloroacetanilides. In: Krieger R (ed). Handbook of Pesticide Toxicology. San Diego, CA: Academic Press; 2001. p. 1543–1558.

[59] Ermler S, Scholze M, Kortenkamp A. Seven benzimidazole pesticides combined at sub-threshold levels induce micronuclei in vitro. Mutagenesis 2013; 28: 417-426.

[60] Kookana RS, Boxal AB, Reeves PT, Ashauer R, Chaudhry Q, Cornelis G, Fernandes TF, Gan J, Kah M, Lynch I, Ranville J, Sinclair C, Spurgeon D, Tiede K, Van Den Brink PJ. Nanopesticides: guiding principles for regulatory evaluation of environmental risks. Journal of Agriculture and Food Chemistry 2014; 62: 4227-4240.

[61] Bergeson LL. Nanosilver: US EPA's pesticide office considers how best to proceed. Environmental Quallity Management 2010; 19 [3]: 79–85. http://onlinelibrary.wiley.com/doi/10.1002/tqem.20255/pdf (Accessed 2 September 2014).

[62] Sekhon BS. Nanotechnology in agri-food production: an overview. Nanotechnology, Science and Applications 2014; 7: 31-53.

[63] Buzea C, Pacheco II, Robbie K. Nanomaterials and nanoparticles: sources and toxicity. Biointerphases. 2007; 2: 17-71.

[64] Mostafalou S, Abdollahi M. Pesticides and human chronic diseases: Evidences, mechanisms and perspectives. Toxicology and Applied Pharmacology. 2013; 268: 157-177.

[65] Gallo MA, Lawryk NJ. Organophosphorus pesticides. In: Hayes WJ Jr.; Laws ER Jr. (Eds) Handbook of Pesticide Toxicology. San Diego: Academic Press. 1991. 2: 917-1123.

[66] Shen, L.; Wania, F. Compilation, Evaluation, and Selection of Physical-Chemical Property Data for Organochlorine Pesticides. J. Chem. Eng. Data, 50, p. 742 – 768, 2005.

[67] Bjorling-Poulse M, Andersen HR, Grandjean P. Potential developmental neurotoxicity of pesticides used in Europe. Environmental Health. 2008; 7-50.

[68] MacBean C. The Pesticide Manual. 6a. Ed. British Crop Production Council. 2012. 557p.

[69] Jokanovic M. The Impact of Pesticides. 1a Ed. The Academy Publish, Cheyenne. 2012. 417p.

[70] Farenhorst A, Saiyed IM, Goh TB, McQueen P. The important characteristics of soil organic matter affecting 2,4-dichlorophenoxyacetic acid sorption along a catenary sequence. Journal of Environmental Science and Health, Part B. 2010; 45:204-13.

[71] Mackay D, Shiu WY, Ma KC, Lee SC. Handbook of Physical-Chemical Properties and Environmental Fate for Organic Chemicals. 2. Ed. Taylor & Francis Group, New York. 2006. 3201p.

[72] Almeida EA, Bainyb ACD, Dafrec AL, Gomesa OF, Medeirosa MHG, di Mascioa P. Oxidative stress in digestive gland and gill of the brown mussel Perna perna exposed

to air and re-submersed. Journal of Experimental Marine Biology and Ecology. 2005; 318: 21–30.

[73] Halliwell B, Gutteridge JMC. Free Radicals in Biology and Medicine, 3ª ed. Oxford University Press, Oxford. 1999.

[74] Lushchak VI. Environmentally induced oxidative stress in aquatic animals. Aquatic Toxicology 2011; 101: 13-30.

[75] Pereira LC, Souza AO, Pazin M. Dorta, DJ. A mitocôndria como alvo para avaliação da toxicidade de xenobióticos, Revista Brasileira de Toxicologia 2012; 25: 1-14.

[76] Kelly SA, Havrilla CM, Brady TC, Abramo KH, Levin ED. Oxidative Stress in Toxicology: Established Mammalian and Emerging Piscine Model Systems. Research Reviews 1998; 106: 375-384.

[77] Griffiths HR, Dias IHK, Willetts RS, Devitt A. Redox regulation of protein in plasma. Redox Biology 2014; 2: 430-435.

[78] Wallace KB. Target organ toxicology series. Taylor & Francis Ltd, Washington 442p. 1997.

[79] Valavanidis A, Vlahogianni T, Dassenakis M, Scoullos M. Molecular biomarkers of oxidative stress in aquatic organisms in relation to toxic environmental pollutants. Ecotoxicology and Environmental Safety 2006; 64: 178-189.

[80] Abdollahi M, Ranjbar A, Shadnia S, Nikfar S, Rezaie A. Pesticides and oxidative stress: a review. Medical Science Monitor 2004;10:141-147.

[81] Wafa T, Nadia K, Amel N, Ikbal C, Insaf T, Asma K, Hedi MA, Mohamed H. Oxidative stress, hematological and biochemical alterations in farmers exposed to pesticides. Journal of Environmental Science and Health, Part B 2013; 48: 1058-1069.

[82] Milatovic D, Gupta RC, Aschner M. Anticholinesterase toxicity, oxidative stress. Science World Journal 2006; 6:295-310.

[83] Sayeed I, Parvez S, Pandey S, Bin-Hafeez B, Haque R, Raisuddin S. Oxidative stress biomarkers of exposure to deltamethrin in freshwater fish, Channa punctatus Bloch. Ecotoxicological and Environmental Safety 2003; 56: 295-301.

[84] Hai DQ, Varga SI, Matkovics B. Effects of diethyl-dithiocarbamate on antioxidant system in carp tissue. Acta Biologica Hungarica 1997; 48: 1-8.

[85] Bergman A, Heindel JJ, Jobling S, Kidd KA, Zoeller T. State of the Science of Endocrine Disrupting Chemicals – 2012. United Nations Environment Programme and the World Health Organization 2013. http://www.who.int/ceh/publications/endocrine/en (Accessed 3 September 2014).

[86] USEPA - United States of Environmental Protection Agengy. Special Report on Environmental Endocrine Disruption: An Effects Assessment and Analisys, U.S. Environmental Protection Agency, Report No. EPA/630/R-96/012, Washington D. C, 1997.

http://www.epa.gov/raf/publications/pdfs/ENDOCRINE.PDF (Accessed 27 August 2014).

[87] Fortin MC, Bouchard M, Carrier G, Dumas P. Biological monitoring of exposure to pyrethrins and pyrethroids in a metropolitan population of the Province of Quebec, Canada. Environmental Research 2008; 107: 343-350.

[88] Freire C, Koifman S. Pesticides, depression and suicide: a systematic review of the epidemiological evidence. International Journal of Hygiene and Environmental Health 2013; 216[4]:445-460.

[89] WHO - World Health Organization. Suicide prevention (SUPRE). http://www.who.int/mental_health/prevention/suicide/suicideprevent/en/ (Accessed 16 August 2014).

[90] Kumar A, Kumar A, Murty OP, Gupta VP, Das S. A rare case of homicidal insecticide (organochloro compound) poisoning by intraperitoneal injection. Medicine, Science and the Law. 2012; 52[4]: 231-233

[91] Hour BT, Belen C, Zar T, Lien YH. Herbicide roundup intoxication: successful treatment with continuous renal replacement therapy. American Journal of Medicine 2012; 125[8]: e1-2.

[92] Van Der Berg F, Kubiak R, Benjey WG, Majewski MS, Yates SR, Reeves GL, Smelt JH. Emission of pesticides into the air. Water, Air & Soil Pollution. 1999; 115: 195-210.

[93] Lourencetti C, Marchi MRR, Ribeiro, ML. Determination of sugar cane herbicides in soil and soil treated with sugar cane vinasse by solid-phase extraction and HPLC-UV. Talanta 2008; 77: 701-709.

[94] Agriculture and Natural Resources. Water quality: Controlling Nonpoint Source (NPS) Pollution. Pesticide Management To Protect Water Quality. Understanding Pesticides And How They Affect Water Quality 1999. Available from http://www.aces.edu/pubs/docs/A/ANR-0790/WQ4.5.1.pdf (accessed 2 September 2014).

[95] Bedos C, Cellier P, Calvet R, Barriuso E, Gabrielle B. Mass transfer of pesticides into the atmosphere by volatilization from soils and plants: overview. Agronomie 2002; 22: 21–33.

[96] Akcha F, Spagnol C, Rouxel J. Genotoxicity of diuron and glyphosate in oyster spermatozoa and embryos. Aquatic Toxicology 2012; 106-107: 104-113.

[97] ÇAVAS TC, KONEN S. Detection of cytogenetic and DNA damage in peripheral erythrocytes of goldfish (Carassius auratus) exposed to a glyphosate formulation using the micronucleus test and the comet assay. Mutagenesis 2007; 22: 263-268.

[98] Van Dyk JS, Pletschke B. Review on the use of enzymes for the detection of organochlorine, organophosphate and carbamate pesticides in the environment. Chemosphere 2011; 82: 291-307.

[99] Jarrard HE; Delaney KR; Kennedy CJ. Impacts of carbamate pesticides on olfactory neurophysiology and cholinesterase activity in coho salmon (Oncorhynchus kisutch). Aquatic Toxicology 2004; 69: 133-148.

[100] Kitamura S, Sugihara K, Fujimoto N. Endocrine Disruption by Organophosphate and Carbamate Pesticides. In: Gupta RC (ed.) Toxicoly of Organophosphonate and Carbamate Compounds. Elsevier Academic Press, New York, 2006. p. 481-194.

[101] Sirotkina M, Lyagin I, Efremenko E. Hydrolysis of organophosphorus pesticides in soil: New opportunities with ecocompatible immobilized His6-OPH. International Biodeterioration & Biodegradation 2012; 68: 18-23.

[102] Vorkamp K, Rigét FF. A review of new and current-use contaminants in the Arctic environment: Evidence of long-range transport and indications of bioaccumulation. Chemosphere 2014; 111: 379-395.

[103] Durmaz H, Sevgiler Y, Üner N. Tissue-speciWc antioxidative and neurotoxic responses to diazinon in Oreochromis niloticus. Pesticide Biochemistry and Physiology 2006; 84: 215–226.

[104] Llasera MPG, González MB. Presence of carbamate pesticides in Environmental waters from the northwest of mexico: determination by liquid chromatography. Water Research 2001; 35 [8]: 1933-1940.

[105] Tien CJ, Lin MC, Chiu WH, Chen CS. Biodegradation of carbamate pesticides by natural river biofilms in different seasons and their effects on biofilm community structure. Environmental Pollution 2013; 179: 95-104.

[106] Li Y, Niu J, Shen J, Zhang C, Wang Z, He T. Spatial and seasonal distribution of organochlorine pesticides in the sediments of the Yangtze Estuary. Chemosphere 2014; 114: 233-240.

[107] Singh B.K, Walker A. Microbial degradation of organophosphorus compounds. FEMS Microbiol Reviews 2006; 30: 428-471.

[108] Pérez-Fernández V, Garcia MA, Marina ML. Characteristics and enantiomeric analysis of chiral pyrethroids. Journal of Chromatography A 2010; 1217: 968–989.

[109] Anadón A, Martínez-Larrañaga MR, Martínez MA. Use and abuse of pyrethrins and synthetic pyrethroids in veterinary medicine. The Veterinary Journal 2009; 182: 7-20.

[110] Albaseer SS, Nageswara Rao R, Swamy YV, Mukkanti K. Analytical artifacts, sample handling and preservation methods of environmental samples of synthetic pyrethroids. Trends in Analytical Chemistry 2011; 30 [11]: 1771-1780.

[111] Cai Z, Wang D, Ma WT. Gas chromatography/ion trap mass spectrometry applied for the analysis of triazine herbicides in environmental waters by an isotope dilution technique. Analytica Chimica Acta 2004; 503: 263–270.

[112] Fenoll J, Vela N, Garrido I, Pérez-Lucas G, Navarro S. Abatement of spinosad and indoxacarb residues in pure water by photocatalytic treatment using binary and terna-

ry oxides of Zn and Ti. Environmental science and pollution research international. 2014; *In press.*

[113] Nwani CD, Nagpure NS, Kumar R, Kushwaha B, Kumar P, Lkra WS. Mutagenic and genotoxic assessment of atrazine-based herbicide to freshwater fish Channa punctatus (Bloch) using micronucleus test and single cell gel electrophoresis. Environmental toxicology and pharmacology 2011; 31 [2]: 314-322.

[114] Cserháti T, Forgács E. Phenoxyacetic acids: separation and quantitative determination. Journal of Chromatography B 1998; 717: 157-178.

[115] Grabinska-Sotaa E, Wisniowska E, Kalka J. Toxicity of selected synthetic auxines—2,4-D and MCPA derivatives to broad-leaved and cereal plants. Crop Protection 2003; 22: 355-360.

[116] Peterson HG, Boutin C, Freemark KE, Martin PA. Toxicity of hexazinone and diquat to green algae, diatoms, cyanobacteria and duckweed. Aquatic Toxicology 1997; 39: 111-134.

[117] Roberts T R, Dyson JS, Lane MCG. Deactivation of the Biological Activity of Paraquat in the Soil Environment: a Review of Long-Term Environmental Fate. Journal of Agriculture and Food Chemestry 2002; 50: 3623-3631.

[118] Padhye LP, Kim JH, Huang CH. Oxidation of dithiocarbamates to yield N-nitrosamines by water disinfection oxidants. Water research 2013; 47: 725-736.

[119] Kubrak OI, Atamaniuk TM, Husak VV, Drohomyretska I Z, Storey JM, Storey KB, Lushchak V. Oxidative stress responses in blood and gills of Carassius auratus exposed to the mancozeb-containing carbamate fungicide Tattoo. Ecotoxicology and Environmental Safety 2012; 85: 37-43

[120] Van Wezel AP, Van Vlaardingen P. Environmental risk limits for antifouling substances. Aquatic Toxicology 2004; 66: 427-444.

[121] Osano O, Admiraal W, Klamerc HJC, Pastor D, Bleeker EAJ. Comparative toxic and genotoxic effects of chloroacetanilides, formamidines and their degradation products on Vibrio fischeri and Chironomus riparius. Environmental Pollution 2002; 119: 195-202.

[122] Abass K, Reponen P, Turpeinen M, Jalonen J, Pelkonen O. Characterization of diuron N-demethylation by mammalian hepatic microsomes and cDNA-expressed human cytochrome P450 enzymes. Drug Metabolism and Disposition. 2007; 35: 1634-1641.

[123] Narciso ES, Nakagawa LE. Análise de praguicidas por bioensaio com mosca drosophila melanogaster e cromatografia em camada delgada. Arquivos do Instituto Biológico 2009; 76[2]: 313-316.

[124] Niessen WM. Fragmentation of toxicologically relevant drugs in negative-ion liquid chromatography-tandem mass spectrometry. Mass Spectrometry Reviews 2012; 31[6]: 626-65.

[125] Wen Y, Fu Z, Xu J, Tang S, Wang Q, Li H, Xie G, Zhu Y, Gu Y, Tan F. Determination of 2, 4-dichlorophenoxyacetic acid in air of workplace by high-performance liquid chromatography. Zhonghua Lao Dong Wei Sheng Zhi Ye Bing Za Zhi 2014; 32[6]: 458-459.

[126] Martins JG, Amaya Chávez A, Waliszewski SM, Colín Cruz A, García Fabila MM. Extraction and clean-up methods for organochlorine pesticides determination in milk. Chemosphere 2013; 92[3]: 233-46.

[127] Santaladchaiyakit Y, Srijaranai S, Burakham R. Methodological aspects of sample preparation for the determination of carbamate residues: a review. Journal of Separation Science 2012; 35[18]: 2373-2389.

[128] Skoog D, Leary J, Principles of Instrumental Analysis, 4th Edition, Saunders College Publishing. 1992.

[129] Andreu V, Picó Y. Determination of currently used pesticides in biota. Analytical and Bioanalytical Chemistry 2012; 404[9]:2659-81.

[130] Assunção NA, Bechara EJH, Simionato AVC, Tavares MFG, Carrilho E. Capillary electrophoresis coupled to mass spectrometry (CE-MS): twenty years of development. Química Nova. 2008; 31: 2124-2133

[131] Poole CF. Derivatization reactions for use with the electron-capture detector. Journal of Chromatografy A 2013; 1296: 15-24.

[132] Di Stefano V, Avellone G, Bongiorno D, Cunsolo V, Muccilli V, Sforza S, Dossena A, Drahos L, Vékey K. Applications of liquid chromatography-mass spectrometry for food analysis. Journal of Chromatography A 2012; 1259: 74-85.

[133] Oliveira, G.A.R.; Lapuente, J.; Leme, D.M.; Ferraz, E.R.A, Meireles, G.; Oliveira, D.P. New paradigms for the environmental assessment: an ecotoxicological and genetic approach. 2012. In: Advances in Environmental Research. Nova Science Publishers.

[134] Hernke MT, Podein RJ. Sustainability, health and precautionary perspectives on lawn pesticides, and alternatives. Ecohealth. 2011; 8:223-32.

[135] Czaja K, Góralczyk K, Struciński P, Hernik A, Korcz W, Minorczyk M, Lyczewska M, Ludwicki JK. Biopesticides - towards increased consumer safety in the European Union. Pest Manag Sci. 2014; In press.